Occupational Health Practice

Occupational Health Practice

Fourth edition

H.A. Waldron PhD MD MRCP FFOM MAE
Consultant Occupational Physician
Occupational Health Department,
St Mary's Hospital, London, UK

C. Edling PhD MD
Professor
Department of Occupational and Environmental Medicine,
Uppsala University Hospital, Sweden

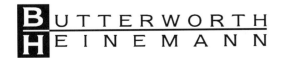

Butterworth-Heinemann
Linacre House, Jordan Hill, Oxford OX2 8DP
A division of Reed Educational and Professional Publishing Ltd

ℛ A member of Reed Elsevier plc group

OXFORD BOSTON JOHANNESBURG
MELBOURNE NEW DELHI SINGAPORE

First published 1973
Reprinted 1975, 1977
Second edition 1981
Reprinted 1982, 1986
Third edition 1989
Reprinted 1993, 1995
Fourth edition 1997

British Library Cataloguing in Publication Data
A catalogue record for this book is available from the British Library

Library of Congress Cataloguing in Publication Data
A catalogue record for this book is available from the Library of Congress

ISBN 0 7506 2720 4

Printed and bound in Great Britain by Hartnolls Ltd, Bodmin, Cornwall

Contents

Contributors

A Anttila PhD
Epidemiologist, Finnish Institute of Occupational
Health, Department of Epidemiology and
Biostatistics, Helsinki, Finland

O Axelson MD
Professor of Occupational and Environmental
Medicine, University Hospital, Department of
Occupational and Environmental Medicine,
Faculty of Health Sciences, Linköping, Sweden

A Bernard PhD
Industrial Toxicology and Occupational Medicine
Unit, Catholic University of Louvain, Brussels,
Belgium

P Sherwood Burge DIH MFOM FRCP FFOM
Consultant Physician; Director of Occupational
Lung Disease Unit; Lecturer of Occupational
Health, Department of Respiratory Medicine,
Birmginham Heartlands Hospital, Birmingham,
UK

N Carter
Department of Occupational and Environmental
Medicine, Uppsala University Hospital, Sweden

P-J Coenraads MD MPH
Professor of Occupational and Environmental
Dermatology, Groningen University Hospital,
The Netherlands

VT Covello PhD
Center for Risk Communication, New York, USA

C Edling PhD MD
Professor, Department of Occupational and
Environmental Medicine, Uppsala University
Hospital, Sweden

K Ekberg PhD
Department of Occupational and Environmental
Medicine, Centre for Public Health Sciences,
Linköping, Sweden

V Haufroid Pharm.
Pharmacist, Industrial Toxicology and
Occupational Medicine Unit, Catholic University
of Louvain, Brussels, Belgium

B Hellman PhD
Toxicologist, Department of Occupational and
Environmental Medicine, Uppsala University
Hospital, Sweden

P Hoet MD MIH MSc
Industrial Toxicology and Occupational Medicine
Unit, Catholic University of Louvain, Brussels,
Belgium

A Kjellberg PhD
Professor, National Institute for Working Life,
Solna, Sweden

R Lauwerys MD DSc
Professor of Occupational Medicine and
Industrial Toxicology, Catholic University of
Louvain, Brussels, Belgium

M-L Lindbohm DrPH
Epidemiologist, Finnish Institute of Occupational
Health, Department of Epidemiology and
Biostatistics, Helsinki, Finland

Ch Mellner MD
Medical Adviser, Pripps Brewery AB, Stockholm,
Sweden

E Menckel PhD
Associates Professor; Specialist in Occupational
Health Psychology, National Institute for
Working Life, Solna, Sweden

M Sallmén MSc
Epidemiologist, Finnish Institute of Occupational
Health, Department of Epidemiology and
Biostatistics, Helsinki, Finland

SJ Searle MD MSc MBA FFOM
The Post Office, Occupational Health Service,
Birmingham, UK

E-P Takala MD
Specialist in Physiatrics, Finnish Institute of
Occupational Health, Musculoskeletal Research
Unit, Helsinki, Finland

H Taskinen MD
Professor of Occupational Health, Department of
Occupational Medicine, Finnish Institute of
Occupational Health and Tampere University
Public School of Health, Helsinki, Finland

T Theorell MD PhD
Professor and Director, National Institute for
Psychosocial Factors and Health, Stockholm,
Sweden

C Timmer MD
Dermatologist, Occupational and Environmental
Dermatology Unit, University Hospital,
Groningen, The Netherlands

H Vainio MD
Chief, Unit of Chemoprevention, International
Agency for Research on Cancer, Lyon, France

KM Venables MD FRCP FFOM MFPHM
Senior Lecturer, Department of Occupational and
Environmental Medicine, Imperial College School
of Medicine at the National Heart and Lung
Institute, London, UK

HA Waldron PhD MD FRCP FFOM MAE
Consultant Occupational Physician, Department
of Occupational Health, St Mary's Hospital,
London, UK

Preface to the fourth edition

Occupational medicine is changing, especially in the countries of the western world where exposure to toxic substances has generally been greatly reduced over the years and this has had a considerable effect on the types of occupational diseases which are now seen. These days occupational physicians need to know a great deal about stress-related illnesses; they will need a good knowledge and understanding of epidemiology and the manifestation of disease in populations; they will be required to know about the causes of musculoskeletal disorders; their knowledge of toxicology will have to encompass the effects of low levels of potentially toxic materials on the central nervous system, on reproduction and on genetic material. They will also need to be informed about the effects of industry on the general environment and on the health of the general population. In this context we, the editors, note that many departments of occupational health are now in the process of renaming themselves as departments of occupational and *environmental* health. This is a trend which we feel is bound to continue.

We have tried to reflect the changes which have taken place in occupational medicine by concentrating the text on those areas which we consider to be of most relevance to practitioners now and for a few years to come. Thus, there are no chapters on what are sometimes referred to as the 'classic' occupational diseases which few occupational physicians are likely to see; we leave this to some other textbooks which seem more concerned to preserve the history of occupational medicine rather than deal with its actuality.

Since the objectives of this present edition are completely different from its predecessors, the contents have been thoroughly reviewed and not many of the chapters from the previous edition survive; we have recruited many new authors and, indeed, a second editor. Many of the chapters in the previous edition have been omitted, not because we felt that the information which they contained was of no value, but simply for reasons of space and because there was little to add to what was said then. Readers are, therefore, advised, not to discard the old edition (if they have it), but to use it in conjunction with this one, the two together forming a useful whole.

We have directed the book towards the occupational physician rather than towards any of the other professionals who practise occupational health, as they now have textbooks aplenty for their own consumption; we hope, however, that occupational nurses, hygienists and ergonomists may find something of interest in the book, perhaps something of value, and frequently areas for discussion and disagreement. There is not one pure way to practise occupational medicine, and what we present here is one of the many possible ways, one which we consider to be a good reflection of how health and work interact in contemporary occupations and of how occupational physicians can best preserve the health of those for whom they are responsible.

Richard Schilling, the first editor of this book, tells how he was once asked by one of his employers, 'Whose side are you on, doc?' The whole of his life as an occupational physician provided the very clear answer – he was on the side of those whose work put their health at risk; it is our view also that occupational physicians cannot fulfil their duty unless they are on the side of those whose health they are engaged to protect. It is our earnest wish that this book may help them to do their duty, to whatever small degree.

HA Waldron
C Edling

Preface to the third edition

Under the editorship of Richard Schilling, *Occupational Health Practice* quickly assumed a leading place amongst text books in the field and it was with mixed feelings that I accepted the invitation to take over the responsibility for the third edition. I felt very honoured and flattered to have been asked to do so, but I also had some trepidation about the task, knowing how much the first two editions had become identified with Richard and how much their success owed to him.

These 15 years have seen apparently better control of toxic hazards and a new emphasis on reproductive and behavioural toxicology, stress and the promotion of health. Many of these changes in emphasis have been prompted by research activities in Europe, particularly in some of the Nordic countries where standards of occupational health practice are especially high. Occupational health is also assuming more importance in the developing countries and nowhere is this upsurgence more evident than in China where great strides are being taken.

To the outsider, occupational health appears to be becoming more proactive and less reactive. These changes and improvements, however, may have less substance than seems obvious at first sight. In the United Kingdom the inspectorates and EMAs have been cut back to a point where their effectiveness must be seriously called into question; far too many men and women lose their lives or sustain serious injuries in accidents at work; large companies have been engaged in reducing their occupational health departments as part of the general economic 'rationalization'

and small companies have, at best, inadequate provision for their employees.

The state of academic occupational health in the United Kingdom is also giving some cause for concern with serious cutbacks in staff and inadequate funding for research. Some departments are under threat of closure and were this to happen, the harm which would befall academic occupational health would be incalculable and the speciality itself would be harmed since without research of a high quality, the discipline will not be held in the regard which it should by the rest of the medical profession.

The authorship of the present edition has been drawn to only a limited extent from amongst those who were involved in previous editions. The involvement of some new contributors reflects the changes which have occurred and the different emphasis of the new edition. Its aim is to be of direct use to those actively engaged in occupational health practice. Its aim is to be of direct use to those actively engaged in occupational health practice wherever they may be, and as far as possible, to the problems which may arise from the complex interaction between work and health. Suggestions as to how the occupational health professional should deal with perturbations in the health of the worker and workplace are also included.

I am conscious there are some gasp in the material presented here but I hope that there will be a chance to rectify these in the future.

I hope that occupational health practitioners will find something of value in this new edition. I hope also that they will find something of the spirit of the earlier editions which always placed an emphasis on the duty of those in the profession to safeguard the health and well-being of those for whom they have responsibility and see to it that working lives may be spent without coming to harm.

HA Waldron

Preface to the first edition

The need for a book describing what the physician, hygienist and nurse actually do to protect and improve the health of people at work has become increasingly obvious to the staff of this Institute. Although many books have been written on occupational health, there are none in English which deal comprehensively with its practice. We teach the principles of occupational health practice to postgraduate students in occupational medicine, nursing and hygiene, and the lack of a standard work of reference has made the task of both teaching and learning more difficult.

Our academic staff and visiting lecturers have attempted to fill this gap, which is repeatedly brought to our notice by students. While our primary aim is to meet a need in formal course programmes it is hoped that the book may also be useful to the many whose interests encompass occupational health but who cannot attend a course, and that it will be of some value to medical and non-medical specialists in related fields.

Our students come from all over the world, many from countries undergoing rapid industrialization. We have therefore tried as far as possible to offer a comprehensive, up-to-date, account of occupational health practice, with some emphasis on the special needs of work people in developing countries. Eastern European countries attach great importance to occupational health and provide comprehensive occupational health services and training programmes. We refer to their methods of practice and training as well as to those of the western world because we believe both East and West have much to learn from each other,

and the developing countries from both. Terms such as occupational health, medicine and hygiene often have different meanings, particularly in the eastern and western hemispheres. Occupational health in the context of this book comprises two main disciplines: occupational medicine, which is concerned primarily with man and the influence of work on his health; and occupational hygiene, which is concerned primarily with the measurement, assessment and control of man's working environment. These two disciplines are complementary and physicians, hygienists, nurses and safety officers all have a part to play in recognizing, assessing and controlling hazards to health. The terms industrial health, medicine and hygiene have a restricted meaning, are obsolescent, and are are not used by us.

The three opening chapters are introductory; the first gives an account of national developments, contrasts the different forms of services provided by private enterprise and the State; and discusses factors which influence a nation or an industrial organization to pay attention to the health of people at work. The second is about a man's work and his health. Everyone responsible for patients needs to realize how work may give rise to disease, and how a patient's ill health may affect his ability to work efficiently and safely. It is as important for the general practitioner or hospital consultant as it is for the occupational physician to be aware of the relationship between work and health. The third chapter outlines the functions of an occupational health service. The chapters which follow describe in more detail the main functions, such as the provision of treatment services, routine and special medical examinations, including 'well-person' screening, psychosocial factors in the working environment and the mental health of people at work. There are chapters on occupational safety and the prevention of accidents and occupational disease which are often the most important tasks facing an occupational health service. Methods used in the study of groups of workers are outlined in sections of epidemiology, field surveys and the collection and handling of sickness absence data; these chapters are of special importance, as it is essential that those practising occupational health think in terms of 'groups' and not just of the individual worker. Epidemiological expertise enables this extra dimension to be added to the investigation and control of accidents at work.

One chapter is devoted to ergonomics while five on occupational hygiene deal with the physical and thermal environments, airborne contaminants, industrial ventilation and protective equipment and clothing. There are concluding chapters on ethics and education in occupational health. Undergraduates in medicine and other sciences frequently lack adequate teaching on this subject and we hope that this book may be useful to them and their teachers.

Although it is not possible to cover fully the practice of occupational health in 450 pages, we hope to convey the broad outlines of the subject to a wide variety of people.

I owe many thanks to many people for help in producing this book, especially to the contributors and to those who assisted them in preparing their manuscripts, and to the publishers for their patience and understanding. For the illustrations I am particularly grateful to Mr C.J.Webb, Miss Anne Caisely and Miss Juliet Stanwell Smith of the Visual Aids Department at the London School of Hygiene and Tropical Medicine, and also to the Wellcome Institute of the History of Medicine, to the Editors of many journals, and to Professors Kundiev and Sanoyski of the USSR.

Manuscripts were read by members of the Institute staff and others who made valuable suggestions; the latter include Professional Gordon Atherley, Professor R.C. Browne, Dr J. Gallagher, Dr. J.C. Graham, Dr Wister Meigs, Mr Wright Miller, Mr Andrew Papworth, Miss Brenda Slaney, Professor F. Valic, my wife and my daughter Mrs Erica Hunningher—I am indebted to them all; I am also grateful to Dr Gerald Keatinge and Dr Dilys Thomas for reading proofs, and to my secretary, Miss Catherine Burling for her help and enthusiasm throughout the long period of preparation.

Richard Schilling

Chapter 1

The medical role in occupational health

C Edling and HA Waldron

Introduction

Occupational diseases have existed since humans began to utilize the resources of nature in order to equip themselves with the tools and the materials with which they could achieve a better and more comfortable standard of living. Some occupational diseases, especially those associated with mining and metalworking, were well recognized in antiquity. For example, Pliny writing in the first century AD described the health hazards which lead and mercury miners experienced and recommended that lead smelters should wear masks made from pig's bladder to protect themselves against fumes from the smelters. The diseases of miners became increasingly to be recognized during the medieval period, but it was not until the publication of Ramazzini's *De Morbus Artificum* in 1713 that occupational medicine became in any sense formalized. Ramazzini stressed the importance of asking patients not only how they felt, but also, what was their occupation? This is a lesson which many doctors have still to learn and is emphasized by a recent 'position paper' from the American College of Physicians describing the internist's role in occupational and environmental medicine [1]. In that paper, a short form for the routine recording of the history of occupational and environmental exposures is presented and a guide is given to help the internist decide whether a complete occupational history should be taken or consultation arranged with a specialist in occupational medicine.

As industry has grown and expanded, new products and new processes have been developed and with them a multitude of occupational diseases. The detection and treatment of what are often now called the 'classical' occupational diseases – lead poisoning, mercury poisoning, toxic jaundice and so on – formed the basis for the development of occupational medicine and many of the early occupational physicians were, in reality, general physicians whose sphere of operations was the factory rather than the hospital. However, in some notable cases – Donald Hunter, for example – hospital physicians who had never held a post in industry contributed significantly to the speciality by virtue of having many individuals with occupational diseases as their patients. As conditions in industry have improved there has been less emphasis on treatment and more on prevention; and prevention is, of course, the most desirable and most successful approach towards improving and protecting workers' health.

Over the years there has been a tendency to divide this area of preventive medicine into two separate disciplines: occupational medicine and occupational health. Occupational health carries with it the implication of a multidisciplinary health service and team work performed at the plant by, for example, ergonomists, nurses, doctors, hygienists and safety officers. By contrast, occupational medicine refers solely to the training and work of the occupational physician.

The doctor is frequently, but not invariably, the manager of the team, but whether this is so or not, it must be clear that only the doctor has the required knowledge and training to pronounce on matters of health – by which is usually meant disease. The health effects of exposures, of whatever sort, on people at work can only be discussed authoritatively by doctors since only they have the expertise in that area; they are also generally much better trained in epidemiology and interpretation of data than other members of the occupational health team and they must insist on maintaining this function and not allow anyone from another discipline to abrogate it. By the same token, it is important for doctors to recognize the limits of their own competence and not venture opinions in areas in which they have no special expertise.

Occupational health concerns are to a large extent universal, with much in common in both industrialized and developing countries. There are considerable differences in the setting of priorities for occupational health needs in different countries, however, which depend greatly upon their stage of development. Occupational health activities are always predicated on the needs of the workers, but the health problems which workers may experience are determined by the kind of industrial activity in which they are engaged. Thus, occupational health needs differ by type and size of company at any given time in an area or a country. The degree of industrialization is the factor which probably has the greatest influence on occupational health needs, however.

The twentieth century has seen a steady improvement in the health and safety of the working population in the developed countries: there are now fewer serious or fatal accidents, a decrease in the relative frequency of accidents, a reduction in the incidence of occupational diseases, and an increase in life expectancy. The decrease in disorders caused by work is partly explained by the shift from manufacturing to service industries that has taken place in the western countries, but also to improvements in working conditions in the manufacturing industries.

In the developing countries, on the other hand, the conditions of the working population may be by no means so congenial. Some of the improvements in working conditions in the developed countries have been brought about by transferring dangerous processes to developing countries and with them their attendant hazards [2]. The developing countries, therefore, will have to face the 'old' problems of occupational medicine for some time to come. The training of occupational physicians in these countries must, therefore, reflect that fact and they may not be best prepared for their future work by attending courses in western countries, where the practice of occupational medicine is often very different from their own.

Occupational medicine has also become fragmented and has gone in different directions in different countries, and even in different industries. There are great differences between the problems facing the physician who works at a coal mine and one employed in a service industry, and their day-to-day activities may have few points of similarity. The role of occupational physicians may show the greatest differences when one compares the developing and developed countries. In the former they are more likely to act as general practitioners, frequently dealing not only with workers but their families as well, and individually may be the only primary care physician available to the workers in an industry. The occupational physician in the developing countries, therefore, will need training not only in occupational medicine but also in general medicine, paediatrics, tropical medicine and probably obstetrics; occupational medicine itself may be only a minor part of the work. In the developed countries, the occupational physician is by way of becoming a consultant in organizational medicine and is increasingly removed from the treatment of sick patients. The treatment of work-related diseases in the western countries is, for the most part, carried out by other specialists and not by occupational physicians – by chest physicians and dermatologists, for example. This, and the tendency to regulate exposure to toxic hazards and to control exposure by biological measures, is likely to weaken the need for the medical input into occupational health care and this in turn may dilute the role of the physician and possibly strengthen the status of other professionals in the field, such as the occupational nurse, hygienist or ergonomist.

The World Health Organisation (WHO) has recently published five recommendations for the overall objectives of an occupational health service, using the terminology from the discussion on the targets for *Health for All by the Year 2000*. The five points raised by WHO are to:

- protect workers from hazards at work
- adapt work and the work environment to the capabilities of the workers
- enhance the physical, mental and social well-being of workers
- minimize the consequences of occupational hazards and occupational and work-related disease

● provide general health care services for workers and their families, both curative and preventive, at the workplace or from nearby facilities.

Despite the improvements that have undoubtedly taken place in working conditions, the scope of occupational health and safety remains wide and many-sided. For example, it has been estimated that about 100 000 chemicals are used at work, that workers are exposed to about 50 physical factors, more than 200 biological agents and dozens of forms of ergonomic and psychological workloads, all of which – in high doses and following long-term exposure – may have an adverse effect on health. This is one reason that the role of occupational physicians is crucial and they must not neglect the 'traditional' elements of their speciality which may assume greater importance if ever there is a requirement for occupational health cover to be given to those working in small industries – the majority now in many countries – where presently there is none, and to home workers as recently proposed by the International Labour Organisation. The traditional aspects of occupational medicine are also important when considering environmental hazards; it is not a cause for surprise that many departments of occupational medicine (or health) have recently renamed themselves as departments of occupational and *environmental* medicine. There has been an increasing trend for occupational physicians to become involved in environmental medicine because many of the issues which cause concern relate to toxic exposure of one sort or another, and the only large repository of expertise relating to these matters resides within occupational medicine. The perception that the role of the physician in occupational health is diminishing has also caused some occupational physicians to seek other areas in which their special skills can usefully be deployed.

In what follows we will briefly discuss some of the areas in which we feel the occupational physician has a key role to play; many of the remaining chapters in this book will discuss them in greater detail.

Chemical hazards

Although exposure to chemicals has changed in significant ways in the industrialized countries, great concern is still expressed about their poten-tial for harm, although exposure to chemicals is a concomitant of life and, indeed, life itself depends upon it. We believe that this must be made clear to the public, since there is a very strong opinion current that chemicals are necessarily dangerous to health. It must never be forgotten, however – and should be widely stated – that, to paraphrase Paracelsus, toxicity is a question of dose. The notion that toxicity is a simple, inherent property of a substance is simplistic and is the cause of much confusion in the public mind, much played upon by the media and others for sensational or political purposes. For example, great alarm has been engendered among the general public about the hazards of asbestos, some ill-informed or mischievous persons propounding the notion of the 'single fibre carcinogen'. This has led to the wide-scale removal of asbestos from public and other buildings when there was no need to do so, or when other measures such as sealing would have been efficacious. The result has been that a cohort of workers has been exposed to asbestos unnecessarily and this may be reflected in an outbreak of asbestos-related diseases many years in the future. Had advice been sought from occupational physicians, this unnecessary intervention might have been averted.

Among occupational health professionals, discussions nowadays are focused, not so much on the risks of a single substance as on the problems associated with mixed chemical exposure at very low levels. To investigate and control these risks, better methods for measuring exposure will have to be developed, using various forms of biological monitoring. The measures of effect will include not only such gross events as death or cancer, but much more subtle effects such as those which can be measured by specific tests of genotoxicity, such as measuring rates of sister chromatid exchange (SCE) or levels of DNA adducts, for example. (See also Chapter 10.)

The conventional approach to conducting occupational cancer epidemiology is gradually being replaced by what has become known as molecular epidemiology, in which molecular biology and gene technology are used to measure both exposure and effect, taking individual susceptibility into account, so far as is possible. Enthusiasm for these new methods may have got rather out of hand, however, and the fact that we still do not know enough about the normal background variation with respect to, for example, DNA adducts, has not been taken fully into account. Nor do we know whether these new methods will actually give us more or better information than the 'old' ones and really help to predict outcome any more successfully than conventional methods. The ethical implications of the use of biomarkers in occupational health also need careful consideration. For example, there is a fear that the test results could be used to discriminate against individuals with regard to employment or insurance, and these matters must be more fully debated by occupational health personnel and the general public, so that preventive medicine does not become predictive medicine. (See also Chapters 6 and 10.)

Another method used to study the effects of chemical exposure is to compare the occurrence of certain symptoms, particularly psychological symptoms, in exposed and unexposed groups as an index of 'comfort'. This technique has been used to some extent in field investigations of the sick building syndrome and in exposure chamber studies of solvent exposure. The increased use of computerized tests has suggested that we now can detect an increasing number of subtle neurotoxic effects at lower exposure levels than before. Recent studies on manganese with this technique have shown effects on the central nervous system at exposure levels far below those currently permitted in industry. These new neuropsychological tests are extremely sensitive but they are not specific, so the results must be interpreted with caution. Perhaps the important question to consider is – here as in all areas of occupational medicine – should we frighten workers with results that will probably have no effect on their health or longevity, or are we duty bound to tell them regardless? Perhaps one of the most important tasks for the occupational physician is to discuss the concept of acceptable risk with the workers. There is plenty of evidence that there is a much greater risk to health from unemployment than from exposure to low levels of chemicals at the workplace. No thanks will be given to those who are supposed to have the welfare of workers most at heart, if they succeed in establishing standards for exposure levels which are so expensive to achieve that small businesses are driven to the wall and jobs are lost.

Physical hazards

Exposure to electromagnetic fields (EMF) has become a great concern during the past few years. These fields have two components – the electric and the magnetic – and both are capable of generating an induced current in those exposed to them. In recent years, interest in the biological effects and possible health outcomes of weak electric fields has increased and studies have been carried out to look at the relationship between EMF and cancer, reproduction and neurobehavioural reactions. Epidemiological studies on childhood leukaemia and residential exposure to EMF from nearby power lines have indicated a slight increase in risk. An excess risk of leukaemia, brain tumours and male breast cancer have all been reported in 'electrical occupations'. In spite of a large number of experimental laboratory studies, however, no plausible or comprehensible mechanism has been presented by which to explain the carcinogenic effect of EMF, although the predominant view is that EMF may act as promoters in the process of carcinogenesis. It must also be pointed out that despite the fact that exposure to electromagnetic fields has increased many tens of times in the past few years, the incidence of leukaemia has remained more or less static. The results of studies on reproduction, including adverse pregnancy outcomes and neurobehavioural disorders, are generally considered insufficiently clear and consistent to constitute a scientific basis for restricting exposure. (See also Chapters 11, 13 and 14.)

The old problem of noise is still a matter of concern in the work environment and, increasingly, in the general environment. Noise–induced hearing loss is the most important adverse effect, but non-auditory effects are also reported, including effects upon efficiency, sleep and blood pressure (Chapter 18).

Biological hazards

Biological hazards are a special risk to those working in the health care professions. Tuberculosis was formerly the disease which presented the greatest risk to doctors, especially to pathologists, but in recent years there has been much more concern about hepatitis B and HIV. Several doctors contracted hepatitis B from their patients before the advent of an effective vaccine, but nowadays there is more concern that patients may contract the disease from their surgeons than vice versa. In England, a small number of surgeons who were highly infectious carriers of hepatitis B were found to be still operating and this led to large – and costly – exercises in which their patients were traced. As a consequence the Department of Health introduced new requirements that all those who were engaged in what were called exposure-prone invasive procedures must be able to demonstrate that they were not hepatitis B carriers. Those who were found to be highly infectious carriers on screening would not be permitted to continue carrying out invasive procedures. No provisions were made for the redeployment, retraining or compensation for surgeons who might suddenly have found themselves without any means of earning their living because they had a condition which they may well have contracted in the first place as a consequence of their work, and these regulations are – to the best of our knowledge – the first designed to protect a government department rather than the professionals for whom they ought ultimately to feel responsible.

Hepatitis B is not regarded as much of a risk now by health care professionals as they have mostly been successfully vaccinated and they tend to be more concerned about HIV. This virus is found in nearly all body fluids but its presence in blood raises most concern for health care workers. The virus is not readily transmitted from a patient to staff in accidents involving contaminated needles and scalpels, nor does it survive outside body temperature for much longer than three to four hours, thus reducing the risk from discarded needles and, mercifully, relatively few health care workers have become infected. A moving account by one doctor who was infected as the result of a needle-stick injury has recently been published [3].

Both hepatitis B and HIV infection are preventable occupational diseases if safe working practices are performed and the role of the occupational physician is paramount here, especially in trying to educate medical colleagues who often seem highly resistant to the blandishments of the occupational health staff. The availability of an effective vaccine for hepatitis B should not blind anyone to the fact that it is a fallback and no substitute for a safe system of work; there are many more infections which are blood borne, including a seemingly endless variety of hepatitis viruses for which there are, as yet, *no* vaccines.

Ergonomics

During the past few decades much interest has centred on the ergonomic problems of heavy lifting and the techniques required to minimize them. In many cases, however, mechanization and automation have led to the introduction of more monotonous work and to new work-related problems. This is a good illustration of the maxim that improvements in the work environment may themselves introduce new hazards, although hopefully with a lower risk than those they have replaced. At present, musculoskeletal disorders, particularly those affecting the back and upper limbs, are among the most important occupational health problems in the industrialized countries. In Sweden, about 60% of all reported occupational diseases are musculoskeletal disorders. They rarely result in serious disability, but they may considerably impair the quality of everyday life and they incur a considerable financial burden due to loss of productivity and sick leave. It has been shown in several studies, however, that affected workers improve more rapidly if they stay at work, contrary to the common belief. To be put off sick is not good treatment and occupational physicians should try to ensure that their colleagues in other specialities, especially in primary care, are made aware of this fact.

Interest in epidemiological research on musculoskeletal disorders has increased and the trend now is to develop better means of defining exposure and disease and to look at such simple measures as prevalence and incidence, since very little is known about the 'true' relationship between occupational physical workload (exposure) and musculoskeletal disorders (effect). There is reasonable agreement between different studies, however, that frequent lifting of heavy loads and lifting while rotating the trunk increases the risk of low back pain and disc herniation, whereas prolonged sitting increases the risk of low back pain. Furthermore, repetitive forceful manual work seems to be associated with an increased risk of hand–wrist tendon syndromes and carpal tunnel syndrome and repeated manipulation of light components for extended periods is associated with an increased risk of developing shoulder–neck disorders. (See also Chapter 17.)

The complex stresses which different lifting techniques impose on the lower back are not fully understood. A safe lifting technique may depend on such factors as leg strength, weight of the load, size and shape of the load and workplace geometry. NIOSH has developed an equation as a methodological tool for safety and health practitioners who need to evaluate the lifting demands of manual handling jobs. This equation can be used to determine the relative risk for low back pain associated with lifting jobs. The most appropriate way to establish the link between a knowledge of ergonomics and an improvement in working conditions is to organize local action through the direct participation of the workforce. The involvement of managers and workers who know the local working conditions best and who can influence decisions for change is essential and this process is best facilitated by the occupational physician.

Psychology

In modern western society the impact of psychosocial factors at work on well-being, sick leave, symptoms and disease has become a matter of concern. There is now a great deal of evidence to indicate the causal effect of work organization upon the occurrence of back problems. Work organization, and in particular the ability of workers to influence their own work pattern, is important when discussing work stress and the risk of certain other diseases, cardiovascular disease, for example. More emphasis must be given to the effects of occupation on the incidence of cardiovascular disease, since not only are work organization and exposure to some chemicals important contributory factors but cardiovascular disease is also a major contributor to morbidity and mortality within the workforce.

A simple model to evaluate 'job strain' has been developed by Karasek and Theorell (Chapter 19). This model takes into account both the psychological demands of the job, the ability of the worker to control his pattern of work, and social support at the workplace. These measures of exposure are easily assessed by the administration of a simple questionnaire to the workers. Using the model, many studies have shown that psychosocial factors are associated with the risk of heart disease, those with high demands and poor control and support having the greatest risk. It also seems that various psychosomatic problems, sleep disturbances and musculoskeletal disorders are also related to these work characteristics and one chal-

lenge which the occupational physician faces in the future is to work to try to ameliorate these risks.

Work and pregnancy

Employment of women has increased everywhere, but to an extent that has varied with culture, religion, political system and economic development. In the Scandinavian countries and the UK, women comprise about 50% of the workforce, mostly in part-time and low-paid jobs. In developing countries from 20% to 60% of the women work in either agriculture or manufacturing, with reproductive hazards in both. Epidemiological studies, which have been performed mostly in the industrialized countries, suggest that employment during pregnancy carries a small risk of fetal death but little if any risk of preterm birth. Most excess fetal deaths have been reported in nurses, waitresses, cleaners, laundry and dry-cleaning workers and women in certain manufacturing jobs. With regard to specific risk factors, physical exertion and ergonomic requirements and solvents are associated with a slightly increased risk of fetal death. (See Chapter 14.)

Although most studies have understandably concentrated on female workers, there is evidence to suggest that the exposures which some men experience may have an adverse effect on fertility and, perhaps, the outcome of pregnancy; these matters are considered further in Chapter 13.

Environmental health

Those concerned with health must be aware not only of the influence of exposures at the workplace but they must also consider the influence of exposure from sources within the general environment, for example food additives, exhausts, passive smoking, dust, noise and mercury in amalgam. In other words, the *total environment* is an important determinant of health. Over the years, occupational health practitioners have accumulated a profound knowledge of the relation between chemical, physical and biological exposures and health effects. In most cases, no other human data on the effect of a certain environmental factor are available other than those obtained from the study of a working population. In practice, environmental issues and occupational health issues are often difficult to separate. Preventive strategies used in environmental and occupational health are clearly similar; in both, the emphasis is on primary prevention. Therefore, it seems natural that departments of occupational medicine should also take responsibility for problems arising outside the 'factory gate' and become departments of occupational and environmental medicine. This will, of course, considerably enlarge the amount of work to be done and will have a considerable impact on the training of future practitioners in the field.

Training

The changing pattern of industrial life and of the nature of preventive occupational medicine must clearly result in a different pattern of activity and consequently in different training for occupational health personnel. This training should reflect local needs rather than try to cover all the topics in the field. Training in occupational medicine must be adjusted to the differing needs in developed and developing countries. The training of occupational physicians in developing countries must be carried out where the problems present themselves, not miles away in a developed country where teachers lack the first-hand experience of local problems, medical, technical and economic. To what extent training in developed countries can be varied and adopted strictly to local needs is questionable. In the short term it may be helpful, since the problems facing the staff in different industries may have little in common. In the long term, however, too narrow a training may limit the desirable mobility on the part of the staff in different units unless they undergo a period of further training beforehand.

The training of an occupational physician must be such as to meet all the demands which may be encountered in the field of occupational and environmental medicine. It must give the doctor biological and medical knowledge of the relationship between exposure and disease, complemented by a sound grounding in biostatistics and epidemiology. The ability to conduct population-based studies and to direct health education programmes are skills without which no occupational physi-

cians in the future can expect adequately to undertake their work.

Medicine in the future will not be about blood and guts but about bits and bytes. More and more communication between people will take place through telecommunication. Nation-wide computer networks are already an established part of health care in many countries, and many authorities and departments in the field of occupational and environmental health have their own home pages on the Internet. We have used the Internet in the training of medical students in occupational and environmental medicine and both teachers and taught have found it of benefit.* It must be emphasized, however, that there will still have to be interaction between the novice and the expert, since the ability to practise occupational medicine depends upon more than the ability to read and to click a mouse button. Another aspect of telecommunication which is particularly important in medicine is that of confidentiality. A solution that has recently been suggested is the use of public key cryptography, where the sender and recipient can encrypt and decipher a secret message by the use of an algorithm.

Future trends

Developments in technology and changes in the methods of production will ensure that there will continue to be changes in the patterns of working life. It seems very likely that new industries will be established on a small scale, employing relatively few people, and that people will increasingly work at home, linked to each other by modems. The average age of the workforce is increasing and chronic morbidity and related disability are likely to increase. Solutions need to be sought to questions such as the maintenance of working capacity, the prevention of musculoskeletal disorders, the reduction of psychological workloads and the assessment of risks from new chemicals and materials. In future, the difference between occupational health and occupational medicine is likely to become more distinct. The term 'occupational health' will describe the team work carried out at the occupational health unit in a plant, where the tasks on an individual level will be directed towards health screening,

* A list of useful addresses on the World Wide Web can be found in the Appendix.

biological and environmental monitoring and rehabilitation. More emphasis will have to be given to preventive aspects and less to the medical treatment of the sick patient, a task which will be more suitable for the general practitioner. Preventive action should take place at national, community and individual levels. Since people spend about a third of their waking hours at work, the occupational health service should facilitate preventive activities at the workplace. It is, therefore, important to increase the access of workers to occupational health services. In Sweden, for example, about 80% of the labour force has access to an occupational health service, whereas in the UK the figure is only about 30%. The association between workers and the occupational health service has to be made on a voluntary basis as part of an agreement between employers' associations and trade unions. However, if more and more people are going to work at home, a trend already seen in the western world, this will almost certainly decrease their access to an occupational health service. The solution then may be to increase the training of general practitioners and have a more flexible system of occupational health services in which only the large companies will have an 'old-fashioned' occupational health unit with specialists in occupational medicine.

The ultimate goal of the occupational health service should be to cover all branches of economic activities, including the small-scale, construction and agriculture sectors. However, even where occupational health services have been in situ for many years, very little is known or documented about their impact on the health of the workforce. Therefore, the audit of occupational health services must become a priority in the future. In a world of shrinking economic resources it is very important to show, in economical terms, the advantages of preventive medicine at the occupational health level. Guidelines which can be used for the implementation of a medical audit have been defined and published. Every occupational health department should have an agreed statement of its purpose and goals as well as its strategy and objectives. It is important that this statement is discussed and agreed by all members of the occupational health team and the management to whom they are responsible.

The future development of occupational health will probably lead to an increase, not only in nurse-based but also nurse-led services, since these are considerably cheaper than those which depend upon doctors. The occupational health area will be more attractive for nurses than doctors, since they can enjoy a greater degree of autonomy and take on a much more extended role than is possible in many other areas of nursing. There will be little medical practice as generally understood in occupational health units of the future; instead the staff will scrutinize working conditions and work organization in close association with both employers and employees. This participation must involve all aspects of occupational health, not only research.

Occupational medicine will be based on hospitals and/or universities and practised in departments of occupational and environmental medicine, departments with an interdisciplinary staff of physicians, occupational hygienists, toxicologists, psychologists and ergonomists. The main activities will be research, training and teaching. The basic tools for research will still be toxicology and epidemiology, and it is important that the research is carried out in close collaboration with the occupational health units so that the findings can constitute the basis for the units' work with regard to monitoring and prevention. Training and teaching will be particularly aimed towards those who are either already in or about to enter the occupational health units, and, as already said, should reflect local needs.

There will be closer links between occupational and environmental health. This will lead to an improved use of resources, better insight and better management concerning the range of factors that affect human health. Surveillance data, case reporting and research in occupational medicine will expand to become more useful to the population at large. International cooperation will play an important role in promoting workplace improvements.

Epilogue

Developments during the past few decades have shown that occupational health hazards can be reduced and managed if sufficient expertise is available, if collaboration is well organized, if common goals are clearly defined and if there is a commitment to achieve these goals. The goals of occupational medicine and occupational health remain as they have always been, that is:

- to study the health effects of the work environment
- to prevent the negative effects of work on health
- to promote the positive health effects.

To achieve these goals there must be a policy and a programme by which health care can be provided to the working population through an occupational health service, a policy which requires the setting of relevant exposure levels in the work environment, a national policy on research in occupational health, and a programme by which an adequate number of competent occupational physicians are trained.

References

1. American College of Physicians. *Annals of Internal Medicine*, **113**, 874–982 1990
2. *Technology Review*, July (1991)
3. Logie, A.W., 'Coming out' – a personal dilemma. *British Medical Journal*, **312**, 1679 1996

Chapter 2

Preplacement screening and fitness to work

HA Waldron

Introduction

Preplacement (or pre-employment) screening has a long history in occupational health practice and formerly took up a great deal of the occupational physician's time. In recent years it has become increasingly clear that the wholesale clinical examination of predominantly healthy men and women has little to commend it, although this is a view which is not always shared by employers whose faith in the doctor's ability to foretell the future state of health of an individual is touching but misplaced.

A discussion of preplacement screening has to recognize that for the three groups of people involved – the occupational health practitioner, the employer and the prospective employee – it has widely differing objectives. The doctor or nurse undertaking the screening wishes to ensure that individuals are both physically and mentally suited for the job for which they have applied, so far as is reasonably practicable. This by no means requires them to be in perfect health, since this is not a necessary prerequisite for many jobs. The employer, however, wishes the pre-employment screen to act as a guarantee that all workers newly engaged *are* in perfect health and will continue in this state for as long as possible in order to maximize efficiency and minimize time lost for reasons of illness. Finally, prospective employees tend to view pre-employment screening as a hurdle to be overcome on their way to a job, and if they are aware of anything in their medical history which may be thought of as a hindrance to achieving that

end, they will neglect to mention it when they come to fill in the questionnaire or answer direct questions put to them by a doctor or nurse. In some cases, their own doctor may collude with them by minimizing the effects of an existing medical condition, seeing as his first duty to secure the job for his patient in the belief that the work will be therapeutic. Anecdotally, it is said that psychiatrists are more prone than many to suggest to their patients that they should not reveal too much of their psychiatric history for fear that this may count against them when it comes to applying for a job. It is, therefore, obvious, that the objectives of these different participants in pre-employment screening may have little in common.

Reasonable objectives

The most reasonable objective of pre-employment screening from the point of view of occupational health practitioners is to ensure that individuals and their jobs are as well suited, in all respects, as possible. It should always be remembered that the occupational physician or the occupational nurse is in no position to deny or to promise an individual a job, except when it is within their own department and they are actually making the appointment. The responsibility of the occupational health department is to give advice in general terms to management on the suitability or otherwise of a candidate and it is the prerogative of management to accept or disregard that advice as they think fit.

The approach

There are few conditions which are an absolute disbarment to any kind of work, and what is required of the occupational health practitioner is first to determine as completely as possible the physical and mental state of the applicant and then see how this measures up against the requirements of the job. In order to do this it should be obvious that those requirements must be well known to those making the assessment; this calls for an intimate knowledge of the working practices within the organization which is not likely to be achieved by a doctor or nurse who does not regularly visit the various places of work. Any legal requirements, such as those (in the UK) which relate, for example, to exposure to lead or asbestos, diving, driving, working with video display units or lifting and handling, for example, will necessarily have to be taken into account. In some cases the doctors making pre-employment assessments must be appointed by the appropriate regulatory authorities in the countries in which they practise.

For each type of work within an organization any physical, chemical or biological hazards must be known and, where possible, quantified. It is hardly likely, however, that any occupational health practitioners would overlook these, so long as they were as familiar as they ought to be with the working practices in their individual company.

There may be other requirements which are not so obvious, however, and occupational health practitioners must have a set of job descriptions for their organization and also the manager's assessment of those attributes which are considered to be essential for someone applying for a particular post. For example, is it a job which requires a great deal of manual dexterity or of physical strength; is it a task which requires considerable mental agility; is colour vision essential? Drawing up what one might call a managerial protocol requires a good deal of collaboration between the occupational health department and the management, but it provides an opportunity to clarify thought and to develop strong ties between the occupational health department and the heads of other departments. Moreover, each side has the opportunity to educate the other about their own approaches to the task of selection. Out of such deliberations may come some written policies in relation to individuals with particular medical

conditions. There has been much heart searching in recent years about the suitability of employing those who might be HIV positive or have AIDS. Some companies still consider that the risks of employing such individuals are too great and will not take them on, whereas others take a more relaxed view and have a policy which does not discriminate against them. Whatever policies are arrived at, however, it is important that the occupational health department has an input into their formulation, especially if they have implications for pre-employment screening. For example, some companies will not accept individuals who abuse drugs or alcohol, and require prospective employees to undergo biological screening to detect evidence of either. It would hardly be sensible for such a company to formulate a screening policy without the best advice from its occupational health professionals.

Having a thorough knowledge of the working conditions, of the requirements of management and of any written policies, the occupational health department must choose how to implement its pre-employment screening procedures. There are, broadly speaking, three choices: by questionnaire alone; by questionnaire and health interview with a nurse; and by questionnaire and clinical examination. Until comparatively recently the third option was widely used, with the result that occupational physicians spent much time in examining well people to no great advantage to the application, the company or themselves. Scarcely anyone would advocate such an approach nowadays, except under special circumstances.

There is a fourth possibility, but one which will almost certainly not be viewed with much approbation by occupational health practitioners, and that is, to do nothing. In my own view, there is a good deal to be said for abandoning pre-employment screening altogether, except where there are legal requirements to do otherwise or very clear medical criteria for particular jobs, and take on all employees on a short-term contract of, say 3–6 months, in the first instance. If health problems arise during this period, then the contract will not be renewed; if they do not, but do so after the initial 6 months, then it is not very likely that they would have been foreseen by any kind of pre-employment screening. My own experience suggests that only a tiny minority of individuals are turned down for a job on medical grounds, and those who find themselves vehemently disagreeing with my suggestion should perhaps conduct a survey in their own departments to determine their own rates of rejection; I doubt if they would be sufficiently high to justify the work involved in pre-employment screening.

The questionnaire

On the assumption that most occupational health practitioners (not to mention *their* employers) will wish to continue with screening prospective employees, the simplest and most cost-effective method for doing so is by the use of a simple questionnaire. An almost infinite variety of these must have been developed over the years, but none can be considered absolutely satisfactory since companies vary in the specific requirements of those they wish to take on their payroll. An example of a screening questionnaire is shown in *Figure 2.1*; it is not meant to be a definitive model, but is one which has worked reasonably well in practice in one occupational setting, a large teaching hospital. Prospective employees should be sent a questionnaire to complete only when they are being seriously considered for a post. This point is worth emphasizing. If questionnaires are sent to *any* individual who applies for a job, the occupational health department will find itself assessing a large number of assessments on individuals who have no prospect of being appointed.

The forms may be sent to applicants by the personnel department or by departmental heads; it does not matter who, so long as they are sent at the appropriate time. They must always be returned – preferably in a reply paid envelope – to the occupational health department, however. It is absolutely essential that applicants are assured that the information in the questionnaire is entirely confidential to the occupational health department, that specific information will not be divulged without written consent, and that management are advised about health matters in general terms only. Some forms require the applicant to sign a declaration that the information given is true and that they understand that falsehoods may lead to dismissal. This quasi-legal declaration appears to be included on the basis that it will induce the applicant to provide more honest answers, but an applicant who wishes to conceal information will almost certainly not be dissuaded from doing so because he has to put his name to the document and, since such a declaration has no standing in law, it is much better to leave it out altogether. What the applicant should

be asked to sign, however, is a form of consent to allow further information to be obtained from his own medical advisers if this is considered necessary to provide a fully informed opinion to management. Most applicants will agree to this.

If it is possible for management and the occupational health department to agree about conditions which are an absolute disbarment to employment in a particular occupation, a simpler procedure could be employed. The form being sent to a prospective employee would state that no one who has now (or had in the past, perhaps) the conditions noted on the form could be employed in the post under consideration, and the applicant would be asked to state that he had none of these. It would not be necessary to ask about other aspects of the medical history, but the applicant would be required to give an unequivocal declaration about those aspects of his health which were considered vital to his being able to carry out the duties attached to the post satisfactorily. Where there were no absolute health requirements there need be no form, but there might be a number of different jobs with different requirements which would mean that several forms would be needed to meet all cases and this would undoubtedly complicate the issue somewhat.

On their return, the forms – of whatever kind – can be scanned by an occupational nurse who should have the authority to advise that an applicant is *suitable* for employment. At times there may be some urgency in advising a manager about the suitability of a candidate and it is reasonable to give a verbal opinion; this must always be confirmed in writing, however.

Where there is any doubt about a candidate's fitness for the post, the form should be referred to the occupational physician. At this stage it will be possible to advise management against employment in some well-defined cases. For example, it would generally be unwise to consider anyone with neurological or renal disorders as suitable for exposure to heavy metals; for those with neurological or hepatic disorders to be exposed to solvents; those with a history of epilepsy would not be suitable for driving; and those with a history of contact dermatitis should not be exposed to skin sensitizers. In such cases, although further information may be required from the applicant's own doctor to confirm a diagnosis, it may not be necessary for the occupational physician to see the individual concerned. When the matter is not entirely clear

<u>IN STRICT CONFIDENCE</u>

Surname .... First names...............................

Address ....

Date of birth .... Marital status ....

Proposed employment ....

Proposed employer ....

Please complete this form as fully as possible and return it as soon as you can in the envelope provided. All the information is strictly confidential and will not be disclosed to anyone without your written permission.

Have you *ever* had any of the following conditions? Please give further details where appropriate.

	Yes or No	*Date*	*Details*

1. Persistent, productive cough?
2. Asthma or hay fever or any other condition?
3. Any skin disorders?
4. Unusual shortness of breath on exertion?
5. Persistent chest pain?
6. Palpitations?
7. Any other heart disease?
8. Fits or faints?
9. Any nervous or mental illness?
10. Jaundice?
11. Kidney or bladder infections?
12. Dysentery, food poisoning or gastroenteritis?
13. Stomach or duodenal ulcers?
14. Persistent pain in the joints?
15. Severe back pain?
16. Diabetes?
17. Do you have any problem with your hearing?
18. Do you have good vision?
19. Do you wear glasses?
20. Have you ever had any illness which required admission to hospital?
        YES/NO

If 'YES', please give further details: ....

....

21. Have you ever had any major operations? YES/NO

If 'YES', please give further details: ....

....

22. Have you ever had an accident which required admission to hospital?
        YES/NO

If 'YES', please give further details: ....

....

Figure 2.1 Pre-placement health questionnaire

23. Are you *at present* having any treatment from your doctor?
                                YES/NO

If 'YES', please give further details: ....

....

24. Are you on the Disablement Register?   YES/NO

If 'YES', what is your disability? ....

....

25. When did you last have a chest X-ray? ....

26. Do you consider that you are in good health at present? YES/NO

27. Have you had a medical examination in the last five years for an insurance policy or for any other purpose?   YES/NO

If 'YES', what was the outcome? ....

28. Do you smoke?   YES/NO

If 'YES', how many cigarettes, or how much tobacco do you smoke a day? ....

....

29. Do you drink alcohol?   YES/NO

If 'YES', how much do you drink per week? ....

Figure 2.1 (*continued*)

cut, however, the applicant must be seen before advice can be given one way or the other.

The majority of cases can be dealt with satisfactorily in this way. Where there are special risks, or where the health and safety of others may be affected, an interview with the occupational nurse as a follow-up to the questionnaire may be advisable. The health interview should be used to obtain specific information. For example, what are the standards of personal hygiene of those who are going to be employed as food handlers? Is the vision of prospective crane drivers adequate? As before, the nurse should have the authority to recommend acceptance, but must refer doubtful cases to the doctor. It is preferable to conduct the health interview on the day of the applicant's job interview, but in busy departments this may not always be possible.

From what has been said so far, it will be clear that pre-employment medical examinations should be the exception rather than the rule. Some are obligatory in order to obtain a licence to undertake the job in question – airline pilots

and heavy goods vehicle drivers or public service drivers, for example – while the demands of some other occupations may make a medical examination desirable. Candidates for the fire and police services come within this category since their job requires a high standard of personal fitness. Some employers may require it for some or all new employees; this is particularly the case for senior appointments, and the occupational physician will have to comply in those instances. He may choose to try to influence against such a policy if he feels that nothing useful is served by it, but in the end, the employer must be free to exercise his preference.

Pre-employment testing

Pre-employment tests may be required as part of the assessment of fitness for a particular job to ensure that the applicants meet certain prescribed standards or to exclude some prescribed conditions such as alcohol or drug abuse, or hepatitis B in those who are going to carry out invasive procedures. Where exposure to potentially toxic materials is involved, it may be considered necessary to undertake some examinations in order to exclude those who may have conditions which would be exacerbated by exposure to the material in question. Thus a chest X-ray might be suggested for those whose job would involve exposure to fibrogenic dusts, or liver function tests for those who will experience solvent exposure. As a general rule, pre-employment tests should only be carried out when there is a clear aim and a clear decision about what result will disbar an individual from employment – blunderbuss screening has nothing at all to commend it.

Some individuals who have exposure to toxic materials will need to be entered into a programme of biological monitoring or some other form of surveillance and others will need to have a series of immunizations to protect them from hazards at work. It is best if any baseline tests which are done prior to continuous monitoring – lung function tests for those exposed to sensitizers, for example – and work protection immunizations are carried out soon after the individual has started work, rather than at the time of pre-employment screening.

Psychometric testing

There has been some discussion in the UK about the role of psychometric testing in the recruitment of children's nurses following a notorious case in which a young woman was found to have caused the deaths of some children in her care. Although some such tests may pick out those with personality disorders, they are blunt instruments and may have little predictive power. They do not, in any case, pick out those who appear normal now, but may develop problems in the future.

Even when it seems appropriate to use psychometric tests as part of a process for selecting new employees, it is extremely doubtful that the occupational health practitioners would have the expertise necessary to apply and interpret them and they are much more likely to provide a false sense of security than to prevent the actions of an occasional mentally disturbed person.

Summary of pre-employment screening

Pre-employment screening, like any other form of screening, should have a clearly defined aim, in this case, to try to ensure the best fit between employees and their jobs. If it is to be carried out, occupational health practitioners must be familiar with the demands of each job and they must be aware of any special hazards associated with them and with any particular requirements of management. It is this special knowledge about the nature and the demands of work which makes occupational health practitioners in any sense different from their colleagues in other specialities and which makes them the best fitted professionals to carry out this task.

Routine medical examinations are unnecessary in the majority of cases which can be dealt with adequately by a questionnaire supplemented, where necessary, by an interview with an occupational nurse. The nurse should be authorized to accept but not to reject candidates; rejection should be the prerogative of the occupational physician.

Pre-employment testing should be carried out only when there is a good and sufficient reason for doing so.

Confidentiality must be assured at each stage of the process and prospective employees must be made to feel that the occupational health department has their best interests foremost in its deliberations while, at the same time, not abrogating responsibilities to other employees and to the employer.

Fitness to work

The assessment of the fitness or otherwise of an individual to work in a particular post is the basis of pre-employment screening, but it also arises in another context in occupational health practice and that is, following return to work after an illness. When making this assessment the same rules as before apply; that is, there must be a good working knowledge of work practices and a good fit between work and worker must be ensured. It is also necessary to determine whether the illness has left any sequelae which may impair the ability to carry out all the tasks normally allotted to the employee, although this is generally straightforward and may often not need the input of an occupational physician. In some cases it will be clear that an individual has become so incapacitated that work is beyond them, but this is usually rare. Most often, there will have been complete recovery, and a brief consultation with a nurse or doctor will confirm this. Other cases may be more problematic and here three different hurdles may present themselves, any or all of which may have to be overcome. These hurdles are placed in the path of the occupational health practitioner by the employee, the manager and the employee's own doctor.

The employee

The employee may be apprehensive about returning to work before being 'ready'. Often it is not clear what is meant by this nebulous concept and it seems to be found most frequently in those recovering from a chronic, debilitating illness such as ME in which convalescence may be prolonged and improvement almost indiscernible on a day-to-day basis. It is useful to encourage a return to work as quickly as possible in these cases, stressing the likely therapeutic benefit to be expected, and the disadvantages that too long an absence from work may have on job security. (It is surprising how many people – in the UK at least – think that their contract cannot be terminated if they are on sick leave.) If possible, a gradual return to work, phased over a few days or weeks, may be helpful, provided that the individual's manager agrees. Redeployment may be another means whereby an employee may be persuaded to return to work, but in the streamlined economies of western Europe this option is becoming rather constrained.

Most employees want to return to their work, however, and it is – in most cases – actually beneficial for them to do so, not only for the financial advantages which may accrue. If the doctor is in any doubt about an individual's readiness to return to work, the best means of dispelling any doubts is to ask the employee if they feel able to go back. If the answer is in the affirmative, then they should be allowed to do so, even if this is on the understanding that it may be on a trial basis (a 'trial of labour'); such employees should be followed up by the occupational health department regularly to ensure that they are truly able to cope. (If the answer to the question about readiness to return to work is 'no', the occupational physician

may need to adopt the strategy suggested in the previous paragraph of this section.)

The employee's manager

The second hurdle to overcome is that placed by the employee's manager. There seems to be a widespread belief among managers that 'fitness' is a dichotomous variable, such that an individual is either 'fit' or 'unfit', with nothing in between. If the occupational physician says that an employee is recovered sufficiently enough to return to work, but that some restrictions may initially have to be placed upon him, the response may be that the manager declines to have the employee back until the worker is 'completely fit'. It seems to me to be very important that occupational health practitioners should educate managers into viewing fitness as a continuous variable and that we are all towards one or other end of the scale at different times, and that our position on the scale is not necessarily a good index of our ability to work satisfactorily.

When an employee has been off sick, the occupational physician is sometimes asked if the illness which caused the absence will affect future attendance and – allowing for some obvious exceptions – it is generally not possible to predict this with any certainty. The occupational physician should try to act as educator by explaining that the present state of health is the result of events which have taken place in the past and may have no value whatsoever in foretelling how the state of health will be in the future. Unfortunately much of the demand for routine medical examinations is predicated on precisely the opposite view and seems only to have value for those who charge for undertaking them.

The employee's own doctor

In many countries occupational health occupies a minuscule part of the undergraduate medical syllabus. My own most recent experience was in teaching medical students for a single three-hour lesson – this was all the formal teaching they had in the subject. It should not be a surprise, then, that doctors outside the speciality have little knowledge of the demands of their patients' work. My experience suggests that doctors generally advise their patients *against* an early return to work and may even give them advice which is entirely counter-productive. One sees this particularly with patients who have back pain who are frequently advised to have time off work and go to bed until the pain subsides, during which time they lose their muscle tone and delay their recovery substantially. The results of the studies which have been carried out on the problem suggest an entirely opposite course of action and show that, unless there are neurological complications, a prompt return to work speeds up recovery, especially if combined with some form of rehabilitation at the workplace (see also Chapters 17 and 22).

Despite advice from their occupational physician, some individuals may feel obliged to accept the advice of the doctor who is treating them, even though this may lead to the loss of their job, which certainly does them no favour at all (see Chapter 1). It is important for occupational physicians to liaise with both general practitioners and hospital specialists in order that the best interests of their mutual patients are served, at least so far as their working life is concerned.

Further reading

Cox, R.A.F., Edwards, F.C. and McCallum, R.I. (eds) *Fitness for Work: The Medical Aspects*, 2nd edn. Oxford University Press, Oxford (1995)

Chapter 3

Basic toxicology

B Hellman

Introduction

An occupational health practitioner meeting patients with a work-related exposure to chemicals should be familiar with the fundamental principles of toxicology and the basis of toxicology testing. The fact that most toxicological data derive from studies on experimental animals reinforces the importance of knowing something about the premises for toxicity testing, and how toxicological data are used in risk assessment. When evaluating the 'toxicological profile' of an industrial agent, information is gathered about its rates and patterns of absorption, distribution, metabolism and excretion, and of its immediate and delayed adverse health effects, target organs of toxicity, clinical manifestations of intoxication, mechanism(s) of action and dose–response curves. Skimming through a rather enormous field, the present chapter focuses on some of the basic concepts in toxicology necessary for the understanding of how toxicity data are used in human risk assessments.

Toxicology – a science and an art

Toxicology deals with chemically-induced adverse effects on living organisms. These chemicals include both man-made, non-naturally occurring agents ('toxicants', 'xenobiotics' or 'foreign compounds'), and naturally occurring substances such as the poisons produced by bacteria, animals and plants (often referred to as 'toxins'). Toxicology is a multidisciplinary science including methods and traditions from several other disciplines (e.g. analytical chemistry, biochemistry, cell biology, pathology, pharmacology and physiology). One particular branch in toxicology, ecotoxicology, is oriented towards the environmental impacts of chemicals, but the mainstream is focused on describing and evaluating toxicity from the human health perspective. Occupational toxicology is only one of several branches of applied toxicology anticipating human health hazards by using fundamental toxicological principles.

Toxicity is often defined as the intrinsic ability of an agent to harm living organisms. This definition is not unequivocal because it will ultimately depend on how the term 'harm' is defined. Toxicity can also be defined as an adverse health effect associated with a change, reduction or loss of a vital function, including an impaired capacity to compensate for additional stress induced by other environmental factors. Changes in morphology, physiology, development, growth and life span leading to an impairment of functional capacities are typical examples of 'toxic', 'deleterious', 'detrimental', 'harmful', 'injurious', 'damaging', 'unwanted' or 'adverse' effects, but should an itchy nose, a subtle change in blood pressure or a small change in a subset of lymphocytes be regarded as adverse effects? Most toxicologists would probably not think of these effects as being significant evidence of toxicity, but rather as non-specific biological indicators of exposure.

The concept of toxicity is indeed rather complex. Is hyperplasia a sign of a healthy physiological adaptation or a pathological process? Should an inflammatory reaction be regarded primarily as an adverse effect or a normal defence mechanism of the body? Moreover, an effect which is adverse to one individual may in some situations be desirable to another. Toxicologists generally discuss toxicity following from exposures exceeding tolerable doses, but harmful effects can also be induced by a state of deficiency, if this deficiency affects an essential element. Toxicologists are experts on the adverse effects of chemicals, but toxicity can also be induced by ionizing radiation and other physical agents. Toxic agents do interact with one another, and these interactions can result in both increased and decreased responses, and biological diversity can explain why a chemical may induce clearly adverse effects in one species but not in another. Certainly, man-made as well as naturally occurring chemicals can induce a broad spectrum of undesired health effects, some of which are clearly deleterious, whereas others are not.

Chemical and physical properties

Toxic agents can be classified in terms of their physical state, chemical and physical properties, origin, mechanism of action, toxic effects, target organ or use, but no single classification will cover all the aspects of a given chemical. The work-related toxicants include most type of agents (metals, dusts, gases, solvents, pesticides, explosives, dyes, etc.), producing different types of adverse effects (skin and eye irritation, skin sensibilization, asphyxiation, tumours, genotoxicity, reproductive toxicity, kidney and liver damage, behavioural changes, etc.), by various mechanisms of actions (e.g. by interfering with the cellular energy production or calcium homeostasis, by binding to various cellular macromolecules, by disturbing the endogenous receptor–ligand interactions, etc.). Agents belonging to a certain class of compounds (e.g. organic solvents) often have some adverse effects in common (e.g. a CNS depressant effect after acute high-dose exposure), but as a general rule, each individual compound has its own unique 'toxicological profile' which, to a large extent, is dependent on its chemical and physical properties.

Consequently, knowledge about the chemical and physical properties is one of the most important prerequisites when testing and evaluating the toxicity of a chemical. The toxicant should be characterized with regard to its chemical identity, molecular weight, physical state, purity, solubility, stability, melting point (for solids), boiling point and vapour pressure (for liquids), particle size, shape and density distribution (for aerosols and dusts), pH and flash point. The identity and concentration of possible impurities and degradation products should also be known. Largely depending on its chemical and physical properties, a toxicant will mainly induce either local or systemic adverse effects. Most toxicants express their deleterious effects after they have been absorbed and distributed in the body, but some chemicals (e.g. strong acids and bases, or highly reactive compounds such as epoxides) primarily act at the first site of contact. Typical examples of effects occurring at the first site of contact are the severe burns on the eyes and the skin following a splash in the face with a strong alkaline agent, the gastric ulcers following the ingestion of a corrosive agent, and the inflammatory reactions in the respiratory tract following the inhalation of an irritant agent.

The concept of 'dose'

By dose, most people intuitively mean the amount of substance entering the body on one specific occasion. This definition of dose is relevant for single exposures but less appropriate when discussing the effects of repeated exposures over an extended period of time. Ideally, dose should be defined as the total amount of toxicant taken by, or administered to, the organism. Typical measures for the dose when testing for toxicity are mg/kg body weight and $\mu mol/cm^2$ body surface area. Often it is more beneficial to talk about the dosage instead of the dose. Dosage (also referred to as the dose–time integral) can be defined as the amount of toxicant taken by, or given to, the organism over time. A typical measure for the dosage when testing for toxicity is mg/kg body weight per day. Finding the appropriate dosage is rather important when designing a toxicity study. For ethical, practical and economic reasons, toxicity testing is usually performed using a restricted number of animals. Critical health effects may be overlooked if the dosage is too low. If the dosage is too high, this may also lead to unfortunate consequences, especially when the interpretation of the outcome of the study is dependent on a reasonable survival of the animals.

One of the most fundamental concepts in toxicology is that it is the dose that makes the poison. This means that all chemicals will become toxic at some dosage. Whereas some compounds are lethal if ingested in minute quantities (e.g. botulinum toxin and plutonium), others will induce their adverse effects only if ingested in relatively large quantities. Disregarding the possible effects of conditioning, a chemical cannot induce any adverse effects unless it reaches a critical site (by itself or in the form of a toxic metabolite), at a sufficiently high concentration, for a sufficiently long period of time. From this follows that even an extremely toxic substance will be harmless as long as it is kept in a closed container, and that a relatively non-toxic chemical can be rather hazardous if handled carelessly.

The concentration of the ultimate form of the toxicant at the site of action will in general be directly proportional to the dosage. However, the final 'target dose' (i.e. the amount of ultimate toxicant present at the critical site for the necessary period of time) is also governed by several other factors such as the actual exposure, the fate of the toxicant in the body once it has been absorbed, and the susceptibility of the individual exposed to the toxicant. Intra- and interindividual variations in susceptibility depend on several factors such as the species, genetic constitution, age and sex, health condition and nutritional status, previous and ongoing exposures to other toxicants, and climate conditions. All these factors should be considered when using data obtained under one set of conditions to predict what the outcome would become under another.

Obviously, the concept of dose is not easy to define unequivocally. 'Dose' can relate both to the 'pharmacological dose' (i.e. the amount actually inhaled, ingested, injected or applied on the skin) and the 'target dose' (i.e. the amount of ultimate toxicant actually present at the critical site for a sufficient period of time), but it can also relate to the 'exposure dose' and the 'tissue dose'. The 'exposure dose' is the amount or concentration of toxicant present in the surrounding environment. In the working environment, a threshold limit value can be defined as an 'exposure dose' that should not be exceeded. The way of expressing the latter type of dose varies depending on the environmental medium, but it is typically expressed in terms of mg/m^2 (e.g. for air contaminants), ppm (parts per million; e.g. for air, water, soil and food contaminants), ppm-hours (e.g. for air contaminants), $\mu g/l$ (e.g. for

air and water contaminants) or mg/kg (e.g. for soil and food contaminants). The 'tissue dose' (or 'organ dose') is the amount or concentration of the toxicant in various organs and tissues after absorption, distribution and metabolism. The 'tissue dose' (usually expressed as the total amount of toxicant per weight of organ, or the amount present in the tissue during a specified time interval), typically varies between various organs.

'Acute exposures' and 'chronic effects'

An 'exposure' is not only characterized by the 'exposure dose' but also by the frequency, duration and route of exposure. In the past, a compound was often considered harmless if it was without immediate adverse health effects when administered in a large single dose. Nowadays it has been recognized that some toxicants accumulate in the body and that the 'tissue dose' will eventually become critically high if the exposure to such agents continues for a sufficiently long period of time, at sufficiently high doses. It has also been recognized that a short-term exposure to some type of toxicants (e.g. potent genotoxic agents) may be sufficient to induce delayed adverse effects (e.g. malignant tumours or genetic diseases).

Toxicologists often use the terms 'acute' and 'chronic' to describe the duration and frequency of exposure in toxicity tests, but these terms can also be used to characterize the nature of the observed adverse health effects in the various types of tests. Consequently, although a single dose exposure in most cases is associated with acute effects (i.e. immediately occurring adverse effects manifested within a few minutes up to a couple of days after the exposure), it can also induce delayed adverse effects manifested only after a lapse of some time. Long-term chronic exposures are usually associated with chronic effects, but they can also induce acute effects typically manifested when a sufficient amount of toxicant has been accumulated in a critical target organ.

Depending on the duration and frequency of exposure, experimental studies on the general toxicity of chemicals are usually referred to as either short-term toxicity studies or long-term toxicity studies (chronic studies). The maximum duration of exposure in an acute study is limited to 24 h. The compound is administered either orally (in most cases as a single dose), by inhalation (usually for 6 h) or cutaneously (usually for 24 h on a shaven area of the skin). The maximum duration of exposure in a short-term repeated dose study (previously referred to as a 'subacute' study) is limited to 1 month, and in a subchronic toxicity study to a time period corresponding to 10% of the normal life span of the animal (usually 90 days). The duration of exposure in a long-term toxicity study should be at least 10% of the normal life span of the animals (usually 1 or 2 years). In the long-term repeat dose toxicity studies, the test compound is usually given via the diet, but it can also be administered in the drinking water (continuous exposure), by gavage or capsule (usually 1 oral dose/day, 5 days/week), on the skin (usually 1 daily application, 5 days/week), or in the inhaled air (usually for 6 h/day, 5 days/ week). In some studies, the animals are exposed for several generations (e.g. in the two-generation reproduction toxicity studies).

'Route of entry' and bioavailability

The bioavailability of a toxicant (i.e. the rate at which the chemical passes from the site of administration into the systemic circulation) depends on several factors. The chemical and physical properties of the toxicant are obviously important. Another, often closely related factor, is the ability of the toxicant to be released from its environmental matrix (i.e. from the material that was injected, ingested, inhaled or applied on the skin). The route of entry (i.e. the way a compound enters the body) is also important for determining the bioavailability of most toxicants.

Maximum bioavailability (and therefore the most intense and rapidly occurring toxic response) should be expected after an intravenous injection. In general, the bioavailability for a given toxicant gradually decreased in the following order: inhalation > intraperitoneal injection > subcutaneous injection > intramuscular injection > intradermal injection > oral administration > dermal application. Workers are typically exposed to dusts or volatile products entering the body via the lungs or by skin absorption, but they can also be exposed to non-volatile materials entering the

body orally or via the skin. Toxicity data generated in inhalation studies and/or after dermal application are therefore of particular value when evaluating the toxicological profile of industrial compounds. Oral toxicity data may also be relevant, especially for agents inhaled as dusts reaching the gastrointestinal tract after mucociliary clearance.

Toxicokinetics

Studies on the rates and patterns of absorption, distribution, metabolism and excretion of toxicants are known as pharmacokinetic or toxicokinetic studies. When studying the toxicokinetics of a chemical in experimental animals, the compound can be administered either as it is, or labelled with a radioactive isotope (e.g. tritium or carbon-14). The concentration of the toxicant (and/or its metabolites) is then usually determined after various time intervals in different body fluids, organs and/or excreta, using gas or liquid chromatographic methods, mass spectrometry or other analytical methods such as liquid scintillation counting for radiolabelled compounds.

Toxicokinetic studies should ideally be performed using both high and low doses, single and repeated exposures, different routes of exposures, both sexes, different ages, pregnant and non-pregnant animals, and different species. Knowledge about the 'fate' of a toxicant in the body under different exposure conditions, facilitates the selection of appropriate testing conditions when designing the subsequent toxicity studies. Toxicokinetic studies can also be of great help when extrapolating animal toxicity data to human health hazards because, often, they will provide important information on, for example, the potential binding to various plasma proteins and/or intracellular macromolecules, and possible interactions with various receptors and/or enzyme systems, under different exposure conditions for different species.

The kinetic parameters determined in the toxicokinetic studies are often used in various mathematical models to predict the time course of disposition of the toxicant (and/or its metabolites) in various 'compartments' of the organism. By using 'one-compartment', 'two-compartment' or 'physiologically' based pharmacokinetic (toxicokinetic) models it is, for example, possible to predict various absorption and elimination rate constants, hepatic, renal and total body clearances, biological half-lives, the degree of plasma protein binding, apparent volumes of distributions, and steady-state concentrations of the toxicant in various organs.

Absorption

The process(es) by which a substance enters the body after being ingested, inhaled or applied on the skin is rather important when discussing the toxicological profile of a given chemical. One way of measuring the absorption in experimental animals is to measure the total amount of toxicant (and/or metabolites) eliminated in the urine, bile, faeces and exhaled air, and compare the excreted amount with that remaining in the body. There are several barriers a toxicant may have to pass before it can induce its systemic toxicity. The skin, lungs and alimentary canal are obvious biological barriers, but there are also others, such the 'blood–brain' barrier and the placenta.

Toxicants are absorbed by the same processes as essential substances. Since most toxicants are absorbed by simple diffusion, small, lipid-soluble and non-ionized molecules will in general be more readily absorbed than bulky, less lipid-soluble, ionized molecules. However, there are no rules without exceptions. Whereas small hydrophilic molecules (e.g. ethanol) easily will pass any biological barrier through the aqueous pores in the membranes, extremely lipid-soluble compounds (e.g. the highest chlorinated polychlorinated biphenyls) may have some difficulties because of their poor solubility in blood and other body fluids. Toxicants can also use various specialized transport systems in order to enter the body. They can, for example, be transported by forming complexes with membrane-bound carriers that usually are involved in the transportation of nutrients, electrolytes, oxygen and other essential elements.

Many substances given orally will never reach the general circulation. When ingested they can, for example, be detoxified by enzymes in the intestinal mucosa. They can also decompose to harmless products. A third possibility is that they are so tightly bound to the material ingested that the whole complex is excreted unabsorbed via the faeces. If an ingested compound is actually absorbed in the gastrointestinal tract, it will immediately be transported to the liver where typically it will be taken care of by various enzymes (the so-called first-pass effect). As long as the tissue dose

in the liver is handled by detoxifying enzymes, the toxicant will not be able to reach the general circulation. However, if the same substance enters the body via the lungs, or through the skin, it will be taken up by the general circulation and have the opportunity to induce systemic toxicity if it accumulates in sufficiently high concentrations in the critical organs.

Distribution

Although some locally induced adverse health effects indirectly may lead to systemic effects (e.g. the kidney damage following from severe acid burns), systemic toxicity cannot be induced unless the toxicant (and/or its toxic metabolites) is present in a sufficiently high concentration in the target organs. For example, a chemical mutagen cannot induce critical germ cell mutations leading to an increased risk for genetic disease in the offspring, unless this mutagen actually reaches the germ cells of a fertile and reproductive individual. Studies on the distribution of a toxicant deals with the process(es) by which an absorbed toxicant (and/or its metabolites) circulates and partitions in the body. There are at least three different types of distribution that are of interest: that within the body, that within an organ, and that within a cell. If a compound is labelled with a radioactive isotope, it is possible to study its actual distribution using whole-body autoradiography (*Figure 3.1*) and/or micro-autoradiography. The concentration of an unlabelled test substance (and/or its metabolites) can also be measured in various organs, tissues and cells using various traditional analytical chemical methods.

After absorption has taken place and the compound has entered the blood it is usually distributed rapidly throughout the body. The rate and pattern of distribution depends on several factors, including the regional blood flow, the solubility of the compound in the blood, and the affinity of the toxicant to various serum proteins and tissue constituents. Whereas some toxicants accumulate in their target organs (e.g. cadmium in the kidneys, chloroquine concentrating in the retina, carbon monoxide binding to haemoglobin, and paraquat accumulating in the lungs), others will concentrate in tissues not primarily affected by toxicity (e.g. lead accumulating in bones and teeth, and polychlorinated biphenyls accumulating in fat depots).

Lung Liver Adrenal cortex

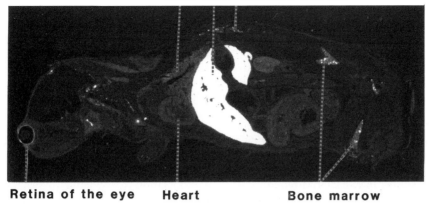

Retina of the eye   **Heart**   **Bone marrow**

Figure 3.1   Whole-body autoradiogram showing the distribution of radioactivity (light areas) in a pigmented mouse, 7 days after an intravenous injection of [^{14}C]DMBA   (i.e. dimethylbenz(a)anthracene, a genotoxic polycyclic aromatic hydrocarbon). The autoradiogram shows a particularly high accumulation of radioactivity in the liver, adrenal cortex, bone marrow and in the retina of the eye (by courtesy of A. Roberto, B. Larsson and H. Tjälve)

Metabolic biotransformation

In physiology, metabolism includes all the anabolic (i.e. synthetic) and catabolic (i.e. degenerative) transformations of the normal constituents of a living organism. These transformations can be disturbed by toxicants, acting, for example, as metabolic inhibitors. In toxicology, the concept of metabolism has become equivalent to the biotransformation of xenobiotics, i.e. the metabolism of any foreign chemical that does not occur in the normal metabolic pathways of the organism. Obviously, the rate and pattern of metabolic biotransformation is one of the most critical factors determining whether or not or a given chemical will be able to induce its toxicity under otherwise standardized exposure conditions. There are a number of factors influencing the biotransformation of a given toxicant. Variations in genetic constitution, age, sex, species, strain, nutritional status, underlying diseases and concomitant exposures to other xenobiotics with enzyme-inducing and/or enzyme-inhibiting activities, can often explain differences in toxicity observed in different species or populations exposed to a particular toxicant at a given dosage.

During evolution, mammals have developed rather specialized systems to deal with the plethora of foreign substances entering the body every day. The purpose of metabolic biotransformation is to convert the xenobiotics to more water-soluble products so that they can more readily be eliminated from the body via the urine and/or faeces. This will usually require at least two different metabolic steps. The first step (a phase I reaction) usually involves the introduction of a reactive polar group into the foreign molecule. In the second step (a phase II reaction), the polar group is generally conjugated with a water-soluble endogenous compound. Metabolic biotransformation is usually equivalent to detoxification leading to an increased rate of elimination of foreign compounds, but sometimes this process can lead to metabolic bioactivation, i.e. to an increased toxicity of xenobiotics.

Phase I reactions include microsomal, mitochondrial and cytosolic oxidations, reductions, hydrolysis, epoxide hydrations and prostaglandin synthetase reactions. The microsomal cytochrome P$_{450}$ system (also known as the mixed-function oxygenase system) is the most important oxidative phase I enzyme system, both in experimental animals and in humans. It comprises a whole family of enzymes involved both in the detoxification and bioactivation of toxicants. So far, at least 70 different cytochrome P$_{450}$ genes have been identified in various species, and there are at least eight different mammalian cytochrome P$_{450}$ gene families present in various organs. The liver is the major metabolizing organ in the body, but cytochrome P$_{450}$s and other microsomal phase I enzymes are present in most other organs (e.g. the lungs, kidneys, intestines, nasal mucosa, skin, testis, placenta and adrenals). There are also different types of phase II enzymes present in most organs. The most important conjugation reaction, at least in humans, is the one involving glucuronic acid which is present in the endoplasmic reticulum of the liver cells, and in most other tissues.

There are numerous ways of studying the process(es) by which a particular toxicant is structurally changed in the body by enzymatic and/or non-enzymatic reactions. In an experimental context, the details of the various steps in the phase I and phase II reactions are often studied using different *in vitro* systems. It may be worth noting that many toxicity tests based on cultured cells and/or prokaryotic organisms (e.g. bacteria) require the addition of a mammalian metabolic activation system. This metabolic system is typically a so-called S9-mix, which is a cofactor-supplemented postmitochondrial fraction from the livers of rodents treated with phenobarbital or other enzyme-inducing agents. When interpreting toxicity data from *in vitro* studies supplemented with an S9-fraction, one should be aware of the fact that these test systems are characterized by a high 'phase I capacity', but a low 'phase II capacity'.

Excretion

The process(es) by which a toxicant is eliminated from the body is usually studied by measuring the concentration of the toxicant (and/or its metabolites) in the excreta (typically urine, faeces and/or expired air). These measurements are usually performed until approximately 95% of the administered dose has been recovered. Sometimes it may be necessary to measure the amounts in the milk, sweat, saliva, tears and hair, in order to get a complete picture of the rate and pattern of elimination for a given toxicant. The kidney is the most important organ when it comes to the elimination of xenobiotics. The elimination processes via the kidneys are rather complex and there are at least three different pathways that are of interest: glomerular filtration (the most important pathway), tubular excretion by passive diffusion (of minor importance), and active tubular secretion (mainly for organic acids and bases and some protein-bound toxicants). Compounds that are small enough to be filtered with the plasma at the glomeruli can be reabsorbed in the tubuli.

Elimination through faeces aggravates the summation of excretion from the liver, intestinal excretion and excretion of non-absorbed ingested material. Hepatic (biliary) excretion is the second most important route of elimination for toxicants. Agents metabolized in the liver can either enter the blood stream or be excreted from the system into the bile. Excretory products with a rather high molecular weight (above 300–500 in rats, guinea pigs and rabbits, and above 500–700 in humans) are primarily excreted in the bile, whereas those with lower molecular weights are primarily excreted in the urine by glomerular filtration. Toxicants excreted in the bile can also be reabsorbed. This process is known as the enterohepatic circulation, and it occurs in the small intestine. Pulmonary excretion can be an important route of elimination for volatile toxicants (e.g. for many organic solvents). The rate of elimination via the respiratory system depends on several factors, the most important being the solubility of the compound in the blood, the blood flow to the lungs and the rate of respiration.

A toxicant will accumulate in the body if the rate of absorption exceeds the rates of metabolic biotransformation and/or elimination. The biological half-life ($t_{1/2}$) of a toxicant is usually defined as the time needed to reduce the absorbed amount in the body by 50%, but it can also represent the elimination half-life required for the concentration of toxicant in plasma (or in a specific organ) to decrease by one-half. The biological half-life varies considerably between various toxicants, from hours (e.g. for phenol), to years (e.g. for some dioxins) or even decades (e.g. for cadmium). The process of 'biomagnification' ('bioamplification') is a special case of bioaccumulation representing the systematic increase of the concentration of an environmental pollutant in various food chains. Biomagnification occurs when a persistent toxicant (e.g. methyl mercury) is transferred from one trophic level to another in the food chain (i.e. from the 'food' to the 'consumer').

Basic principles in toxicity testing

Toxicity testing is an important part of hazard identification. The main purpose is to identify the 'toxicological profile' of a given chemical, i.e. to characterize its 'inherent' potential to act as a toxicant. The spectrum of adverse health effects ('toxicological end-points') that can be induced by a chemical includes both reversible and irreversible effects, local and systemic toxicity, immediate and delayed effects, organ-specific and general adverse effects. Toxicity testing provides information about the shape of the dose–response curves for the various types of toxic effects identified, including the so-called 'no observed adverse effect levels' (NOAELs) and 'lowest observed adverse effect levels' (LOAELs). The most valuable information about the toxicity of a given chemical derives from observations made in exposed human populations, but most people would probably agree that *deliberate toxicity testing* on human subjects is out of the question. Of necessity, toxicity data are therefore usually generated in studies on experimental animals. The results obtained in these studies are then extrapolated to human exposure.

The whole concept of toxicity testing is based on the assumption that experimental animals can be used to identify potential health hazards for humans. The fact that vinyl chloride, an industrial solvent, induces liver tumours in both experimental animals (rats, mice and hamsters) and humans is only one piece of evidence indicating that the same type of adverse effects can be observed in both humans and experimental animals. Another fundamental assumption underlying the toxicity

testing is that the rate of adverse health effects increases as the dosage (exposure) increases.

The toxicity tests used when testing for the potential adverse health effects of chemicals can be separated into two major categories: those designed to identify general toxicity, and those designed to identify specific types of adverse health effects (*Table 3.1*). For most toxicity tests there are internationally accepted guidelines available describing how each individual test should be performed in order to obtain a well-defined framework for both the testing and the evaluation of toxicity (e.g. the OECD Guidelines for Testing of Chemicals). The guidelines specify the prerequisites, procedures (preferred species, group sizes, limited tests, etc.), testing conditions (dosages, routes of administration, clinical observations, haematology, pathology etc.), statistical procedures, and how the test report should be formulated. The guidelines have also been developed in order to minimize unnecessary suffering for the experimental animals. To protect the animals from unnecessary stress following from pain and

Table 3.1 Toxicological end-points measured in a complete battery of toxicity tests

Adverse health effect	*A representative sample of tests for which there are internationally accepted guidelines*
Acute toxicity and lethality	Acute oral toxicity study on rats Acute inhalation toxicity study on mice Acute dermal toxicity study on guinea pigs
Short-term repeat dose and subchronic toxicity	14 days oral toxicity study on mice 21 days dermal toxicity study on rats 90 days diet study on rats 90 days inhalation toxicity study on guinea pigs
Chronic toxicity	12 months oral toxicity study on dogs 24 months inhalation toxicity study on rats
Local effects on the skin	Acute dermal irritation and corrosion study on rabbits
Local effects on the eye	Acute eye irritation and corrosion study on rabbits
Allergic sensitization	Skin sensitization study on guinea pigs
Genotoxicity and mutagenicity	HPC/DNA repair test *Salmonella typhimurium* reverse mutation assay Micronucleus test Sister chromatid exchanges in peripheral lymphocytes
Tumourigenicity	18 months dietary cancer bioassay in mice 24 months inhalation cancer bioassay in rats
Embryotoxicity and teratogenicity	Teratogenicity study on pregnant rabbits
Reproductive toxicity	Two-generation reproduction study on rats
Neurotoxicity	(No specific testing guidelines available for neurotoxicity or behavioural toxicity; indirect evidence in general toxicity studies)
Immunotoxicity	(No specific testing guidelines available; thymus toxicity can be monitored in general toxicity studies)

discomfort is not only important from a humane point of view, but also because of the fact that this type of stress may interfere with the 'true' toxic responses induced by the chemical under test.

It should be emphasized that all toxicity tests are designed to reveal potential toxicity, not to prove the harmlessness of chemicals. The various tests are therefore usually designed to be as sensitive as possible. In order to compensate for the limited number of animals in most regular toxicity tests, it is absolutely necessary to use relatively high dosages. However, 'high' doses do not necessarily mean lethal doses. For example, the highest dosage in a chronic cancer bioassay is often referred to as the 'maximum tolerated dose' (MTD). This is unfortunate because many people will then think of the MTD as an almost inevitably lethal dosage, killing most of the animals. It would be better if MTD was comprehended as a 'minimally toxic dose', because according to most guidelines the highest dosage in cancer bioassay should be high enough to induce some signs of toxicity (e.g. a slightly reduced body weight gain), but it should not substantially alter the normal life span of the animals due to effects other than tumours.

The possible limitations of toxicity testing on animals and cultured cells must always be considered when evaluating the results from these tests, and experimental exposure can never exactly mirror true human exposure. The latter is typically characterized by simultaneous exposure to varying concentrations of a complex mixtures of chemicals by various routes. When evaluating animal toxicity data, one should also be aware of the fact that there are several factors that can influence the outcome in a toxicity study. Important modifying factors are the species, strain, sex, age, body weight, health condition, nutritional status, route of exposure, duration and frequency of exposure, climatic conditions, and, as in many other situations, the human factor. It is not unusual for different laboratories to report different results from a specific toxicity test of a given test chemical, and this rather frustrating situation can often be explained by differences in laboratory conditions and experimental procedures. Despite all the possible limitations with toxicity studies and the undeniable fact that different animals species may respond differently to various toxicants, it still seems to be a general consensus that these limitations and differences are not so great that interspecies comparisons are impossible.

Studies on general toxicity

Acute toxicity

Testing for acute toxicity is often considered to be equivalent to studies on lethality. In most cases it is indeed possible to calculate approximate median lethal doses after various routes of exposures (i.e. oral or dermal LD_{50} doses, and/or inhalation LC_{50} concentrations), but the main purpose of acute toxicity testing is to gather some basic toxicological information before the further toxicity testing. After exposing a restricted number of animals (orally, cutaneously or by inhalation), these are examined at least once a day for 14 days. Animals showing severe signs of intoxication are killed in advance in order to reduce unnecessary suffering, and all animals are necropsied at the end of the study.

Acute toxicity studies provide not only important information on immediate health hazards and clinical signs of intoxication, but they can also identify potential adverse effects, possible target organs, and conceivable modes of actions, for the further toxicity testing. Obviously, the results from these tests are valuable when establishing the dosage regimens in repeat dose toxicity studies. The results can also be used to classify chemicals in terms of various types of toxicity ratings. For example, depending on its estimated median lethality (LD_{50} or LC_{50}), a chemical can be classified as being 'practically non-toxic', 'slightly toxic, 'moderately toxic', 'very toxic', 'extremely toxic' or 'super toxic'. Many recommendations regarding protective measures and need for medical attention are based on such acute toxicity classification systems.

Short-term repeated dose and subchronic toxicity

Short-term repeated dose and subchronic toxicity studies can provide rather detailed information on both immediate and delayed adverse effects, possible bioaccumulation, reversibility of damage and development of tolerance. The clinical and histopathological examinations are rather extensive and it is therefore often possible to establish NOAELs and LOAELs that can be used when establishing the dosage regimen in other toxicity studies. If no data are available from chronic toxicity studies (not unusual for many industrial agents), these dose levels can also be used when establishing threshold limit values and other types of guideline levels and safety criteria for human exposures.

Chronic toxicity

The main purpose of chronic toxicity testing is to identify adverse effects requiring long periods of latency and/or bioaccumulation, and to establish dose–response relationships for these effects. The chronic toxicity studies can provide important information on various types of biochemical, haematological, morphological, neurological and physiological effects. Using rodents, each dose group (including a concurrent control group) should include at least 20 animals of each sex. When non-rodents are used (less common), a minimum of four animals (usually dogs or primates) of each sex is recommended per dose. The test compound should be administered on a daily basis in at least three different doses for at least 12 months. A careful clinical examination should be made at least once a day, and all clinical signs of toxicity (changes in body weights, food consumption, etc.) should be recorded. Measurements of clinical chemistry, haematological examinations and urinalysis should be performed on a regular basis, and all animals should be subjected to a complete gross examination at necropsy. The histopathology should include at least a complete microscopic examination on most of the organs and tissues from the animals in the highest dose group and the control group, including all animals that died or were killed during the study period. The NOAELs and/or LOAELs obtained in a chronic toxicity study are typically used when establishing various threshold limit values and other types of guideline levels and safety criteria for human exposures.

Studies on various types of specific adverse health effects

Skin and eye irritation

The main purpose of the testing for local toxicity on skin and eyes is to establish whether or not a chemical induces irritation (i.e. reversible changes) or corrosion (i.e. irreversible tissue damage) when applied as a single dose on the skin, or to the anterior surface of the eye. As with all other toxicity studies, this type of testing should be performed using common sense. Obviously, there is no point in testing strongly acidic (with a demonstrated pH of 2 or less) or alkaline (with a demonstrated pH 11.5 or above) agents for local toxicity on the skin and eyes, and if an agent has been shown to be corrosive to the skin, it seems rather pointless to proceed with an acute eye irritation/corrosion study. The testing for local effects on the skin or eye is usually performed on albino rabbits (each animal serving as its own control). The degree of skin (or eye) reaction is read and scored at various time intervals (up to 14 days after the application). Depending on the degree of erythema and oedema on the skin, or the degree of various types of ocular lesions (on the cornea, iris and conjunctivae), the test chemical is either classified as a non-irritant, irritant or corrosive agent.

Sensibilization and sensitization

Skin sensitization, i.e. allergic contact dermatitis, is an immunologically mediated reaction requiring an initial contact with a sensitizer inducing sensibilization. Sometimes it can be difficult to distinguish between an allergic contact dermatitis caused by skin sensitization, and an 'ordinary' contact dermatitis following from skin irritation, because the symptoms (typically involving erythema and oedema, sometimes also including vesicles) are quite similar (see Chapter 16). However, when sensibilization has occurred, the responses are often more severe and elicited by rather low, non-irritating doses without apparent thresholds. Being the most sensitive species, the guinea pig seems to be the preferred species when testing for skin sensibilization and sensitization. There are several alternative tests available (e.g. Freund's complete adjuvant test, the guinea pig maximization test and the open epicutaneous test), but most follow the same general outline. In order to make the animals hypersensitive, they are first exposed to a rather high dose of the test compound. After an 'induction period' without exposure, the animals are then exposed a second time to a low, non-irritating dose. After this challenge dose, the animals are examined with regard to the possible development of allergic contact dermatitis. Sensitization can occur also after other routes of exposure (notably inhalation), but so far, internationally accepted testing guidelines have only been developed for allergic contact dermatitis.

Phototoxicity

Tests have also been developed to evaluate the combined dermal effect of chemical exposure and light. These tests (measuring either 'phototoxicity' or 'photoallergy') are modified skin irritation and skin sensibilization tests. The animals (usually rabbits or guinea pigs) are first exposed to the chemical and then to light (usually ultraviolet light). The phototoxic and photoallergic reactions are probably mediated by reactive species ('free radicals') formed when the chemical is hit by the light. These radicals can either cause direct damage to the skin, or, by binding to endogenous proteins, form antigens provoking an allergic reaction.

Genotoxicity

'Genetic toxicity' is a diversity of genetic end-points including primary DNA damage (DNA adducts, cross-linking, intercalation, DNA strand breaks, etc.), point and gene mutations (changes in the nucleotide sequence at one or a few coding segments within a gene), structural chromosomal aberrations (e.g. translocations and inversions following from chromosome or chromatide breakages), and numerical chromosomal aberrations (e.g. aneuploidy and other genomic mutations). If primary DNA damage is not repaired correctly before DNA replication and cell division, it can become manifest as a mutation. All mutations are, by definition, permanent alterations of the genetic material leading to a change in the information coded by the nucleotide sequence.

Most mutations are either associated with cell death (which is of minor importance for the whole organism) or without biological effects whatsoever. However, some mutations can be critical, at least if they occur in an unfortunate position of an important gene. If such mutations occur in somatic cells they may contribute to the development of malignant tumours or other somatic diseases. If a critical mutation occurs in a germ cell it may, at least in the worst case, be associated with an increased risk for embryonic death, malformations, childhood cancer and genetic diseases in the offspring and/or later generations. It is not only the potential health impacts of mutations that makes genotoxicity such an important toxicologi-

cal end-point, but also the shape of the dose–response curve in the low-dose region. A single molecule of a chemical mutagen interfering directly with the genetic material may be sufficient to induce a critical gene mutation, indicating at least theoretically that there is only one absolutely safe exposure level for this type of agent, and that is zero.

There are numerous (> 200) test systems available detecting various types of genetic end-points, using a broad spectrum of 'indicator' organisms (from plants, bacteria, yeast, insects and cultured mammalian cells, to intact experimental animals). So far there are internationally accepted testing guidelines for approximately 15–20 of these test systems. The main purpose of genotoxicity testing is to establish whether or not a given compound has the 'inherent' ability of being mutagenic (usually with the aim of identifying potential carcinogens and germ cells mutagens). This issue is usually resolved using a limited battery of *in vitro* tests. This battery can, for example, consist of the following four 'short-term' tests: the *Salmonella*/mammalian microsome reverse mutation assay, better known as the Ames test (to detect point mutations in bacteria); the CHO/HGPRT assay (to detect gene mutations in cultured mammalian cells); a cytogenetic assay on mouse lymphoma cells arrested in metaphase (to detect chromosomal aberrations in cultured mammalian cells); and the HPC/DNA repair assay (to detect DNA damage in primary cultures of rat hepatocytes). Compounds found to be mutagenic *in vitro*, are usually also tested *in vivo* (e.g. in the mouse micronucleus test registering chromosomal aberrations in bone marrow cells). If necessary, the further mutagenicity testing should also include an assay for germ cell mutations (e.g. the mouse heritable translocation assay registering structural and numerical chromosome mutations).

Carcinogenicity

Tumour development is a multistage process involving both permanent genetic alterations (i.e. mutations) and other, 'epigenetic', events. The neoplasms (tumours, cancers, malignancies, etc.) are a family of diseases characterized by an aberrant control of cell proliferation and cell differentiation. Most malignant diseases are multifactorial in origin, and obviously there are several factors that are of importance for their development. Among those are environmental factors (i.e. various chemical, biological and physical factors), lifestyle and cultural factors (e.g. smoking habits, alcohol consumption, diet and sexual behaviour) and various host factors (e.g. inheritance, age, sex, endocrine balance, immunological factors, capacity of DNA repair and balance between the various phase I and phase II enzyme systems).

The process of tumour development is obviously extremely complex, but the definition of a chemical carcinogen is actually rather simple. Basically, a chemical carcinogen is an agent that has been shown to increase the tumour incidence, and/or shorten the period of latency for tumour development in humans and/or experimental animals. The main purpose of a chronic cancer bioassay is to study the potential development of tumours in experimental animals exposed for the major portion of their life span. Typical evidence of carcinogenicity include: development of types of neoplasms not observed in controls; increased incidence of types of neoplasms also observed in controls; occurrence of neoplasms earlier than in the controls; and/or increased multiplicity of neoplasms in animals exposed to the test compound. Chronic cancer bioassays are usually performed on at least two different species (typically mice and rats), using at least 50 males and 50 females per dosage for each species (including an unexposed group of control animals).

Reproductive toxicity

Reproductive toxicity can be the result of a disrupted spermatogenesis or oogenesis (i.e. gametogenesis), or adverse effects on the fertilization, implantation, embryogenesis, organogenesis, fetal growth, and/or the birth. In a broad sense, reproductive toxicity studies include single- and multigeneration studies on fertility and general reproductive performance (segment I studies), studies on embryotoxicity and teratogenicity (segment II studies; see below), and peri- and postnatal studies on effects occurring during the late pregnancy and lactation (segment III studies).

The main purpose of a typical one- or two-generation reproduction toxicity study (i.e. a segment I study) is to provide information on chemically-induced adverse effects on the male and female reproductive performance. By studying, for example, the parturition, duration of gestation, number and sex of pups, stillbirths, live births, microscopic alterations in the gonads of the adult animals and gross anomalies in the offspring, information can

be obtained on adverse effects on the gonadal function, oestrogenous cycle, mating behaviour, conception, parturition, lactation and weaning.

These studies should also be able to provide some information on the developmental toxicity, including neonatal morbidity and behaviour. In a typical segment I study, both sexes (usually rats) are exposed to graduated doses of the test compound. The males should be exposed for at least one spermatogenic cycle, and the females for at least two oestrogen cycles. After mating, the females are continuously exposed during the pregnancy and nursing period. In a two-generation study, the test compound is also given to the offspring (the F_1 generation), starting at weaning and continuing until the second generation (the F_2 generation) is weaned.

Embryotoxicity, teratogenicity and fetotoxicity

Chemicals may affect the developing embryo or fetus, without inducing any overt signs of maternal toxicity. For example, depending on the stage of embryonic or fetal development, a toxicant may induce both early embryonic death, fetal death, malformations, slowed maturation, low birth weights, as well as various metabolic and physiological dysfunctions, and cognitive deficiencies in the offspring. In the broadest sense, embryotoxicity can be defined as all types of adverse effects exhibited by the embryo (i.e. toxicity occurring from the formation of the blastula until the completion of the organogenesis). Fetotoxicity (i.e. the adverse effects exhibited by the fetus) is induced after the completion of organogenesis. Typical examples of such effects are increased lethality at birth, low birth weights, various types of physiological and psychological dysfunctions, and cognitive disturbances manifested after birth.

In order to be able to distinguish between the various types of adverse health effects that may follow from a chemical exposure during pregnancy, 'embryotoxicity' has come to mean the ability of a chemical to induce either embryonic growth impairment or embryonic death. Teratogenicity, which in the broadest sense can be defined as the potential of a chemical to induce permanent structural or functional abnormalities during the embryonic development, has become equivalent to the specific ability to induce external malformations (e.g. exencephaly, hydrocephaly and cleft palate), skeletal abnormalities (e.g. poly-dactyly and fused ribs), and/or visceral anomalies (e.g. enlarged heart, undescended testes and hydronephrosis). The main purpose of teratogeni-city testing is to provide information on the poten-tial hazards to the unborn following from an exposure during pregnancy. Embryotoxic and ter-atogenic effects occurring without apparent mater-nal toxicity are then particularly alarming. The test compound is given in different doses to preg-nant animals (usually rats or rabbits), including the period of organogenesis. As in most other toxi-city studies, the highest dose administered should elicit some maternal toxicity and the lowest dose should be without apparent signs of toxicity. The pregnant animals are sacrificed shortly before the expected delivery, and the offspring are then examined for various embryotoxic, and terato-genic effects.

Neurotoxicity and behavioural toxicity

Neurotoxicity can be defined as any chemically-induced adverse effect on any aspect of the central and peripheral nervous system, including various supportive structures. From this it follows that 'neurotoxicity' is associated both with various types of pathological, physiological, biochemical and neurochemical changes in the nervous system, and various types of functional and neurobeha-vioural changes. Obviously, neurotoxicity is not a single end-point that can be evaluated in a single test system. Pathological changes in various regions of the brain and/or clinical signs of intox-ication deriving from CNS toxicity (e.g. piloerec-tion, tremor or coma) can be monitored in the acute and repeated dose toxicity studies. Chemically-induced behavioural changes (often rather subtle effects) are more difficult to monitor. This usually requires a completely different type of testing procedure, not always familiar to a 'traditionally' trained toxicologist.

Despite the absence of internationally accepted testing guidelines for the testing of behavioural effects in experimental animals, there are several test systems available measuring various types of subtle CNS effects (e.g. changes in the reflexive or schedule-controlled behaviours, or reduced perfor-mances in different learning and memory tasks). The whole concept of behavioural toxicology is based on the notion that behaviour is the final functional expression of the whole nervous system (indirectly including also the endocrine system and other organs). The general idea is that behavioural changes can be used as sensitive indicators of che-mically-induced neurotoxicity, both in adult ani-mals and in animals exposed *in utero*, or shortly after birth ('neurobehavioural teratology').

Behavioural toxicity tests are based on changes either in an internally generated behaviour of the animals (e.g. their natural social or exploratory behaviours), or a stimulus-oriented behaviour. The latter tests are either directed towards an operant conditioned behaviour (the animals are trained to perform a task in order to avoid a pun-ishment or to obtain a reward), or classical con-ditioning (the animals are learned to associate a conditioning stimulus with a reflex action). Typical responses recorded in the various types of behavioural toxicity tests are: 'passive avoid-ance'; 'auditory startle'; 'residential maze' and 'walking patterns'. It is not always easy to inter-pret the results from behavioural neurotoxicity tests. Apart from the obvious problems associated with the functional reserve and adaptation of the nervous systems, there is also an inherent large variability in behaviour. Since neurobehavioural testing usually involves multiple testing, using multiple measurements in several different test sys-tems, there is an obvious risk for 'mass signifi-cance' which sometimes can make the statistical analysis rather dubious.

Immunotoxicity

Toxic effects mediated by the immune system are sometimes referred to as immunotoxicity. However, from a toxicological point of view, immunotoxicity is defined in most cases as chemi-cally-induced adverse effects on the immune sys-tem. The immune system is a highly complex and cooperative system of cells, tissues and organs, protecting the organism from infections and neo-plastic alterations. Immunotoxic agents can inter-act with the immune system in many ways. They can, for example, interfere with the function, pro-duction or life span of the B- and T-lymphocytes, and/or interact with various antigens, antibodies and immunoglobulins. Basically, immunotoxic agents are either functioning as 'immuno-suppressive' agents or as 'immunostimulants'. Consequently, like several other toxicological 'end-points', immunotoxicity is not a single end-point that can be monitored with a single test sys-tem.

So far, there are no internationally accepted guidelines for the specific testing of the immunotoxicity of chemicals. Tests of the immune system in intact experimental animals usually involve either the weight and morphology of lymphoid organs, or the capacity of the organism to respond to challenge doses of mitogens (e.g. concanavalin A or phytohaemagglutinin), or various antigens. Thymus toxicity and other types of adverse effects on lymphoid organs can be monitored in various studies on general toxicity. During the past few years, several *in vitro* tests have been developed, measuring various types of 'immunological' parameters (e.g. inhibition of macrophage migration, lymphocyte transformation by antigens and mitogens, leukocyte function and differentiation, and production of various antibodies). It is not always easy to interpret the results from the immunotoxicity testing. A change in the differential leukocyte count may indicate that the immune system is a potential target for toxicity, but a small change in a subset of lymphocytes is not equivalent to immunotoxicity. Thymus atrophy is often associated with immunosuppression, but is not an absolute proof of immunotoxicity.

Mechanisms of toxicity

Most toxicants (genotoxicants, chemical carcinogens, neurotoxicants, sensitizers, immunotoxicants, reproductive toxins, teratogens, liver poisons, etc.) induce their adverse effects by interacting with normal cellular processes. Many toxic responses are the ultimate result of cell death leading to loss of important organ functions. Other responses follow from interactions with various biochemical and physiological processes, not affecting the survival of the cells. Common mechanisms of 'toxic action' include receptor–ligand interactions, interference with cellular membrane functions, disturbed calcium homeostasis, disrupted cellular energy production, and/or reversible or irreversible binding to various proteins, nucleic acids and other 'biomolecules'. Toxicity can be the result of one specific physiological change in a single target organ, or follow from multiple interactions at different sites, in several organs and tissues. In a review such as this, it is not possible to go into details about the mechanisms of actions underlying various types of 'toxicological end-points', so what follows is a brief description of some of the most important mechanisms of toxicity.

Many toxicants induce their adverse effects by binding to an active site on a biologically active molecule. This molecule can be a protein (e.g. a 'high-affinity' receptor, a bioactivating or detoxifying enzyme, a DNA-repair enzyme, a channel protein or a transport protein), a nucleic acid (DNA or RNA), a lipid, or other macromolecules with important biological functions. A 'receptor' is usually referred to as a high-affinity binding site interacting with an endogenous ligand. Typical examples of such receptors are those interacting with various neurotransmittors in the CNS, and the intracellular receptors interacting with, for example, calcium or various steroid hormones. However, in a broad sense a receptor can be defined as any binding site available for a particular ligand. Toxicants interfere with both type of receptors. When a toxicant binds to a high-affinity receptor for endogenous ligands, it can either 'activate' the biological responses mediated by the receptor or block its function. An 'agonist' is an agent interacting with the receptor in the same way as the endogenous ligand. The agonist can act directly by binding to the receptor or indirectly by increasing the concentration of the endogenous ligand at the receptor (e.g. by inhibiting its degradation). Agents blocking the normal function of the receptor are known as antagonists.

There are numerous examples of toxicants acting by binding to various macromolecules. For example, many genotoxic agents form various types of DNA adducts by binding covalently to DNA (increasing the risk for critical mutations). The anoxia following from the high-affinity binding between carbon monoxide and haemoglobin is another example of an adverse effect which is due to binding (in this case a non-covalent binding). 'Metabolic poisons' interfere with the biological activity of various enzymes (e.g. various phase I and phase II enzymes). Some toxicants do this by binding to the enzymes, thereby changing their structure. Other types of 'metabolic poisons' interfere with the metabolic pathways by competitive inhibition. Toxicants can also interfere with the cellular energy production. One way of doing this is to inhibit the oxidative phosphorylation in the mitochondria, interfering with the production of high-energy phosphates such as adenosine triphosphate (ATP). Other toxicants act as 'cellular poisons' by interfering with various membrane-bound functions and transport processes. Among those are many potent neurotoxins acting as ion channel blockers by binding to various channel proteins.

Many toxicants form reactive intermediates during the metabolic biotransformation. The electrophilic intermediates formed can bind directly to various cellular macromolecules, but they can also induce 'oxidative stress' in the cells. This will eventually lead to the formation of various reactive oxygen species, including highly reactive hydroxyl radicals interacting with, for example, DNA (causing DNA damage) and unsaturated fatty acids in the cell membrane (causing lipid peroxidation). Oxidative stress has been implicated as an important factor in many biological processes, including ageing, inflammatory reactions and tumour development. Lipid peroxidation (which is associated with an increased fluidity of cell membranes, membrane disruption and cell necrosis) has been implicated as a mechanism of action for many hepatotoxic agents inducing centrilobular liver necrosis.

Dose response in toxicity testing

One of the most fundamental concepts in toxicology is the quantitative relationship between the 'dose' (i.e. the magnitude of exposure) and the 'response' (i.e. the magnitude of the induced adverse effect). It is often useful to make a distinction between 'dose effect' (the graded response after exposure to varying doses of a toxicant) and 'dose response' (the distribution of a 'quantal' response in a population exposed to varying doses of the toxicant). Death and clinical manifest tumours are rather obvious quantal responses (i.e. 'all-or none' effects), but all types of adverse effects can be classified as quantal if a cut-off procedure is used when distinguishing between an adverse response and a 'normal' response. Consequently, whereas the dose effect expresses the extent of response on an individual level (exposure to 10 ppm of toxicant A is associated with a 15% reduction of 'liver function'), the dose response expresses the incidence of responses on a population level (reduced liver function was observed in 15 out of 100 mice exposed to 10 ppm of toxicant A).

When evaluating toxicological data it is generally the relationship between the 'dose' and the 'population-based' response that is of interest. It is then assumed that there is a causal relationship between an observed response and the adminis-tered toxicant. It is also assumed that the response is related to the exposure. This implies that the adverse effect is induced by the toxicant and not by some unrelated factor. It also implies that there is some kind of a 'critical receptor' which the toxicant can interact with in order to induce its toxicity, that the degree of response is related to the concentration of the toxicant at this 'receptor', and that the concentration of the toxicant at the 'receptor' is related to the administered 'dose'. The relationship between 'dose' and 'response' is often illustrated graphically as a dose–response curve, using the population-based definition of dose response. The magnitude of exposure is plotted on the x-axis and the magnitude of response as a cumulative percentage on the y-axis (*Figure 3.2*). The only absolute requirements when establishing a dose–response curve in a toxicity study are that the toxicant can be administered accurately and that the means of expressing the toxicity are precise.

Dose–response relationships are closely associated with a related issue in toxicology, i.e. whether or not thresholds exist for various types of adverse effects. Using the population-based definition of dose response, a threshold dose is equivalent to a 'minimally effective dose' that evokes a stated 'all-or-none' response. Most acute and chronic adverse effects are associated with threshold doses. This means that there is an exposure below which no health risk exists. The true threshold dose for a particular adverse effect is impossible to determine experimentally, but as indicated in *Figure 3.2b*, dose–response curves can be used to determine NOAELs and LOAELs. It should be pointed out that the NOAELs and LOAELs are not absolute effect levels, and that they are highly sensitive to the testing conditions (the number of animals, dosages, methods for registration of responses, number of surviving animals, number of animals and organs subjected to histopathological examinations, etc.).

For some types of adverse health effects (notably neoplasms and genetic diseases induced by mutagens interacting directly with the genetic material), the absence of true thresholds cannot be excluded. At least theoretically, one single molecule may be sufficient to induce the critical response. However, this is indeed a complex issue and the discussion on whether or not there are threshold levels for genotoxic agents will inevitably involve questions about the importance of various DNA repair mechanisms (e.g. the balance between the error-free, high-fidelity excision repair

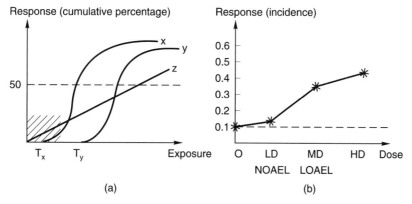

Figure 3.2 (*a*) Dose responses for three different chemicals. Chemicals x and y are toxicants with threshold doses and typical sigmoid dose–response curves. Chemical x is a more potent toxicant than chemical y, as indicated by its lower threshold dose (T_x), lower median effective dose and by its higher efficacy (maximum response). The no-threshold dose–response relationship shown for chemical z, represents a typical dose response for a genotoxic carcinogen, assuming a linear relationship in the low-dose region (shadowed area) which cannot be studied experimentally. (*b*) A typical dose–response curve obtained in a repeated dose toxicity study using control animals (0), and three different groups of animals exposed to a 'low' (LD), 'medium' (MD) or 'high' (HD) dose of the toxicant. NOAEL represents the 'no observed adverse effect level', and LOAEL the 'lowest observed adverse effect level'

pathways and more error-prone pathways). One should also be aware of the fact that there is a constant and unavoidable exposure to 'endogenous mutagens', and that virtually all cells are subjected to spontaneous mutations and 'naturally' occurring DNA damage. This issue is further complicated if there is an effect of 'hormesis' of genotoxic agents, where for example, a low-level exposure stimulates the activity of the high-fidelity DNA repair. 'Hormesis' is when exposure to a chemical, known to be toxic at higher doses, is associated with a beneficial effect at low doses.

The enormous scope of toxicology

The evaluation of toxicological data is often straightforward when it comes to immediate adverse health effects following from a well-characterized chemical exposure. However, when it comes to low dosages, exposures to complex mixtures, thresholds, and the significance of various types of chemically-induced biochemical and physiological changes, toxicological evaluation can become rather complicated. One complicating factor is the development of tolerance, i.e. a decreased responsiveness towards the toxicity of

a chemical resulting from a previous exposure. Tolerance is an adaptive state which becomes obvious when it is necessary to increase the dosage in order to obtain a given response. One example of acquired tolerance is that following from the induction of the cytochrome P_{450} system. By inducing this enzyme system, many chemicals stimulate both their own detoxification and that of others. An increased activity of this enzyme system is also associated with markedly increased metabolism of endogenous compounds. A complicating factor is that the induction of cytochrome P_{450} also can increase the bioactivation of many toxicants (leading to an increased concentration of reactive species in the cells). Another classical example of an acquired tolerance is the development of cadmium tolerance due to the induction of metallothionein, a metal binding protein.

The fact that chemicals can interact with each other is indeed a complicating factor when discussing the toxicity of industrial chemicals and dose–response relationships. This issue is usually not addressed in conventional toxicity testing, which focuses on one chemical at the time. The interaction between chemicals can result in an additive effect (the combined effect equals the sum of the effect of each individual agent given alone), a synergistic effect (the combined effect is much greater than the sum of the effect of each agent given alone), a potentiating effect (one of the agents is without toxic effects of its own to the particular organ system, but when given together with a toxic agent it will multiply the toxic effect), or an antagonistic effect (the combined effect is lower than the sum of the effect of each agent given alone).

Conclusion

Most toxicological data are based on animal experiments. Toxicokinetic studies provide information about the rates and patterns of absorption, distribution, metabolism and excretion of a potential toxicant after various routes of exposures. Toxicity studies identify the nature of health damage that may be associated with a given chemical compound, and the range of doses over which the damage is produced. When reviewing such data, one should always evaluate the methods used. Was the toxicant administered accurately? Were the means of expressing the toxicity precise? Did the study include an adequate num-

ber of animals and dosages? Did the study include a control group? Were the results statistically significant? Were the responses biologically significant? The results from one type of study should be interpreted in conjunction with the results obtained in others. One should also be aware of the fact that a direct extrapolation to a human exposure situation in most cases is valid only to a limited extent.

Further reading

Amdur, M.O., Doull, J. and Klaassen, C.D. (eds) *Casarett and Doull's Toxicology. The Basic Science of Poisons*, 4th edn. Pergamon Press, New York (1991)

Brooks, S.M., Gochfield, M., Herzstein, J. *et al.* (eds) *Environment Medicine*. Mosby Year-Book, St Louis (1995)

Hodgson, E., Mailman, R.B. and Chambers, J.E. (eds) *Macmillan Dictionary of Toxicology*. The Macmillan Press, London (1988)

OECD Guidelines for Testing of Chemicals. OECD, Paris (1989)

Chapter 4

Principles of occupational epidemiology

O Axelson

An historical note

Epidemiology deals with the occurrence of disorders in a population. It probably started in England with John Graunt, a haberdasher, publishing *Natural and Political Observations . . . made upon the Bills of Mortality* in 1662. There was no further development for a long time, but a new interest in the quantitative aspects of the causes of death arose in the earlier part of the nineteenth century and included also occupational aspects. Then, William Farr, responsible for the mortality statistics in England, reported some observations on Cornish tin miners. Some years later Augustus Guy, also in England, took an interest in 'pulmonary consumption' and physical exertion in letterpress printers and other occupational groups [1, 2]. The observations from 1879 of an increased lung cancer risk among Schneeberg miners represent another example of early occupational epidemiology, as well as the report on an excess of bladder cancer among German aniline workers that appeared some decades later [3].

Modern occupational epidemiology may be thought of as starting in the 1950s and early 1960s, involving for example bladder cancer studies in rubber workers and lung cancer among gas workers in the UK, and asbestos workers and miners in the USA [3]. Observations on cardiovascular disease also appeared relatively early regarding, for example, carbon disulphide workers in the UK and Finland. Although cancer studies have continued to be a predominant part of occupational epidemiology, the field has broadened, especially since the 1980s, to encompass the work-related aspects of almost any disorders and no longer only physical and chemical exposures [4].

For example, the interest in cardiovascular disease has shifted from chemical exposures to the effects of shift work and various psychosocial determinants in the work environment. Other recent studies concern disorders such as multiple sclerosis, Parkinson's disease, Alzheimer's dementia, etc., and their possible relationships to different occupational exposures. Ergonomic risk factors and musculoskeletal disorders as well as the reproductive hazards are other fields attracting interest. Occupational aspects of gene–environment interaction phenomena have also come into focus through so-called molecular epidemiology [5]. From the exposure point of view, the possible health effects of electromagnetic fields in particular may be mentioned as one of the most intriguing questions in occupational and environmental epidemiology of the 1990s.

The progress in epidemiology has been efficiently catalysed by methodological progress, along with the development of the now commonly available analytical packages for personal computers. However, it is not only the many important and interesting results published since the late 1970s that deserve interest, but also the ethical aspects and implications for disease prevention [6].

This chapter will not consider any specific results on subject matters; instead, the intention is to provide a relatively brief introduction to some basic principles of epidemiological research, which are shared with many disciplines, although the emphasis here is on the occupational health aspects. To obtain a deeper insight into methodological issues, the reader is referred to some of the many textbooks which are now available [7–14].

General concepts

Character of populations and disease occurrence

The general population of a country or a region, with a turnover of individuals due to births, deaths and migration, is *open* or *dynamic* in character [15]. A group of once-identified individuals without turnover is a *closed* or *static* population, usually referred to as a *cohort* (originally a unit in the Roman army). Individuals in a cohort have something in common, such as working in a certain factory, a similar exposure although in different factories, or exposure to a chemical accident, etc. A defining event could also be birth in a particular year, inclusion in a particular birth cohort, or having been selected by some criterion of a more or less administrative character and enrolled into a particular register or study.

The open or dynamic population, as considered in an epidemiological study, is a circumscribed part of the general population and defined by its temporary state as living in a certain area or belonging to a particular group, occupational or otherwise. Hence, holding a particular state for some time might be used for defining an open population in that time period. In another perspective, this temporary state may also be taken as a group-defining event, transferring the individuals of an open population into a closed one and establishing a cohort for follow-up beyond the period of time when the particular state was held.

A time aspect is always involved in epidemiology, and a population-time segment under consideration forms the *base* for any observation of mortality or morbidity, irrespective of whether the population is open or closed [15]. The population in a base may be referred to as the *base population* or *study population*, being considered during the *study period*.

For a closed population, the measure of morbidity or mortality is the *cumulative incidence (rate)*, which is the fraction or percentage of affected individuals and requires a specification of the time-span involved [16]. Since the numerator of the cumulative incidence is part of its denominator, this means that the closed population formally retains its cases. By contrast, the open population by definition omits the cases or deaths in the turnover process. The measure to be applied to an open population is the *incidence rate* (or *incidence density*), relating the number of cases or deaths to a denominator of subject-time (usually person-years) of healthy persons, that is, the candidates for falling ill or dying. This point is particularly clear for mortality, since those already dead are not contributing any person-years at risk of dying. For example, an open population (say, a small town) with an average of 1000 individuals followed for 5 years (producing, say, 10 cases) would result in 5000 person-years of observation. The incidence rate or incidence density is here 10/5000 or 2 per 1000 person-years [16]. However, cancer registration usually provides cases per mean population per year so that the surviving cases are 'incorrectly' contributing to the person-years in the denominator of a cancer rate. In recurrent disease studies, case subjects would also have to generate person-years after recovery, that is, when candidates for a relapse of the disease.

The time period of the cumulative incidence can also be an age-span; for example, the cumulative incidence may consider cases or deaths from 50 to 59 years. The cumulative incidence corresponds well to the concept of *risk*, that is, the probability of attracting a certain morbidity or mortality during a time period or in an age-span. However, 'risk' is also commonly used as a general term, synonymous with rate. The incidence rate (density) is also applicable to closed populations by observing cases in relation to the accumulation of person-years as used in one type of occupational cohort studies and discussed below. The incidence rate of a closed population takes care of favourable or poor survival (or health), as the person-years under observation are obtained from surviving (or healthy) individuals only, whereas the cumulative incidence is insensitive in this respect. As an extreme example, the mortality from all causes over a long follow-up period would lead to a cumulative incidence approaching 100%, irrespective of whether many died young or survived until old age. However, poor survival would reduce the number of person-years observed, which makes the incidence rate more sensitive, especially if competing mortality risks are operating.

Whether the population is closed or open, a *cross-sectional* study can be undertaken with regard to the occurrence of a disease at a particular point in time, in other words, the study period is reduced to zero. The number of individuals with the disease, out of all individuals observed at the particular point in time, is the *prevalence rate*, that is, a fraction or a percentage. Considering the character of the prevalence rate, there is good reason for viewing the cross-sectional approach as creating a closed study base.

To be meaningful, rates usually have to be considered for both sexes and different age classes, and some relationships between rates are shown in Appendix A [10]. The rates may be thought of as absolute measures of the occurrence of disease or death, but tend to be somewhat abstract and difficult to appreciate. Therefore, the rates are usually compared between populations as a quotient or a difference, that is, by the *rate ratio* (or risk ratio, which is preferable when the cumulative incidence is involved; the rate or risk ratio is also called relative risk) and *rate difference* (or correspondingly, risk difference). These parameters may be taken as relative measures of morbidity or mortality among compared populations, but would also serve as absolute measures of the effect of an exposure when exposed individuals are contrasted against a non-exposed reference population. Excess relative risk is sometimes used and is obtained from the relative risk by subtracting the baseline risk, which by definition is unity.

Disease and its determinants

Disease is usually defined by the medical community rather than by the epidemiologist. It is not uncommon, however, that the criteria for a particular diagnosis vary between countries and even between regions and hospitals in a country. Whenever possible, disease entities should be based on the ICD (International Classification of Diseases) codes, but in studies of symptoms, syndromes and other less well-defined health disorders, a specific case definition may have to be set up in the frame of the study. Histopathological subtypes of tumours may be of interest to study in relation to some exposure. Likewise, case entities may be based on molecular biology data, for example, regarding presence (or not) in the tumour of a mutation in an oncogene [5].

Most disease rates are dependent on age and sex and so is mortality. Therefore, age and sex are

determinants of the morbidity or mortality, but age, for example, would not necessarily increase the risk of disease, since the probability for some conditions developing also decreases with age. As applicable also to preventive factors, 'determinant' is a more general term than 'risk factor'. A 'determinant' can also merely be descriptive in character and is not necessarily a true cause or preventive factor. For example, male sex is a determinant of prostatic cancer but is certainly not its cause.

In principle, aetiological research in epidemiology aims at the identification of such determinants that can be manipulated in terms of preventive measures. In epidemiology at large, some studies may be considering hereditary factors and other determinants embedded in life itself, and this kind of epidemiological research may then be looked upon as part of basic medical science, helping the understanding of some fundamental principles. In occupational health epidemiology, however, the determinants of interest are usually chemical or physical exposures, but workload and various stress factors may also be considered. In addition, general determinants or background variables such as age and sex, smoking, alcohol use and perhaps eating habits may need attention. There may also be an interaction with an industrial factor, for example, smoking increasing the risk of lung cancer among asbestos workers. Other aspects of interaction relate to genetic factors in combination with work-related exposures as discussed below.

Occupational exposures

Occupational epidemiology should aim to be specific in relating health hazards to agents or work processes rather than to job titles, since prevention cannot be directed towards occupations. Great difficulty is always involved in assessing exposure, not only for obtaining exposure information but also conceptually in accounting for both intensity and duration [17,18]. Considerable efforts have been made to improve the quality of exposure assessment in occupational epidemiology [19–22], but there are no simple and general solutions. Usually, the time integral of the concentration or the intensity has been used as measures of exposure, for example, working level-months for radon daughter exposure in mines, fibre-years in the context of asbestos studies, etc. Long-term exposure to a low concentration is not the same as short-term high exposure, however, although indistinguishable in these terms.

In cancer studies at least, recent exposure has traditionally been thought of as playing a lesser role than earlier exposure, suggesting a *latency time* requirement by disregarding exposure for the past few years or about a decade before diagnosis. Considering multistage carcinogenesis, more interest should perhaps be devoted also to exposures occurring later in time. Previous knowledge may sometimes support discarding both remote and late exposure, accepting exposure to be effective only in a 'time window'. Although there have been suggestions of more sophisticated methods for a time-weighing of the exposure [17,18], this is rarely practised, presumably because of the conceptual complexity involved.

In cancer studies, an exposure variable based on some measure of intensity of exposure seems more often to have resulted in monotonically increasing exposure-response gradients and larger relative risks than if based on duration of exposure [23]. Regarding the pharmacokinetic relationships between cumulative exposure and tissue dose for insoluble, respirable dust particles and toxic metabolites of a nonpolar organic solvent, no linear relationship was found for typical exposure intensities [24]. It was suggested that this observation could help explain why a disproportionately high risk of pulmonary effects is commonly seen for workers with relatively short but intense dust exposures. Such, seemingly paradoxical dose–response relationships have also been discussed by others, including the aspect of exposure-driven duration of employment [25].

Peak exposures in terms of intensity might be thought of as particularly relevant for more or less acute diseases. There are also indications, however, that the dose to the tissue and the resulting damage to the susceptible tissue is related to cumulative exposure [22]. This view requires linear kinetics in the metabolism of an agent, which is presumably correct for many but not all potentially hazardous agents in the work environment.

In epidemiological practice, often just the years spent in an occupation have been taken as the measure of exposure, but hygienic standard setting would benefit from a more elaborated assessment of exposure and first and foremost requires information on exposure intensity. Also so-called *job-exposure matrices* have been elaborated and are commonly applied, but can only suggest a specific exposure for a worker on a national or regional probability basis with regard to the job title [26,27]. As direct information as possible about exposure is always preferable, and especially structured questionnaire information is rather valid, although under-reporting of exposures may be a problem rather than the reverse [28,29]. Exposure assessments by an expert team should also be considered and might be more efficient than using a job-exposure matrix [30,31]. Even so, used in a proper way, the job-exposure matrix has turned out to be a valuable tool in many studies, being superior to simply using occupational titles as the measure of exposure [32].

When earlier hygienic measurements are utilized for epidemiological purposes, the sampling strategies should be considered [33], since many if not most samples may have been taken for control measures and tend be biased dependent on whether they were taken before or after changes of an industrial process for hygienic reasons. Also data from *biological monitoring* [34] of exposed workers, such as determinations of lead in blood or mandelic acid in urine as a styrene metabolite, may sometimes be a useful basis for a study, especially when a new effect of an otherwise surveyed exposure is feared. When there are measurements available for some of the exposed individuals, it should be noted that the variance of the exposure within and between worker groups can be considerable, and also between workers from the same factory and with the same job titles [35]. In contrast to indoor work in continuous processes, there may be great day-to-day variations for outdoor workers and when the process is intermittent.

For physical workload there is less experience in exposure assessment than for chemical or physical exposures. Static and dynamic workloads may be identified in terms of lifting or moving weights, walking with burdens, stair or ladder climbing, etc., and also working in twisted or locked positions, kneeling and so forth, along with the number of hours spent in the various activities [36,37]. Again, such epidemiological measures of exposure that can be interpreted in terms of preventive standard setting would be preferable. The problems in this respect are likely to be even more complicated than the use of epidemiological results on adverse health effects of chemical and physical agents for assessing acceptable exposure limits.

Epidemiological study designs

Descriptive versus aetiological studies

Descriptive

For practical and economic reasons, the occurrence of disease in a population (country or region) may be investigated through a representative sample to allow any inference about the total population. When no aetiological questions are involved, the study is descriptive and the information obtained is specifically anchored in time and place.

Aetiological

Aetiological (or analytical) epidemiology, on the other hand, concerns a general, scientific question, for instance, whether or not a particular exposure may cause a disease [10]. No representation of the population of a country or region is required (but any study is obviously bound in time and place and may be thought of as representing a kind of hypothetical 'superpopulation' with just the characteristics of the study population). Instead comparison of the health outcome between individuals with and without the exposure is the key issue, as in the experiment where some animals are exposed and others are kept as controls and the outcome is evaluated without need for any representation of a particular animal population. The important aspect is rather to obtain comparability between the exposed and the non-exposed animals through a random distribution of exposure to individuals. In the absence of any randomization of the exposure in epidemiology, the demand instead is to select a suitable population for study in relation to the relevant determinant, so as to have comparable individuals with and without exposure.

Where an occupational disease is a clearly recognizable and unique effect of an exposure, for example, silicosis due to inhalation of silica dust, it may be sufficient to demonstrate a *dose–response* pattern in comparable worker groups, that is, an increasing disease rate with degree of exposure. However, the disease(s) of interest in current occupational epidemiology are of all kinds, some with known or suspected causes among industrial exposures. With a proper reference population it would be possible to distinguish an effect of the exposure, by an altered rate of the disease compared with the spontaneous occurrence of that disease in the reference population. Any indication of a dose–response phenomenon would also be of interest, strengthening the likelihood of a causal connection.

Aetiological study designs

The most straightforward type of study would be to follow a closed population with both exposed and non-exposed individuals for a period of time, comparing their disease outcome. This design would be a *cohort study*, with the non-exposed individuals as a reference cohort. Similar to the exposed population (or *index population*), the reference population is closed, and the defining event may be taken as just the enrolment of individuals in the study at a given point in time.

In occupational epidemiology it is common to use a variant of the cohort study without any reference, and rely on a comparison with an expected number of cases derived from the rates in the general population [38]. This study design may be thought of as involving the construction of a hypothetical, non-exposed reference cohort, which is similar to the index population with regard to age and sex. Although a common approach in occupational epidemiology, it is applicable only to studies of mortality and cancer incidence, since other rates cannot usually be obtained from general health statistics.

For an aetiological study in an *open population*, all the cases are usually ascertained, but only a sample of healthy subjects (with regard to the disease studied) is drawn from the base population to account for the distribution of the exposure and other determinants of interest in the study base. The cases are then considered in relation to the individuals of the sample with regard to (various categories of) the exposure at issue. This approach, involving only a sample of the base population, is known as a *case-referent* or *case-control study*.

If a sample is drawn from a closed population, that is, within a cohort, then a so-called *nested* case-referent study is obtained. The nested case-referent study is usually to elucidate particular aspects, when cohort data constitute the main study. For example, the combined effect of an industrial exposure and smoking or some other determinant might attract interest. Then, if the distribution of smoking or this other determinant is not known for the cohort members, this characteristic needs to be determined only for the cases and for a sample of the base population, that is, the cohort members.

A drawback with the case-referent approach is that the case-referent ratio in the exposed and non-exposed population sectors only expresses a sort of relative rate, allowing only an estimate of the rate ratio (*Figure 4.1*). There are indirect ways to obtain some other estimates given that the overall rate for the study population is known or can be estimated from some extraneous source [16]. It may be noted in this context that if the number of referents is increased, they may finally encompass all healthy individuals in the study base, so there is

Taking D_1 as the exposure of interest one obtains

	D_1+	D_1-
Cases	13	15
Base	4u	12u
Sample/ referents	4s	12s

Figure 4.1 Study base with two independently (additively) operating determinants, D_1 and D_2. Cases are symbolized with dots in relation to population units (u; the squares), taken as either individuals (including cases, that is, cumulative incidence) or person-years of healthy individuals as also reflected in a sample (s) over time of (healthy) referents in a case-referent study. The rate ratio, *RR*, with regard to D_1 is
$RR = (13/4u)/(15/12u)$, or for case-referent data, the exposure odds ratio, *OR*, is $OR = (13/15)/(4s/12s) = (13 \times 12s)/(15 \times 4s) = (13/4s)/(15/12s) = RR$, where $OR = RR$ becomes an approximation for nested case-referent data involving the cumulative incidence

no longer a sample study but rather a census of the entire base population.

With a continuous census over time in an open study base, a comparison could even be made with regard to incidence rates in regions with a more or less concentrated representation of the type of industry under consideration. Although some studies of this type have been presented, this design cannot be recommended because of the dilution with non-exposed individuals. The design is more useful in environmental epidemiology; for example, studying health effects of air or water pollution and similar aspects. It may be referred to as a *correlation study*, especially when the rates in several areas are correlated with some particular exposure. The fact that studies can involve only a sample of the base population as in case-referent studies, or complete information as in cohort and correlation studies, has led to the view that studies involve either a census or a sample of the study base [10,15]. This is illustrated in *Table 4.1*, where the concept of *aetiological fraction* is also mentioned, as explained in Appendix B. This gives information about the fraction of cases that may be due to the exposure (*preventive* fraction is the corresponding measure in preventive situations [39]).

Comparability and standardization

Ideally the distribution of compared populations should be equal with regard to determinants of the disorder at issue, for example, age and gender but also other background determinants. *Figure 4.1* shows a situation with two determinants, D_1 and D_2, operating symmetrically; that is, the area of the square is assumed to represent the study base in terms of individuals or person-years and the dots are the number of cases appearing in each sector or unit of the study base. Whichever determinant is considered as the exposure, this base has comparability between the sectors with or without the determinant at consideration – the exposure.

By contrast with *Figure 4.1*, consider the populations in *Table 4.2* with a different distribution over age (but any determinant could have been considered). The overall, unadjusted or *crude* rates differ, but the age-specific rates are the same for two of the populations (II and III). For comparison it is necessary to weigh together the age-specific rates from each population in a similar way, either against a particular standard popula-

Table 4.1 Type of approach and epidemiological study designs with reference to character of population along with various measures of morbidity or mortality

	Character of the population		
Type of approach	*Open**	*Closed†*	*Obtainable measures*
Census studies	Correlation study	Cohort study	Rate*† rate ratio and difference; aetiological fraction
Sample studies	Case-referent study	Nested case-referent study	Rate ratio; aetiological fraction

* Incidence rate, prevalence rate and their derivatives.
† Cumulative incidence, incidence rate; prevalence rate and their derivatives (the odds ratio only approximating the risk ratio in nested case-referent studies).

tion (for example, as defined by WHO as 'World population', 'European population', etc.) or against a subpopulation within the study (usually the non-exposed) [40]. This adjustment procedure, shown in the table, is called *direct* standardization and the corresponding rate ratio is called the *standardized rate ratio* (SRR).

There is also an *indirect* standardization, resulting in a rate ratio referred to as the *standard mortality* (or morbidity) *ratio* (SMR); SIR (standard incidence ratio) is usually taken as the corresponding concept when dealing with morbidity. This standardization means that the rates of the standard population (usually that of the country) are weighted by the number of person-years or individuals in the different age groups of the study population. This leads to an expected rate (or number of cases) for the index population, and the quotient between the observed and the expected in the index population is the SMR (the procedure is like calculating the expected number of cases or deaths in an occupational cohort with the national rates as the reference, Appendix C).

Indirect standardization does not provide for comparability between more than two populations at a time, since the standards (that is, the index populations or populations II and III in *Table*

Table 4.2 Example of standardizations: hypothetical populations, of which II and III have the same age-specific rates but a different age structure

	Population I		*Population II*		*Population III*	
Age	*Cases*	*Denominators**	*Cases*	*Denominators*	*Cases*	*Denominators*
40–49	12	1200	8	800	2	200
50–59	16	800	20	500	20	500
60–69	20	400	30	200	120	800
40–69	48	2400	58	1500	142	1500
Crude rate	20	1000	39	1000	95	1000
Crude rate ratio	(1.0)		2.0		4.8	
Standardized rate†	20	1000	43	1000	43	1000
SRR‡	(1.0)		2.2		2.2	
SMR§	(1.0)		2.1		2.7	

* 'Denominators' refers to either individuals, person-years or referents.
† Direct standardization (with population I as the standard), that is, rates from population II applied to population I: $(1200 \times 8/800 + 800 \times 20/500 + 400 \times 30/200)/(1200 + 800 + 400) = 104/2400 = 43/1000$. Similarly for population III.
‡ SRR, the standardized rate ratio, = (standardized rate II)/(standardized rate I) = $(43/1000)/(20/1000) = 2.2$; the reference is indicated by parentheses in the table, that is (1.0).
§ SMR = the standard mortality (or morbidity) ratio. Rates from population I are applied to populations II and III, which gives the expected number; then SMR = (observed)/(expected). Population II gives $58/(800 \times 12/1200 + 500 \times 16/800 + 200 \times 20/400) = 58/(8 + 10 + 10) = 58/28 = 2.1$, and population III gives $142/(200 \times 12/1200 + 500 \times 16/800 + 800 \times 20/400) = 142/(2 + 10 + 40) = 142/52 = 2.7$.

4.2), will otherwise vary in age composition (or other determinant), which influences the numerical value of the SMR as seen in *Table 4.2*. Taking the referents as the denominator, the same standardization procedures can be applied to case-referent data.

Confounding, modification and inference

Two different study bases are shown in *Figure 4.2(a,b)*, with asymmetrical relations between the two determinants for the disease, D_1 and D_2. It is assumed that D_1 increases the back-

ground rate threefold and that D_2 doubles it, and jointly the action is sixfold, that is, a multiplicative interaction [41]. If the crude rate ratio for the presence versus the absence of D_1 is calculated, one gets 3.5 and 2.5 respectively instead of the 'real' rate ratio of 3.0, because D_2 exerts *confounding*. Hence, a confounding factor is a determinant of the disease, not necessarily causal but at least reflecting some underlying causal mechanism, appearing in different frequencies in the populations compared. It may be positively or negatively associated with the exposure, thereby exaggerating or masking the effect of the exposure (D_1 in this case) [42, 43].

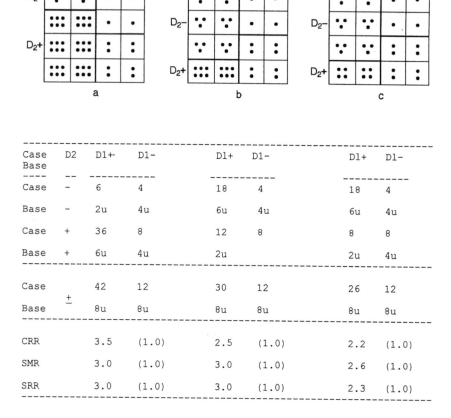

Case Base	D2	D1+	D1-	D1+	D1-	D1+	D1-
Case	–	6	4	18	4	18	4
Base	–	2u	4u	6u	4u	6u	4u
Case	+	36	8	12	8	8	8
Base	+	6u	4u	2u		2u	4u
Case		42	12	30	12	26	12
Base	+	8u	8u	8u	8u	8u	8u
CRR		3.5	(1.0)	2.5	(1.0)	2.2	(1.0)
SMR		3.0	(1.0)	3.0	(1.0)	2.6	(1.0)
SRR		3.0	(1.0)	3.0	(1.0)	2.3	(1.0)

Figure 4.2 The base may be represented either by a census or by a sample (the referents), the census giving full information about the size of the base units (u), whereas the sampled referents only provide relative information. CRR is the crude rate ratio, SMR and SRR calculated as in *Table 4.2*. In bases *a* and *b*, there is a multiplicative effect of the two determinants but also positive and negative confounding, respectively. In base *c*, D_1 adds two cases and D_2 one case per population unit. A measure of confounding (as controlled) is obtained in terms of the confounding rate ratio, CoRR = CRR/SMR, which is >1.0 for positive confounding and <1.0 for negative confounding (the reverse applies when considering prevention, as positive confounding exaggerates the effect looked for and negative confounding masks it)

Standardization, either by the SMR or the SRR, brings back the threefold increase in risk.

If there is independent activity of the two determinants *Figure 4.2(c)*, the rate ratio appears as decreased even after standardization, simply because the stratum specific rate ratio is only 2.0 in the D_2 stratum due to the elevated background among the non-exposed (those without D_1). This phenomenon is usually referred to as a modification of the effect, and is of formal rather than biological character as it is dependent on the model of the risk estimate; here the rate ratio as inherently based on a multiplicative model. The risk difference would take better care of an additive situation, but cannot be derived from case-referent data (see *Table 4.1*).

A difference in the overall, standardized rates between the compared populations would indicate that another determinant is also operating, or the differences could be due to chance (as subject to statistical evaluation). This other determinant is likely to be nothing but the exposure factor, when the compared populations have been defined on the basis of an exposure. Alternatively, control of confounding may be incomplete, or another factor associated with the exposure could be responsible, that is, an unknown confounding factor; this is impossible to account for as only known or suspected factors can be included in data collection and analysis. There is little justification, however, to be too critical and speculate about the operation of various unknown confounding factors as soon as an effect is seen in a study. There should be at least some rationale for such an alternative explanation.

Technical comments on study designs

Cohort studies

Employment records or trade union registers are almost always the starting point for setting up an occupational cohort. Past cross-sectional studies of specific exposures or data for biological monitoring may also offer suitable groups for follow-up. Occupational cohorts are usually historical or retrospective in character, but a cohort may also be prospective (followed into the future). The terms 'retrospective' and 'prospective' have also

been taken to indicate directionality – the cohort being prospective as going from exposure to outcome, and the case-referent study retrospective as looking back into the exposure history of cases and referents.

Tracing cohort individuals

In tracing the individuals of an occupational cohort, a computerized linkage with the registers of the living population and of deaths or registered cancers should be quick and effective if possible. In many countries the use of driving licence registers, telephone directories, writing and calling those with similar family names living in the area of the factory, etc., are a cumbersome way of tracing cohort members. A reasonably successful follow-up should include some 95% of the cohort, but 98–100% may be traced in countries with good registers. If a follow-up with health examinations is required, the participation rate may drop to, say, 80–90% or even lower, causing subsequent uncertainty of the results.

Analysis of cohort material

The analysis of cohort material may be based on either cumulative incidence or incidence density, with a comparison between the exposed and unexposed in terms of a rate ratio or, more rarely, a rate difference. In countries with proper mortality statistics and cancer registries, the observed numbers of specific causes of death or cancer types in a cohort are usually compared to expected numbers as calculated by the 'person-years method' from the national or regional rates [38, 44]. A latency time criterion is usually applied (especially in cancer studies) by disregarding both the new cases and the cumulative person-years for a certain period of time after start of exposure. Alternatively, the cases and the person-years might be given by time periods like 0–4, 5–9, etc., years since first exposure.

Given a hazardous exposure, cohort studies utilizing national or regional rates for the expected number of cases may show an excess of some specific cause(s) of death or of some cancer type(s), but a total mortality that is lower than expected. This phenomenon is referred to as the 'healthy worker effect' [45] and reflects the fact that employment requires better health than average in the general population. The problem of the healthy worker effect may be reduced by adjusting for length of follow-up particularly, as well as employment status if associated with the disease, independent of the exposure [46]. Computer programs have become available to provide appropriate person-time data for such adjustments [47]. Furthermore, by taking employment status into account, an otherwise negative trend in SMR with employment duration may disappear, connected with the healthy worker effect [48]. Should workers leave employment because of the exposure, then the analyses get more complicated, however [48, 49].

The principle for obtaining the person-years distribution is shown in Appendix C along with some statistical calculations [50]. As various statistical packages have become commercially available, Poisson regression analyses are now commonly applied to cohort data and can provide estimates corresponding to either SRR or SMR (SIR); further insights might be obtained from textbooks (for example [11]).

Case-referent studies

Aetiological factors for rare diseases are usually best studied by case-referent studies, given a reasonably common exposure, which may be achieved by choosing the study population in an area or within a company where the particular exposure operates. However, should the exposure of interest be both scattered and rare, the case-referent approach tends to fail; this also happens if the exposure is extremely common.

The study base for a case-referent study is usually open, but may be closed if the study is nested in a cohort. An open *primary* base can be predetermined by selecting the study population in geographical or administrative terms, but the boundaries may also be laid down secondarily by the way the cases are recruited. In the former situation, the cases may be harvested and the referents randomly drawn from a population register, but in the latter case, the study base is *secondary*, and one would have to recruit the referents similar to the cases, usually using other patients to represent the base population, that is, 'hospital referents' [51].

When such other disease entities are used as referents, a possible relation between the exposure and some of these should be considered, so that the exposure frequency of the base population is properly reflected and not misrepresented by the referents; otherwise the risk ratio gets biased. If a mix of other disorders are used as the referents, some disease entities may relate to the exposure and therefore have to be excluded. Should unrelated disorders be misjudged and also excluded, it would not lead to any biased estimate of the rate ratio (historically and formally also taken as the exposure *odds ratio* in all types of case-referent studies; see *Figure 4.1*), as the relation of exposed to non-exposed among the remaining, properly selected referents is not affected but material is lost. However, appropriate exclusions may easily be misunderstood and lead to sceptical comments unless there is a clear argument for leaving out some disorders from the referent series.

Should a secondary study base be used for considering several exposures with regard to the disease under study, the referent disorders may have to be further refined as some of them might be related to some but not all exposures [52]. This concern is not relevant when the referents represent a primary study base and have been randomly drawn from a population register, nor does it apply even to a secondary study base as reflected by hospital referents, if the exposure-related diagnosis was not the reason for admittance to hospital.

Three different types of case-referent studies may be distinguished: those in the open and closed populations, respectively, recruiting the cases and referents over a period of time, and also a type of study based on prevalent cases with a sample of referents drawn at a particular point in time [16,53]. In an open population study, the odds ratio reflects the incidence density ratio. A referent drawn early in the study period may later become a case (although rare in practice), which follows from the fact that the referents should reflect the occurrence over time of the exposure and other determinants in the base population. If the study population is closed, that is, the case-referent study nested, and the referents are drawn from those remaining healthy at the end of the study period, then the disease under study has to be relatively rare if caused by the exposure, since otherwise the relation between still healthy exposed and non-exposed individuals would be distorted relative to the original situation in the base population. The estimate of the risk ratio, in terms of the odds ratio, would now only approximate the cumulative incidence ratio.

When the case-referent study is based on prevalent cases at a particular point in time and a contemporary sample of referents, the odds ratio also equals the incidence rate ratio (given no influence by the exposure on duration of the disease) and not the prevalence rate ratio, as might perhaps be expected [53]. Case-referent studies can also be based entirely on deceased subjects, as further discussed below in terms of the mortality odds ratio study. The practical implications of the fact that there are several types of case-referent studies are usually marginal. Sometimes there are also mixed designs; for example, the cases might have been collected from an open population over some time but the referents are all drawn at the end of the study period. This is acceptable, when there is only little or no change of the exposure pattern over time.

Matching has often been employed in case-referent studies for the control of confounding, but fails in this respect as discussed below (when considering confounding). In some instances, however, matching may improve efficiency [54]. If matching has been undertaken for one reason or another, it is wise to maintain the matched pairs, triplets, etc., in the analysis, unless it can be shown that the matching did not bring about any correlation in the exposure pattern between cases and referents. If there is such a correlation, this would also tend to obscure the effect of an exposure. For example, suppose that the lung cancer and mining relationship is studied in an area, with no other industrial activities but some farming and forestry by self-employed people. If the cases of lung cancer were matched on employee status, then every lung cancer case in a miner would get a miner as a referent and no effect would be seen of mining, not even if every lung cancer case had occurred among miners. This is an (exaggerated) example of so-called overmatching, which appears when matching is undertaken on exposure-related factors in a case-referent study. Furthermore, matching also makes it impossible to evaluate the effect of the matching factor.

A simple analysis of a case-referent material with adjustment for some slight confounding by age is shown in Appendix D. The Mantel–Haenszel statistic has been applied together with a simple calculation of approximate confidence limits for the Mantel–Haenszel estimate of the odds ratio, that is, the incidence density ratio (unless the case-referent study is nested in a cohort, when it becomes an approximation of the cumulative incidence ratio, cf. above) [16]. This estimate might be seen as a suitable weighing of the stratum specific rate ratios.

However, when there is a need for the concurrent adjustment for several confounding factors, the number of strata increases rapidly so that the Mantel–Haenszel estimation becomes inefficient. The choice in such situations is to apply logistic regression modelling by means of some of the commercially available epidemiological package. The principles for this type of analysis can be found in several of the epidemiological textbooks (for example [11,55,56]. Unfortunately there tends to be a loss of insight into the data when such analyses are applied, unless the material is displayed by stratification on some major confounder(s) as well, a procedure that can be recommended both for checking the correctness of the regression modelling and for providing the reader of a study some confidence in this respect.

Proportional mortality studies and mortality odds ratio studies

The proportional mortality study may be seen as a kind of cross-sectional study at the point in time of death, even though the deaths considered are not contemporary in the traditional meaning. Its principle is to take the number of deaths of a particular disease out of all deaths and compare this proportional mortality for exposed and non-exposed individuals in terms of the proportional mortality ratio (PMR). Stratifications on age, etc., and standardizations may be applied. A possibility is also to use national or regional proportions of specific causes of death for comparisons. The proportional mortality study tends to be somewhat insensitive because any excess mortality would not only affect the numerator but also increase the denominator.

The PMR study may also be changed into a case-referent study, in this context called a mortality odds ratio study, namely if the referents are taken as deaths other than those constituting the case entity [57,58]. Thus, the exposed and non-exposed are compared in terms of the odds of the index causes of death and the other deaths, for example, the number of lung cancer deaths to all other deaths in the two (or more) exposure categories. As the case-referent study is a better concept, the mortality odds ratio design is preferable to the PMR study. Should there be a suspicion that some of the potentially eligible referent causes of death are related to the exposure, exclusions might be necessary, as discussed above in the section on case-referent studies.

Cross-sectional studies

A traditional approach in occupational epidemiology has been to examine an exposed and a non-exposed group at a particular point in time and to compare the prevalence of some disease or symptoms in the two groups or over categories of degree of exposure. A weakness with this type of study is that subjects suffering from a disease or symptoms due to the exposure tend to quit the employment or be absent on sick leave, so that the prevalence among the exposed tends to be underestimated. To take an extreme example, the risk associated with an exposure such as to carbon disulphide leading to lethal myocardial infarction would not be seen at all in a cross-sectional study, since a case would hardly appear just at the time of the examination.

In general, the longitudinal studies, either of cohort or case-referent character, are preferable. However, many less serious but economically important health problems may have to be studied by a cross-sectional approach as there is no other realistic possibility. Some of these disorders may be quite common, which should be noted with regard to the analysis of such prevalence data. Hence, odds ratio calculations by means of logistic regression have become common, but for high prevalences among the non-exposed (that is about 10% or more) and two or three times as high, or even higher, prevalences among the exposed, the odds ratio gets considerably increased in comparison to the prevalence ratio and no longer approximates this latter, intelligible measure of risk. Furthermore, confounding is different when considering prevalence data in terms of a prevalence ratio or an odds ratio. The use of logistic regression to adjust the odds ratio for confounding is therefore of little use in cross-sectional studies, where the prevalence ratio is the desirable risk estimate; further aspects on this issue are available elsewhere [59–61].

A new application of cross-sectional studies in occupational health, concerned with molecular biology data regarding DNA or protein adducts, may be mentioned. These adducts may be taken as either a sort of subclinical disorder in relation to some exposure, or alternatively as an indicator of exposure; the latter view involves also a possibility for a cohort follow-up with regard to some final outcome such as cancer. Adduct studies represent a relatively recent and important step forward in risk assessment, and there are both shorter overviews and extensive conference proceedings available on this topic [62–64].

Interaction between exposures and effect of hereditary factors

Although an epidemiological study might focus on the effect of some particular exposure or work process, it might be of interest to investigate also the combined effect with some other factor(s). For such analysis the material is, in principle, divided into several exposure categories with exposure to none of the factors as the reference, and other categories might show the effect of the factors alone as well as in combination. For more than two factors the situation becomes complex and usually requires regression analysis. The synergistic interaction between smoking and asbestos exposure with regard to lung cancer is well known, but there are not too many such examples of interaction in the literature. More studies in this respect can probably be foreseen in the future and may perhaps help explain some inconsistencies between study results from various countries or regions as dependent on the presence of some interacting factor that strengthens or weakens the effect of interest in some of the populations studied.

A new aspect of interaction concerns the utilization of data from molecular biology in combination with occupational exposures. It remains to be seen, however, how important this development might be for occupational health. From a methodological point of view, the case-referent design is a suitable approach when dealing with health effects in relation to an exposure in combination with the polymorphism of an enzyme and related differences in metabolic capacity [5]. To achieve a cost-effective case-referent study in this respect, it is worth noticing that knowledge about the metabolic pattern is needed only for the cases and not for the referents, as it is unlikely that the genetic characteristics regarding metabolism would determine occupational exposure among the referents.

An early example of this kind of interaction study suggested that the extensive debrisoquine metabolizers had a fourfold risk of lung cancer compared to poor metabolizers [65]. A history of exposure to occupational carcinogens increased the risk ratio almost threefold after adjustment for smoking and age. Extensive metabolizers who were smokers and also exposed to asbestos had an 18-fold increase in lung cancer risk. Another related example seems to suggest that so-called gene penetrance for a clearly hereditary disease might also be a matter of a combined effect with some exposure. Hence, a study of familial amyloid neuropathy showed a high risk ratio for solvent exposure, suggesting a gene–environment interaction [66]. Both these examples need confirmation by other studies, but nevertheless illustrate the principle character of this type of study. The ethical consequences of this new kind of research should be noted, namely if the knowledge about genetically determined susceptibility to occupational exposures is used to select workers for risky jobs. Instead, the proper goal should be to create a safe work environment even for those individuals who are susceptible in one respect or another.

Validity in occupational health epidemiology

General remarks

Any findings in epidemiology should be subject to considerations regarding possible errors in design or analysis. If methods and data are well displayed, the reader should be able to develop a view on the quality of the design and to check at least some of the calculations. To some extent, the statistical analysis may even be thought of as a service to the reader, and further analyses might also be undertaken. In this respect, however, the regression methods commonly used in modern epidemiology tend to hide away the data and create hindrances.

When only small-scale studies are available, some kind of combined evaluation is usually needed to reach a more definite conclusion on a health risk that has been indicated. Then, the more or less consistent data from several studies may be considered either on a judgemental basis or taken care of in a formal *meta-analysis*, where a common risk estimate with confidence limits is calculated based on the published information (for some methodological guidance, see, for example, [55]). Alternatively, a *pooled analysis* of the data from various studies can be done, but usually requires a collaboration between authors to get access to the original data and not only to published risk esti-

mates and confidence limits as used in the meta-analysis.

Although the analysis of the data in an epidemiological study is important, the design underlying the data obtained it is even more crucial and is therefore the core issue for the investigator. So, the critique of a study focuses on design rather than on analysis, emphasizing the importance of validity in the design. A good validity means freedom from systematic errors and there are various attempts to describe this issue under a few main concepts; this principle is followed in the next section.

Selection bias

One type of systematic error may be selective in character and distort the study base. For example, dead individuals could have been sorted out from company records or from trade union registers, making them useless for epidemiological purposes. Pre-employment health examinations and other selection of the fittest for employment, particularly in qualified jobs, tend to create a 'healthy worker effect', that is, a lower mortality than the expected, as estimated from the death rates of the general population [45]. A corresponding phenomenon may occur also when more qualified workers are compared to those who are less skilled.

A selection phenomenon will also take place if the exposure somehow becomes part of the diagnostic criteria. For example, a pathologist would probably be more apt to diagnose a mesothelioma when the histology is suggestive and if the case is known to have had asbestos exposure. Similar concerns may arise as soon as there is some suspicion of a relationship, but there is usually little problem in occupational epidemiology because most disorders are diagnosed without much concern about suspected occupational risks.

Another type of selection is that patients attending clinics of occupational medicine are referred conditionally on some kind of exposure and therefore represent only the exposed part of the population, whereas the same kind of patients lacking the suspect exposure will not appear. As a consequence it is impossible to use patient data from such clinics for epidemiological assessment of a suspected association between exposure and disease. A somewhat similar situation may arise if a case registry of some kind enrols only those cases who permit registration, as socioeconomic circumstances, and thereby the potential for a certain occupational exposures, might influence the registration. Such selective registries seem to exist in some countries, and, when considered for epidemiological studies, create problems similar to those connected with the use of a secondary study base in case-referent studies, as discussed above.

There is no satisfactory way to cope with selection bias if present in epidemiological material. By proper measures, the effect of some kinds of selection bias may be eliminated, for example, by adequate selection of referents to represent a secondary study base. Usually it is difficult to get around the problem of a distorted base, however, and it might be wiser to abstain from a study or cancel it in the first phase, if some sort of selection appears to have affected the study base.

Observational problems

Given that no selectional forces have distorted the study base, a further problem is to observe properly the population under study both with regard to exposure and disease outcome. The latter is more crucial in cohort studies, especially when the general population is used as the reference. Then, the case diagnoses should preferably be those given by the authority in charge of the registration in order to achieve good comparability with the number of expected cases calculated from official mortality or cancer rates. However, when the medical files and/or the histopathological preparations are checked, the official diagnosis may sometimes come into question. Comparability would be best served by keeping the official diagnosis, although highly unsatisfactory when such a diagnosis is known to be wrong. There is no solution to this dilemma other than to explain the situation clearly when presenting the study.

Case-control studies are less problematic in comparable diagnostic quality, since the researcher may set up special criteria for the case diagnosis and check both exposed and non-exposed cases, preferably blind with regard to their exposure status. Instead the crucial problem of observation relates to the assessment of exposure, since both the unhealthy individuals themselves and the interested investigator may reveal pertinent exposures more efficiently among cases than among referents (*recall* and *observer bias*, respectively). This is at least the constantly repeated critique but poorly documented weak-

ness of case-referent studies, whereas little is usually said about the opposite phenomenon, namely that random misclassification tends to obscure an effect, although an exaggeration may sometimes occur due to chance [67]. In general, however, questionnaire information on exposure has been found to agree rather well with 'objective' information from company records [68,69]. This latter source of exposure information should preferably be used in case-referent studies of occupational risks whenever available and sufficiently detailed.

Confounding

Concern is often expressed about uncontrolled confounding, for example, when information on smoking or other widely operating risk factors is lacking. However, even a comparison population will include a substantial fraction of smokers, either as a specially selected reference group or as part of the general population. Even at worst, the contribution of an uncontrolled and commonly occurring risk factor would hardly cause a risk ratio of more than about 1.5, not even smoking with regard to lung cancer [43]. *Table 4.3* shows the potential confounding effect for lung cancer with regard to differing smoking habits in the index population. The formula in the table footnote allows adjustments of the expected rate or numbers with regard to any confounding factor for which the risk ratio and the occurrence in the population can be estimated.

Although concerns about uncontrolled confounding in occupational epidemiology often relate to smoking, drinking and other generally operating determinants, there is a more relevant aspect of confounding, namely from other industrial exposures, when the effect of a particular agent rather than an overall, job-related risk is supposed to be evaluated. For example, haematite mining has been associated with lung cancer and haematite itself suspected to be the cause. However, exposure to radon daughters has also occurred in haematite mines and is more likely than haematite to be the main cause of lung cancer. Similarly, silica exposure may be carcinogenic to the lung, but again concomitant carcinogenic exposures are difficult to rule out; for example, soot exposure for foundry workers, radon daughter exposure for miners, etc. Only studies from less complex industrial environments can more clearly elucidate the role of the various exposures. Other

Table 4.3 Estimated effect of confounding from uncontrolled smoking in terms of rate ratios with regard to the fraction of smokers in various hypothetical populations (after Axelson [43])

Percentage and type of smokers in the population			*Rate ratio*
Non-smokers (risk of 1)	*Moderate smokers* (risk of 10)	*Heavy smokers* (risk of 20)	
100	–	–	0.15
80	20	–	0.43
70	30	–	0.57
60	35	5	0.78
50*	40*	10*	1.00*
40	45	15	1.22
30	50	20	1.43
20	55	25	1.65
10	60	30	1.86
–	–	100	3.08

* Compared to the reference population with 50% non-smokers, 40% moderate smokers, and 10% heavy smokers. The model behind the table may also be used for correction of expected numbers, that is $I = RI_0P_{CF} + I_0(1 - P_{CF})$, where I is the overall rate, R the rate ratio of the confounding factor (smoking in this case), I_0 the rate among those without the confounding factor and P_{CF} the proportion of the population with the confounding factor, which can be split up into heavy and moderate smokers, etc., with their respective rate ratios. Solving I_0 and adjusting P_{CF} according to smoking habits in a population provides for the figures in the table and for adjustment of I in a study.

similar examples could be exposure to pesticides or solvents that usually involves an aggregate of several different compounds, and the effect therefore has to be studied in the aggregate, as is done similarly for industrial processes that entail complex exposures.

Even if the effect from confounding is usually smaller than believed, control is desirable as far as possible either by restricting the study to individuals without the confounding factor or through stratification by (categories of) the confounding factor or regression analysis. For a cohort, matching may be an attractive way of creating an 'unconfounded' comparison group. Even if the number of matching factors have to be limited for practical (economic) reasons, relatively little uncontrolled confounding is likely to remain from other factors after matching on a few determinants of the disease. For example, matching on smoking would presumably also take care of much of the potential confounding from alcohol drinking and other associated lifestyle factors.

As already mentioned, matching does not solve the problem of controlling confounding in case-referent studies as it does not create an homogeneous study base. The situation is even more problematic, however, since the selection of referents is influenced by random variation, so that confounding may appear in the data although absent in the base and vice versa, and positive confounding in the base may come up negative in the data or the reverse. So in principle there is no way of fully controlling for confounding in case-referent studies, but a reasonable number of controls, say about 200 at least, would reduce random influence and reasonably well transfer confounding from the study base into the data, allowing some control by the methods mentioned [70].

Comparability of populations

Another issue of validity concerns the general character of the reference population. For example, an industrial population other than that under study could have some totally different exposure causing the same disorder(s) as the exposure at issue. Hence, the choice of a group of copper smelter workers (similar in smoking traits, etc.) as a reference population for miners would fail to reveal fully the excess risk of lung cancer due to radon daughter exposure in the mines, since the copper smelter workers also suffer from lung cancer, although essentially due to arsenic exposure. Nor should the reference group come from an urbanized area, if the index population is rural and if, say, an increased risk of lung cancer is part of the hypothesis under study. Similar considerations are always necessary, but the circumstances may be less obvious than in these examples.

These remarks on comparability of populations may be equally relevant to both cohort and case-referent studies. Although commonly seen, it is questionable to evaluate just one exposure at a time, disregarding other determinants of the disorder operating in the unexposed sector of the study base (that is, a situation that may also be seen as one of negative confounding). Instead it is important to try and identify a population sector of the base, which is free from any *a priori* known determinants of the disease and to use this sector as the reference. For example, when miners and copper smelter workers lived in the same area, it was necessary to identify and separate these categories and to use others as the reference category [71]. Hence, occupational or other well-defined determinants of the disease should not be allowed to operate in the reference population and obscure the effect of the exposure under study. A proper risk estimation also requires that the reference population reflects the characteristic disease rate of the region and the socioeconomic sector in which the exposure takes place.

Because of the problem in identifying an ideal reference group, there is some justification for using national or regional rates in the context of cohort studies [38]. For case-referent studies the corresponding justification would be to have just all non-exposed as the reference, but this disagrees with the principle argued above. In case-referent studies it is certainly easier than in cohort studies to achieve some refinement, at least in socioeconomic terms by excluding, for example, white collar professions from the study population when an industrial exposure is studied. By contrast, national rates, as used for obtaining the expected number of cases in cohort studies, inevitably include not only the adverse health effects of all kinds of occupations but especially the high mortality associated with unemployment, that is, with the resulting incomparability phenomenon – the 'healthy worker effect'.

reasonably high, say at least 5% among the referents. For scattered and rare exposures the cohort approach is the only possibility, picking up a few individuals with exposure from a large number of companies. Since occupational health epidemiology usually deals with relatively high risk estimates, often about 2.0 or above, even rather small populations may be studied.

As a rule of thumb, it is reasonable to have at the very least 50–60 cases in a case-referent study, given an exposure frequency of some 15–20% among the referents. In principle, an equal number of cases and referents would be the most efficient, but with a lack of cases the number of referents might be increased up to about 5 referents per case, though little gain in power is obtained thereafter. To obtain reasonable control of confounding in the base, at least 200 referents would always be required.

Cohorts with the general population as the reference should preferably have a size and age structure so that the expected number of cases would be at least two or three for the disorder of interest. Even so the study would yield uncertain information also when the risk is more than doubled or tripled.

Formal calculations can be made regarding the power of a study; these may be used in the planning stage, and also for the reporting of a negative or non-positive result [72]. The size of a study and its power do not relate to the number of individuals *per se* but rather to the expected number among the exposed, as also reflected in the expected rate ratio. Hence, even a large cohort of young individuals would not give much information about a cancer risk, simply because few if any cases would occur. In deciding whether or not a study should be undertaken, or if a presented non-positive study has power enough to be informative, some guidance may be obtained from power calculations as reflected in *Table 4.4* [8,73,74]. Various priorities and circumstances in addition to power may determine why a study is finally undertaken.

Costs, power and size

Even relatively small studies are expensive, and an estimate of the costs and effectiveness of an intended study is therefore desirable. In general, a case-referent approach tends to be less expensive than a cohort, given that the exposure frequency is

Evaluating study results

When considering the results of an epidemiological study, there is first and foremost a need for evaluating its validity, that is, whether there might be some selectional or observational bias or confounding not adjusted for, that might

Table 4.4 Required numbers in a study for 80% probability (power) of detecting a given rate ratio at 5% significance level (one-tailed)

Cohort studies; no. of expected cases		*Case-referent studies; no. of cases required with a case-referent ratio of 1:2 and different exposure frequencies†*		
Rate ratio	*Expected no.**	*Rate ratio*	*Exposure frequency 5%*	*Exposure frequency 20%*
1.3	75	1.3	2602	808
1.5	40	1.5	1041	332
2.0	12	2.0	327	110
2.8	5	3.0	116	43
3.7	3	4.0	67	27
8.0	1	5.0	47	20

* The required number of person-years is obtained by dividing this number with the (national) rate for a particular disease (or aggregated rates for certain groups of disorders like cancer, cardiovascular diseases etc.).
† The exposure frequency in the population is estimated through the referents as representing the population or, in the planning stage, from other information.

explain the findings either that there is an effect or not. It is important to realize also that lack of any clear effect of an exposure might well depend on poor validity; nevertheless studies not showing much effect often escape proper evaluation. In contrast, studies with positive findings meet heavy criticism, often unduly vague, however, rather than precise and based on careful scrutiny of the available report.

The criticism of an epidemiological study is often of a hypothetical character, implying that there could be deficiencies of one kind or another explaining the results, which does not necessarily mean that there actually are errors present in the study. Still, even suggestions with little foundation concerning an error in a study often seem to attract more credibility than the results in a well-conducted study. It seems proper, therefore, to require that the criticism should be concrete and aim at a quantitative evaluation of the impact of the assumed deficiencies on the risk estimates rather than just being a sort of speculation about qualitative problems with the study. Hence, reasonable assumptions may be made about the degree of misclassification or about the strength of remaining confounding, etc., and subsequently, some sensitivity calculations can then show whether the results are resistant or not towards the assumptions made.

Usually there is some *a priori* suspicion or hypothesis of an adverse (or preventive) health effect that initiates a study. This suspicion may originate from clinical observations, some earlier epidemiological findings or animal data. Sometimes it may be felt that a large worker population has an exposure for which there is simply not enough knowledge regarding health effects. Circumstances of this kind are usually readily apparent with regard to cohorts, as cohorts are defined by the event of being exposed.

In contrast, case-referent studies can easily take many exposures into account, and some of these might have been included on a rather vague basis, perhaps just because of the convenient use of some 'standard questions' in interviews or questionnaires. The result might be a sort of case-referent scrutiny, which is often referred to as a 'fishing expedition', with possibilities for chance findings without any relevance. Sometimes, however, surprising findings may be tentatively explicable by constructing an *a posteriori* hypothesis based on existing facts or experiences of experimental or observational nature. Some authors divide and discuss their findings with regard to one or more *a priori* hypotheses versus results without such background, which seems to be a good practice. Unexpected results certainly provide important clues to epidemiological as well as other research and should therefore not be neglected but should be published, although with a clear indication of their uncertain nature.

To the extent that the result of the study is in agreement with the *a priori* hypothesis, the supporting evidences have obviously increased and the interpretation is relatively straightforward. The situation is more problematic when there is a strong hypothesis, but a study shows no effect or no clear effect. Such outcome of a study usually means that the result is inconclusive, rather than exclusive of an effect, unless the study is very large with narrow confidence limits around unity, say, in the range of 0.9–1.1 or even narrower. A 'large study' refers to the effective size of the study which is essentially dependent on the number of exposed cases. Many if not most studies tend to be too small in this respect to provide such a narrow confidence interval around unity, and a general conclusion of no effect is justified.

A fairly common result of a study is a moderately increased risk ratio (up to about two), and a lower confidence limit just below unity, say, 0.95 or so. The interpretation might then be that there is no convincing effect of the exposure at issue, that is, the study is non-positive rather than negative, as the result does not rule out but rather weakly supports the possibility of an effect [75]. Considerations of the width of the confidence interval and power calculations may also help judging the magnitude of an effect that would be consistent with a non-positive result obtained.

In spite of no immediately clear information in a non-positive study, the result may nevertheless be useful when evaluated together with findings in other studies in a meta-analysis or on a judgemental basis. Furthermore, as there is often some anxiety among workers with a potentially hazardous exposure, a non-positive result in a relatively small-scale study is often (locally) appreciated both by workers and management, especially if the risk ratio is close to unity or even below. Still, such a result should not be trusted as indicating a safe work environment for the future, if there is evidence to the contrary.

Not only the non-positive results but also weakly positive findings are problematic to interpret, that is, when the risk ratio is moderately increased with a confidence interval that does not include unity. Sometimes authors claim that there is no clear effect even in such situations, but this is hardly a correct interpretation [75]. Instead the inevitable conclusion in reporting the study has to be that an effect has been indicated, but if there is little or no supportive information from outside the study it is usually too early to claim that a 'new risk' has been assessed. Indeed, consistent results from several good studies are necessary to establish finally the existence of a health hazard from some particular exposure; it is prudent therefore to distinguish between the reasoning in the discussion section and the conclusion about an effect in any particular study and the general acceptance of an adverse health effect of an exposure.

Appendix A: Relation of rates

$CI = 1 - e^{-a\Sigma I}$, where CI is the cumulative incidence; ΣI is the sum of incidence rates over categories, a is the width of age categories and e the base of the natural logarithms. Example: incidence rates (1960) from Appendix C give a cumulative incidence for the age span 50–64 years as $CI_{50-64} = 1 - e^{-5(230+420+685)/1\,000\,000}$ or 0.007; also approximately $CI = a\Sigma I$.

To obtain the relationship of incidence and prevalence, assume a steady state with n cases in a population of N, that is, n new cases have to appear in a period d, equal to the average duration of the disease. Therefore $n = (N - n)dI$, where $(N - n)d$ are the person-years of healthy individuals, upon which the incidence rate acts. Divide by N and obtain $n/N = (1 - n/N)dI$, where n/N is the prevalence rate, P. Therefore, $P = (1 - P)dI$ and also $P = dI/(1 + dI)$.

Appendix B: Aetiological fraction

The aetiological fraction among the exposed, EF_1, is the fraction of the cases (or of the rate) caused by the exposure, that is $(R_1 - R_0)/R_1$, where R_1 and R_0 are the rates for exposed and non-exposed, respectively. With $R_1/R_0 = RR$, the rate ratio, $EF_1 = (1 - 1/RR)$ or $EF_1 = (RR - 1)/RR$ (also called attributable risk). The aetiological fraction for the total population EF is obtained by multiplying EF_1 with the case fraction, CF, which is the fraction of exposed cases out of all cases, that is, $EF = CF \times (RR - 1)/RR$, an expression showing the relative contribution of cases in the total population as due to the exposure. When the joint effect of two or more exposures is more than additive, the sum of the aetiological fractitons for each exposure may exceed unity, for example, for asbestos (say risk ratio of 5) and smoking (say risk ratio of 10), $EF_a = (5 - 1)/5 = 0.8$ and $EF_s = (10 - 1)/10 = 0.9$ and also $0.8 + 0.9 > 1.0$.

Appendix C: Principal procedure of cohort analysis using national rates

1. Obtaining person-years: Take Mr A. born in 1910, exposed from 1951, died in 1967.

Requiring 10 years of induction-latency time he would contribute half a person-year (the half-year approximating the exact date) at observation in 1961 in the age group 50–54 and will continue with 1 person-year in 1962, 1963, 1964, but in 1965 he contributes to age group 55–59 and continues to do so throughout 1966, with half a person-year assigned in 1967 (the half-year approximating the exact date).

2. By the same token, all individuals in a cohort contribute person-years, so that a (hypothetical) table may be created as follows:

Person-years

	Calendar year								
Age group	1960	1961	1962	1963	1964	1965	1966	1967	1968 etc.
50–54	29	25	24	23	20	15	15	13	13
55–59	16	18	20	17	19	24	24	25	25
60–64	26	21	34	31	45	38	34	29	33

Underlined figures – see point 4 below.

3. National incidence rates (for a particular disease) per 1 000 000 person-years.

Incidence rates

	Calendar year								
Age group	1960	1961	1962	1963	1964	1965	1966	1967	1968 etc.
50–54	230	239	249	243	294	261	252	288	280
55–59	420	431	418	427	416	410	408	421	415
60–64	685	696	711	693	710	712	698	715	731

4. Obtain the expected number of deaths from this disease by multiplying cell by cell in the two tables and sum up $(1/1 000 000)(29 \times 230 + 25 \times 239 + 24 \times 249 + \ldots + 33 \times 731) = 0.33$ and suppose three cases of the disorder were observed.

5. Calculate the SMR with three cases observed and 0.33 expected, that is SMR = 3/0.33 = 9.1. The lower and upper confidence limits for the SMR (SMR_L; SMR_U) may be obtained by means of chi-square (χ^2) table as the confidence limits for the observed divided by the expected number, E. Then $SMR_L = 0.5[\chi^2_{\alpha/2}(2a)]/E$ and $SMR_U = 0.5[\chi^2_{1-\alpha/2}(2a + 2)]/E$, where $(2a)$ and $(2a + 2)$ refer to the degrees of freedom, a being the observed cases, and $100(1 - \alpha)$ indicates the desired confidence interval, for example, with $\alpha = 0.10$, the 90% interval is obtained. Hence, for 3/0.33 one obtains $SMR_L = 0.5[\chi^2_{0.05}(6)]/0.33$ and $SMR_U = 0.5[\chi^2_{0.95}(8)]/0.33$ and by means of the χ^2 table 0.5[1.635]/0.33 and 0.5[15.507]/0.33

or 2.4–23.5 (the limits preferably abbreviated outwards).

Appendix D: Analysis of stratified case-referent data

Stratified data from a study of the relationship between arsenic exposure and cardiovascular disease (after Axelson [76])

Stratum	Age	Case-referent	Non-exposed	Exposed	Total
1	30–54	C	$6 = b_1$	$7 = a_1$	$13 = N_{11}$
		R	$14 = d_1$	$2 = c_1$	$16 = N_{01}$
			$20 = M_{01}$	$9 = M_{11}$	$29 = T_1$
2	55–64	C	$25 = b_2$	$19 = a_2$	$44 = N_{12}$
		R	$16 = d_2$	$6 = c_2$	$22 = N_{02}$
			$41 = M_{02}$	$25 = M_{12}$	$66 = T_2$
3	65–74	C	$45 = b_3$	$27 = a_3$	$44 = N_{13}$
		R	$26 = d_3$	$10 = c_3$	$36 = N_{03}$
			$71 = M_{03}$	$37 = M_{13}$	$108 = T_3$
1–3	Total	C	76	53	
		R	56	18	
Crude rate ratio		(1)		2.2	
SMR		(1)		1.9	
$\chi^2(1)$ (Mantel–Haenszel)				5.52	
Rate ratio (Mantel–Haenszel):					
point estimate				2.1	
90% confidence interval				1.2–3.5	

The crude rate ratio, CRR, taken as an odds ratio, is $(53 \times 56)/(76 \times 18) = 2.2$ (and as in *Table 4.2*) SMR = $(7 + 19 + 27)/(6 \times 2/14 + 25 \times 6/16 + 45 \times 10/26)$ or SMR = $53/(0.86 + 9.38 + 17.31) = 1.9$. Some positive confounding is present, because the confounding rate ratio, CoRR = CRR/SMR, is 2.2/1.9 = 1.2. This value represents the magnitude of the confounding that was controlled through the stratification. The Mantel–Haenszel χ^2 statistic (with 1 degree of freedom) has the structure

$$\chi^2(1) = (\Sigma_j a_j - \Sigma_j N_{1j} M_{1j}/T_j)^2 /$$
$$[\Sigma_j N_{1j} N_{0j} M_{0j} M_{1j}/T_j^2(T_j - 1)]$$

with N_{1j} etc. denoting the exposed and N_{0j} etc. the non-exposed, as shown in the table above (Σ_j means summation over the strata, j; for example $\Sigma_j a_j$ means $a_1 + a_2 + a_3 = a$, or in the example $7 + 19 + 27 = 53$.)

The Mantel–Haenszel estimator of the rate ratio (or odds ratio) is $RR_{M-H} = \Sigma_j(a_jd_j/T_j)/\Sigma_j(b_jc_j/T_j)$.

The calculations can now be made as shown in the following scheme:

Stratum a_j		$N_{1j}M_{1j}/T_j$	$N_{1j}N_{0j}M_{1j}M_{0j}/$ $T_j^2(T_j-1)$	a_jd_j/T_j	b_jc_j/T_j
1	7	4.034	1.590	3.379	0.414
2	19	16.667	3.504	4.606	2.273
3	27	24.667	5.456	6.500	4.167
Σ_j	53	45.368	10.550	14.485	6.854

Hence, $\chi^2(1) = (53 - 45.368)^2/10.550 = 5.52$; $RR_{M-H} = 14.485/6.854 = 2.11$. The approximate Miettinen lower and upper confidence limits (90%) are RR_L, $RR_U = (2.1)^{1\pm1.645/\sqrt{5.52}}$ or RR_L, $RR_U = 1.2$–3.5.

A statistical package for calculations of the Mantel–Haenszel odds ratio, along with better estimates of the confidence interval and other useful calculations, is available free of charge (also on Internet) as developed by the Centers for Disease Control and Prevention in the United States [74]. This package also provides a test for trend of the odds ratios when several exposure categories are involved.

References

1. Rothman, K.J. The rise and fall of epidemiology. *New England Journal of Medicine*, **304**, 600–602 (1981)
2. Lilienfeld, A.M. and Lilienfeld, D.E. A century of case-control studies: progress? *Journal of Chronic Diseases*, **32**, 5–13 (1979)
3. Axelson, O. Some recent developments in occupational epidemiology. *Scandinavian Journal of Work, Environment and Health*, **20** (special issue), 9–18 (1994)
4. McDonald, J.C. *Epidemiology of Work Related Diseases*. BMJ Publishing Group, London (1995)
5. Söderkvist, P. and Axelson, O. On the use of molecular biology data in occupational and environmental epidemiology. *Journal of Occupational and Environmental Medicine*, **37**: 84–90 (1995)
6. Soskolne, C.L. Epidemiological research, interest groups and the review process. *Journal of Public Health Policy*, **6**, 173–184 (1985)
7. Breslow, N.E. and Day, N.E. *Statistical Methods in Cancer Research*, Vol. I, *The Analysis of Case-Control Studies*; Vol. II, *The Design and Analysis of Cohort Studies*. International Agency for Research on Cancer, Lyon (1980 and 1988)
8. Schlesselman, J.J. *Case-Control Studies: Design, Conduct, Analysis*. Oxford University Press, Oxford (1982)
9. Kleinbaum, D.G., Kupper, L.L. and Morgenstern, H. *Epidemiologic Research. Principles and Quantitative Methods*. Lifetime Learning Publications, Belmont, California (1982)
10. Miettinen, O.S. *Theoretical Epidemiology, Principles of Occurrence Research in Medicine*. John Wiley and Sons, New York (1985)
11. Checkoway, H., Pearce, N.E. and Crawford-Brown, D.J. *Research Methods in Occupational Epidemiology*. Oxford University Press, New York (1989)
12. Rothman, K.J. (1986). *Modern Epidemiology*. Little, Brown and Company, Boston (1986).
13. Monson, R.R. *Occupational Epidemiology*, 2nd edn. CRC Press, Boca Raton, Florida (1990)
14. Hernberg, S. *Introduction to Occupational Epidemiology*. Lewis Publishers, Michigan (1992)
15. Miettinen, O.S. Design options in epidemiologic research. An update. *Scandinavian Journal of Work and Environmental Health*, **8** (suppl. 1), 7–14 (1982)
16. Miettinen, O.S. Estimability and estimation in case-referent studies. *American Journal of Epidemiology*, **103**, 226–235 (1976)
17. Axelson, O. Dealing with the exposure variable in occupational and environmental epidemiology. *Scandinavian Journal of Social Medicine*, **13**, 147–152 (1985)
18. Checkoway, H. Methods of treatment of exposure data in occupational epidemiology. *Medicina del Lavoro*, **77**, 48–73 (1986)
19. Heederik, D., Boleij, J.S.M., Kromhout, H. *et al.* Use and analysis of exposure monitoring data in occupational epidemiology: an example of an epidemiological study in the Dutch animal food industry. *Applied Occupational and Environmental Hygiene*, **6**, 458–464 (1991)
20. Axelson, O. and Westberg, H. Introductory note to the concepts of exposure and dose in occupational epidemiology. *American Journal of Industrial Medicine*, (special issue), **21**, 3–4 (1992)
21. Checkoway, H. and Rice, C.H. Time-weighted averages, peaks, and other indices of exposure in occupational epidemiology. *American Journal of Industrial Medicine*, **21**, 25–33 (1992)
22. Rappaport, S.M. Biological considerations in assessing exposures to genotoxic and carcinogenic agents. *Archives of Occupational and Environmental Health*, **65**, S29–S35 (1993)
23. Blair, A. and Stewart, P.A. Do quantitative exposure assessments improve risk estimates in occupational studies of cancer? *American Journal of Industrial Medicine*, **21**, 53–63 (1992)
24. Smith, T.J. Occupational exposure and dose over time: limitations of cumulative exposure. *American Journal of Industrial Medicine*, **21**, 35–51 (1992)

25. Park, R.M., Silverstein, M.A. and Mirer, F.E. Characteristics of worker populations: exposure considerations in the selection of study populations and their analysis. *Applied Occupational and Environmental Hygiene*, **6**, 436–440 (1991)

26. Hoar, S.K., Morrison, A.S., Cole, P. *et al.* An occupation and exposure linkage system for the study of occupational carcinogenesis. *Journal of Occupational Medicine*, **22**, 722–726 (1980)

27. Pannet, S., Coggon, D. and Acheson, E.D. A job-exposure matrix for use in population based studies in England and Wales. *British Journal of Industrial Medicine*, **42**, 777–783 (1985)

28. Joffe, M. Validity of exposure data derived from a structured questionnaire. *American Journal of Epidemiology*, **135**, 564–570 (1992)

29. Roeleveld, N., Zielhuis, G.A. and Gabreëls, F. Mental retardation and parental occupation: a study on the applicability of job exposure matrices. *British Journal of Industrial Medicine*, **50**, 945–954 (1993)

30. Siemiatycki, J. (ed.) *Risk Factors for Cancer in the Workplace*. CRC Press, Boca Raton, Florida (1991)

31. Dewar, R., Siemiatycki, J. and Gerin, M. Loss of statistical power associated with the use of a job-exposure matrix in occupational case-control studies. *Applied Occupational and Environmental Hygiene*, **6**, 508–515 (1991)

32. Hoar, S.K. Job-exposure matrices in occupational epidemiology. *Journal of the National Cancer Institute*, **69**, 1419–1420 (1982)

33. Ulfvarson, U. Validation of exposure information in occupational epidemiology. *American Journal of Industrial Medicine*, **21**, 125–132 (1992)

34. Ate, A., Riihimäki, V. and Vainio, H. *Biological Monitoring and Surveillance of Workers Exposed to Chemicals*. Hemisphere Publishing Corporation, Washington (1984)

35. Kromhout, H., Symanski, E. and Rappaport, S.M. A comprehensive evaluation of within- and between-worker components of occupational exposure to chemical agents. *Annals of Occupational Hygiene*, **37**, 253–270 (1993)

36. Vingård, E., Hogstedt, C., Alfredsson, L. *et al.* Coxarthrosis and physical work load. *Scandinavian Journal of Work and Environmental Health*, **17**, 104–109 (1991)

37. Croft, P., Cooper, C., Wickham, C. *et al.* Osteoarthritis of the hip and occupational activity. *Scandinavian Journal of Work and Environmental Health*, **18**, 59–63 (1992)

38. Gardner, M. Considerations in the choice of expected numbers for appropriate comparisons in occupational cohort studies. *Medicina del Lavoro*, **77**, 23–47 (1986)

39. Miettinen, O.S. Proportion of disease caused or prevented by a given exposure, trait or intervention. *American Journal of Epidemiology*, **99**, 325–332 (1974)

40. Miettinen, O.S. Standardization of risk ratios. *American Journal of Epidemiology*, **96**, 383–388 (1972)

41. Rothman, K.J., Greenland, S. and Walker, A.M. Concepts of interaction. *American Journal of Epidemiology*, **112**, 467–470 (1980)

42. Miettinen, O.S. Confounding and effect modification. *American Journal of Epidemiology*, **100**, 350–353 (1974)

43. Axelson, O. Aspects on confounding in occupational health epidemiology. *Scandinavian Journal of Work and Environmental Health*, **4**, 85–89 (1978)

44. Breslow, N.E. Elementary methods of cohort analysis. *International Journal of Epidemiology*, **13**, 112–115 (1984)

45. McMichael, A.J. Standardized mortality ratios and the 'healthy worker effect': scratching beneath the surface. *Journal of Occupational Medicine*, **18**, 165–168 (1976)

46. Pearce, N. Methodological problems in time-related variables in occupational cohort studies. *Revue d'Epidémiologie et de Santé Publique*, **40**, S43–S54 (1992)

47. Pearce, N. and Checkoway, H. Epidemiologic programs for computers and calculators. A simple computer program for generating person-time data in cohort studies involving time-related factors. *American Journal of Epidemiology*, **125**, 1085–1091 (1987)

48. Steenland, K. and Stayner, L. The importance of employment status in occupational cohort mortality studies. *Epidemiology*, **2**, 418–423 (1991)

49. Robins, J.M., Blevins, D., Ritter, G. *et al.* G-estimation of the effect of prophylaxis therapy for *Pneumocystis carinii* pneumonia on the survival of AIDS patients. *Epidemiology*, **3**, 319–336 (1992)

50. Liddell, F.D.K. Simple exact analysis of the standardised mortality ratio. *Journal of Epidemiology and Community Health*, **38**, 85–88 (1984)

51. Miettinen, O.S. The 'case-control' study: valid selection of subjects (with dissents, comment and response). *Journal of Chronic Diseases*, **38**, 543–558 (1985)

52. Axelson, O., Flodin, U. and Hardell, L. A comment on the reference series with regard to multiple exposure evaluations in a case-referent study. *Scandinavian Journal of Work and Environmental Health*, **8** (Suppl. 1), 15–19 (1982)

53. Axelson, O. Elucidation of some epidemiologic principles. *Scandinavian Journal of Work and Environmental Health*, **9**, 231–240 (1983)

54. Thomas, D.C. and Greenland, S. The efficiency of matching in case-control studies of risk-factor interactions. *Journal of Chronic Diseases*, **38**, 569–574 (1985)

55. Ahlbom, A. *Biostatistics for Epidemiologists*. Lewis Publishers, Boca Raton, Florida (1993)

56. Berry, G. Analysis and interpretation. In: McDonald JC (Ed.) *Epidemiology of Work Related Diseases* (ed. J. C. McDonald), BMJ Publishing Group, London (1995)

57. Axelson, O. The case-referent (case control) study in occupational health epidemiology. *Scandinavian Journal of Work and Environmental Health*, **5**, 91–99 (1979)

58. Miettinen, O.S. and Wang, J.-D. An alternative to the proportionate mortality ratio. *American Journal of Epidemiology*, **114**, 144–148 (1981)

59. Axelson, O., Fredrikson, M. and Ekberg, K. Use of the prevalence ratio v. the prevalence odds ratio in view of confounding in cross-sectional studies. *Occupational and Environmental Medicine*, **52**, 494 (1995)

60. Nurminen, M. To use or not to use the odds ratio in epidemiologic analyses? *European Journal of Epidemiology*. **11**, 365–371 (1995).

61. Zocchetti, C., Consonni, D., Bertazzi, P.A. *et al.* Letters to the Editor. Estimation of prevalence rate ratios from cross-sectional data. *International Journal of Epidemiology*, **5**, 1064–1067 (1995)

62. Hemminki, K. Use of molecular biology techniques in cancer epidemiology. *Scandinavian Journal of Work and Environmental Health*, **18** (Suppl. 1), 38–45 (1992)

63. Vineis, P. Uses of biochemical and biological markers in occupational epidemiology. *Revue d'Epidémiologie et de Santé Publique*, **40**, S63–S69 (1992)

64. Bartsch, H., Kadlubar, F. and O'Neill, I. Biomarkers in human cancer - part II. Exposure monitoring and molecular dosimetry. *Environmental Health Perspectives*, **99**, 2–309 (1992)

65. Caporaso, N., Hayes, R.B., Dosemeci, M., *et al. Lung cancer risk, occupational exposure, and the debrisoquine metabolic phenotype. Cancer Research*, **49**, 3675–3679 (1989)

66. Hardell, L., Holmgren, G., Steen, L. et al. Occupational and other risk factors for clinically overt familial amyloid polyneuropathy. *Epidemiology*, **6**, 598–601 (1995)

67. Sorahan, T. and Gilthorpe, M.S. Non-differential misclassification of exposure always leads to an underestimate of risk: an incorrect conclusion. *Occupational and Environmental Medicine*, **51**, 839–840 (1994)

68. Pershagen, G. and Axelson, O. A validation of questionnaire information on occupational exposure and smoking. *Scandinavian Journal of Work and Environmental Health*, **8**, 24–28 (1982)

69. Joffe, M. Validity of exposure data derived from a structured questionnaire. *American Journal of Epidemiology*, **135**, 564–570 (1992)

70. Axelson, O. The case-referent study. Some comments on its structure, merits and limitations. *Scandinavian Journal of Work and Environmental Health*, **11**, 207–213 (1985)

71. Pershagen, G. Lung cancer mortality among men living near an arsenic-emitting smelter. *American Journal of Epidemiology*, **122**, 684–694 (1985)

72. Hernberg, S. 'Negative' results in cohort studies. How to recognize fallacies. *Scandinavian Journal of Work and Environmental Health*, **7** (Suppl. 4), 121–126 (1981)

73. Beaumont, J.J. and Breslow, N.E. Power considerations in epidemiologic studies of vinyl chloride workers. *American Journal of Epidemiology*, **114**, 725–734 (1981)

74. Dean, A.G., Dean, J.A., Coulombier, D. *et al. Epi Info, version 6*. Centers for Disease Control and Prevention, Atlanta (1994)

75. Ahlbom, A., Axelson, O., Stöttrup Hansen, E. *et al.* Interpretation of 'negative' studies in occupational epidemiology. *Scandinavian Journal of Work and Environmental Health*, **16**, 153–157 (1990)

76. Axelson, O., Dahlgren, E., Jansson, C.-D. *et al.* Arsenic exposure and mortality, a case referent study from a Swedish copper smelter. *British Journal of Industrial Medicine*, **35**, 8–15 (1978)

Chapter 5

Risk assessment

VT Covello

The purpose of this chapter is to describe the processes involved in risk assessment. It describes what to look for in a risk assessment, what to expect from the assessment, and how to evaluate the results.

Basic definitions

Risk

Here *risk* is defined as the possibility of suffering harm from exposure to a risk agent. Risk agents include chemicals, radiation, heavy metals, and other hazardous or toxic materials.

For a risk to exist, three elements must be present: a hazard, a probability of exposure to the hazard, and probability of harm or adverse consequences from the exposure. A complete risk assessment describes (1) a hazard, that is, the risk agent that can cause harm; (2) the event or events that create the possibility of harm; and (3) a statistical estimate of likelihood that the harm will occur.

Hazard

In most texts, the term 'risk' does not mean the same as 'hazard'. Risk is created by a hazard. In the growing body of risk assessment literature, 'hazard' refers only to the source of a risk. By this definition, 'hazardousness' is the inherent property of a risk agent, within a particular context, and not subject to change, whereas 'risk' may be modified by human actions or natural forces. The potential for harm from exposure distinguishes risk from hazard. For example, a chemical or heavy metal that is a hazard to human health does not constitute a risk unless there is human exposure. This issue is discussed in greater depth later in the chapter.

Likelihood

A risk estimate is basically an estimate of the likelihood, or statistical probability, that harm will occur as a result of exposure to a risk agent. Most risk estimates say more than a risk is 'possible', since almost anything is possible.

The risk assessment process

Techniques for analysing risks have evolved from a variety of technical fields and applications, such as medicine, toxicology, industrial hygiene, occupational safety, environmental impact studies, and epidemiology. In recent years, the passage of environmental laws designed to protect public health has generated rapid growth in the development and application of risk assessment techniques. From these efforts emerged a process and framework for analysing many types of risk. The power of the process and framework that has evolved derives primarily from the systematic use of data, assumptions and expert judgements to exploit fully the relatively small amounts of information available to estimate the probability of adverse effects.

Risk assessment and risk management

Much debate has centred on the distinction between risk assessment and risk management. The basic point of contention is the degree to which risk assessment and risk management are different and should be viewed independently.

As noted above, risk assessment involves the systematic analysis of risk-related information to identify and estimate the probability and magnitude of risks associated with a particular hazard. For example, decision-makers use risk assessments in situations where answers are not obvious and available information is ambiguous and uncertain. Risk assessment techniques provide a means of organizing the relevant information and estimating the adverse health consequences of different decisions.

Risk management, by contrast, refers primarily to the integration of risk information with information about social, economic and political values, and various response options to determine what action to take, if any, to reduce or eliminate a risk. A critical factor influencing this determination is the resources and the technical capabilities available. Risk management also includes the design and implementation of policies and strategies that result from this decision process.

In practice, it is often impossible completely to eliminate all risks associated with a particular hazard. Risk management, therefore, involves (1) weighing the risks of alternatives; and (2) weighing trade-offs between the health and environmental benefits of incremental efforts to reduce risks and the costs to society of using its resources to obtain those benefits. Making such trade-offs is usually keyed to a consideration of what constitutes an acceptable level of risk. Issue Summary I (below) discusses the factors involved in trying to establish a risk threshold or *de minimis* risk level, that is, a specific level below which a risk may be so small that it can be ignored. Issue Summary II outlines the issues involved in making the decision, essentially a social and political, rather than a scientific, decision, as to whether a risk is acceptable to society. *De minimis* risk and acceptable-risk deci-

sion-making are both critical aspects of the process of risk management.

Risk-management, therefore, can be highly political. Balancing the costs of risk reduction against the benefits of use is a controversial and value-based process. More generally, the extent to which risk assessment and risk management can be distinct is still unresolved. The controversy revolves around the degree to which, in practice, the scientific assessment is, or should be, kept free from biases or values that typically are part of a management decision. For example, the practice of risk assessment at the Environmental Protection Agency (EPA) has been criticized from both ends of the environmental political spectrum. Proponents of less restrictive environmental regulation have charged that the techniques and assumptions used in EPA risk assessments reflect an unjustified bias in favour of overprotective risk management values. Environmental activists, on the other hand, have argued precisely the opposite, claiming that risk assessments used to support EPA decisions reflect techniques and assumptions that understate risks for the purpose of relieving regulatory burdens on industry.

The classic case in this regard was the controversy about Alar* that erupted in 1989. In this and many similar cases, the public was exposed to inconsistent and contradictory information about the risks of a chemical. Experts from the Natural Resources Defense Council said the risks were high. Experts for Uniroyal, the producer of Alar, said the risks were negligible. An understanding of risk assessment may help sort out the reason for these differences.

Risk assessment and risk perception

When experts talk about environmental health risks, they generally mean risk as estimated by the basic risk assessment process, that is, the likelihood or probability of specific adverse effects. By contrast, there is a commonsense notion of risk, as people perceive it in their everyday lives, that is intricately linked with numerous other social and psychological considerations.

People perceive risks differently, depending upon the nature of the risk and individual experiences. Researches from the fields of psychology,

---

*Alar (diaminizide) is a registered trademark of the Uniroyal company.

social psychology and decision analysis have identified several qualities or dimensions of risk that influence risk perceptions. For example, some people judge the riskiness of risk agents such as chemicals or heavy metals solely on the basis of the likelihood of the risk actually occurring, while others are primarily concerned about the effects of the risk agent – for example, who it affects, how widespread the effects may be, and how familiar and dreadful the effects are. Furthermore, perceptions of risks are influenced strongly by issues of choice and control. Risks often seem riskier to people if they have not voluntarily agreed to bear the risks and if they have no control over the source and management of the risks. In addition, people often incorporate into their perceptions of risks consideration of the benefits derived from accepting the risks. Fairness, equity, and the distribution of risks and benefits are also important factors in risk perception.

These differences between risk perception and risk assessment have important consequences. For example, in the Alar controversy, public response and media coverage were influenced to a significant degree by the perceptual characteristics of Alar. Alar, a growth regulator used on apples, had an exceptionally large number of perceptual characteristics that heighten public perceptions of risk. These included perceptions that Alar was involuntary, unfair, provided few public benefits, posed an imminent risk, affected children, caused a dreaded disease (cancer), could not be controlled by consumers (Alar was a systemic chemical), and contaminated a highly valued cultural symbol of health, motherhood, and country (i.e. apples).

For additional discussion of this issue, see Chapter 6.

Issue Summary I: De minimis risk – what level of risk is insignificant and can be ignored?

To what level should risks be reduced? Should no risk be tolerated? Is some level of risk so small that it can be ignored?

To achieve no, or zero, risk, the activity creating the risk must be banned completely. And when a risk agent is banned, there are usually risks associated with the substitutes.

In practice, zero-risk goals have proven difficult if not impossible to achieve. The classic case in point is the difficulty experienced by the USA Food and Drug Administration in implementing the Delaney Amendment to the federal Food, Drug, and Cosmetic Act, which mandates that no substance that has been found to cause cancer in animals or humans shall be added to the food supply.

Many federal environmental laws and regulations explicitly or implicitly recognize that very small levels of risk are not significant or worthy of attention, but the determination of how small those levels should be is often controversial. The concept of *de minimis* risk refers to a specific level below which risks are so small that they are usually ignored. (The term '*de minimis*' is derived from the legal doctrine *de minimis non curat lex*, 'the law does not concern itself with trifles'.) Proponents of a *de minimis* risk-management principle contend that regulatory agencies should establish *de minimis* levels and regulate only those hazards that pose a risk greater than these.

For many activities, some risk is tolerated to gain the benefits of the activity. People continue to drive automobiles, for example, even though the annual risk of dying in an automobile accident in the USA is about 1 in 4000, and the lifetime risk of dying in an automobile accident is about 1 in 65. In comparison, a *de minimis* risk level of 1 in 1 million for other hazards, such as the risk of cancer from exposure to a chemical, may for some appear quite reasonable (in part because a one-in-a-million risk represents an increase of only 0.000 3% over the current 1 in 3 chance of developing cancer).

There is as yet no consensus within government on what constitutes a *de minimis* level of risk. At the federal level, the Environmental Protection Agency and the Food and Drug Administration have often considered a risk level of one in a million as a *de minimis* level. EPA, for example, has stated that carcinogenic risks from chemicals are considered negligible when they are smaller than 1 in 1 million. Similarly, the Food and Drug Administration has adopted a 'one in a million' *de minimis* criterion in implementing the Delaney Clause of the Federal Food, Drug, and Cosmetic Act. However, it has yet to be settled by the courts whether the Delaney Clause prohibits application of the *de minimis* principle to pesticide residues.

By comparison, regulations associated with California's Safe Drinking Water and Toxic Enforcement Act of 1986 (Proposition 65) states that, for chemicals assessed using appropriate methods:

> . . . the risk level which represents no significant risk shall be one which is calculated to result in one excess case of cancer in an exposed population of 100,000, assuming lifetime exposure at the level in question, except where sound considerations of public health support an alternative level as, for example, where a cleanup and resulting discharge is ordered and supervised by an appropriate government agency or court of competent jurisdiction.

Proponents of the *de minimis* concept argue that a *de minimis* level, if widely accepted and adopted by regulatory agencies, could help agencies decide whether a hazard poses a significant public health risk. It would also help agencies set consistent levels of risk requiring regulatory action. Finally, it would encourage agencies to focus their attention on truly risky activities and avoid spending scarce agency resources on trivial risks.

Critics of the *de minimis* criterion, however, argue that the use of a *de minimis* risk criterion is problematic because of the difficulties of defining a level of risk that is insignificant. *De minimis* risks are typically defined in relation to a probability of experiencing an adverse effect; for example, a one-in-a-million chance of contracting cancer in a lifetime. Critics argue that the probability of experiencing an adverse effect is not the only factor that defines a risk. For example, a risk for which the probability of death is 1 in 1 million may be perceived as trivial if only 100 people are exposed to the hazard, but significant if 1 million or 1 billion people are exposed.

Other aspects of a hazard also affect people's perceptions about the significance of a defined level of risk. These aspects include familiarity, controllability and catastrophic potential. An unfamiliar, involuntary risk, such as living near a hazardous-waste site, is perceived as more risky than a familiar, voluntarily accepted one, such as skiing.

Consequences other than the annual mortality caused by the hazard may also be important. For example, the risk to future generations and effects on ecosystems influence public perceptions of risk.

Finally, a level of risk that is in itself insignificant may not be insignificant if it is part of a cumulative burden of risk. Some analysts argue that the cumulative effect for new risks indicates that stricter *de minimis* standards might be necessary for new risks.

Establishing a *de minimis* risk level will be difficult as long as experts and the public perceive risks differently. Moreover, a risk that at one time was deemed by society to be *de minimis* may not be so in the future.

Despite these reservations, focusing on serious risks first and trivial ones last can save lives. Eventually, society may reach a consensus on a definition of *de minimis* risk that allows agencies to allocate risk-management resources more efficiently, while accounting for all of the dimensions of risk that people consider important.

Issue Summary II: Acceptable risk – how safe is 'safe enough'?

At an individual level, the choice of whether to accept a risk is primarily a personal decision, such as choosing whether to eat foods known to have trace amounts of residual pesticides. On a societal level, where values conflict and decisions have winners and losers, the decision to restrict or allow the use of a risk agent becomes more difficult.

Determining the acceptability of a risk for society is a social and political decision, not a scientific one. Because people value the qualitative dimensions of risks, there is no numerical level of risk – other than zero – that will receive universal acceptance. Unfortunately, trying to eliminate all risks is not only impossible but would force people to give up many things of great social benefit. Thus, except where prohibited by law, decision-makers and risk managers typically face the task of identifying levels of risk that are greater than zero but that are also 'safe enough' in light of other factors such as the costs of risk reduction, the benefits gained from the activity or substance that poses the risk, and the availability of substitutes for that activity or substance.

Several approaches have been used, sometimes in varying combinations, to help decision-makers choose acceptable levels of risk. Historically, decision-makers have relied upon the judgement of technical experts to choose risk levels that will be considered safe. To allow for uncertainties in the experts' knowledge, margins of safety or safety factors have been incorporated into many risk-related decisions.

In an effort to formalize acceptable risk decisions, as well as to quantify the costs and benefits of alternative policy decisions, decision-makers increasingly have turned to techniques such as cost–benefit analysis, cost-effectiveness analysis, and decision analysis. However, use of these techniques is controversial. Like risk assessment itself, these techniques provide insight but are also fraught with uncertainties.

Some analysts have taken a different approach to the problem, arguing for a comparative and precedent-based approach to acceptable risk decisions. Acceptable-risk decisions, under this principle, should be guided by comparison with other risks that people have already chosen to accept. One way to determine an acceptable level of risk would be to identify the level of risk accepted implicitly or explicitly in prior societal decisions and use that as an acceptable level. Another way would be to use the risks of natural hazards as a basis for making acceptable-risk decisions. Each of these approaches has been severely criticized. A closely related idea that has recently received considerable scrutiny is the concept of *de minimis* risks (see above).

Increasingly, decision-makers have encountered opposition to acceptable-risk decisions based on these techniques, especially when large components of expert judgement are required. In some cases, however, acceptable-risk decisions have been upheld by the courts based on the determination that the decision by the federal agency was reasonable. Indeed, the term 'reasonable' – or, more commonly, 'unreasonable' – appears in several federal statutes as the primary criterion for making the difficult decisions about risks and costs. 'Reasonableness' is left undefined in these laws, however, requiring the regulatory agencies and, frequently, the courts, to determine what constitutes a reasonable decision about the acceptability of a risk.

Partially in response to the ambiguous nature of the reasonableness criterion and criticisms of formal methods of analysis, decision-makers have increasingly focused their attention on possible changes in the process by which acceptable risk decisions are made. For example, regulatory agencies have begun to make greater use of negotiation, consensus building, and other strategies designed to broaden outside involvement in acceptable-risk decisions.

Risk assessment methods

Covered here are the basic analytical methods used in risk assessment, along with a discussion on the strengths and limitations of specific tests, studies and models.

Risk assessors typically go through a four-step process to generate a risk estimate. These are:

- hazard identification
- exposure assessment
- dose–response assessment
- risk characterization.

Each is described below.

Hazard identification

Many of the difficulties surrounding the use of results from risk assessments begin with the validity of techniques used to answer the seemingly straightforward question: Does a health hazard exist?

The term hazard is not absolute. Its usage depends on the characteristics of the risk agent being studied and the circumstances of its use. Sometimes, the term incorporates an estimate of the likelihood of exposure. Therefore, the term may hold different meanings for different people. As a result, it is important to clarify the usage in any particular risk assessment. For the purposes of this section, hazard refers only to the potential for a risk agent to cause adverse health effects.

For some risk agents, short-term health effects, such as skin rashes, can be tested by using relatively well-established laboratory techniques. Health effects, however, are often more subtle: effects such as cancer, birth defects and behavioural modifications require more sophisticated detection methods. For an example of the difficulty in the identification of carcinogens, see Issue Summary V (below).

To identify environmental health effects, risk assessors use four types of analytical techniques:

- animal bioassays
- short-term *in vitro* cell and tissue culture tests
- environmental epidemiological studies
- structure–activity relationship analyses.

Each is described below.

Animal bioassays

For most risk agents, adequate data from human studies are not available. As a result, most environmental health risk assessments are based on information from laboratory studies on live animals. For example, most studies of acute effects have been done using guinea pigs, mice, rats and some primates. Most studies of chronic effects such as cancer have been done using rats and/or mice.

Test procedures for animal bioassays fall into three general categories: acute exposure tests, subchronic exposure tests and long-term chronic exposure tests (including carcinogenicity).

Acute exposure tests

Tests for acute (short-term) effects generally involve exposure of one or more species of test animals to the risk agent being studied. The route of exposure typically depends on the exposure route or routes of concern in humans, be it through ingestion, inhalation or contact with the skin. For practical reasons, however, many risk assessors use different exposure routes in their animal tests.

In oral toxicity studies, researchers administer a single oral dose to each test animal and a placebo (or no dose) to a control group. When the concentrations of the test chemical or toxic material cannot be carefully controlled in the test animals' food, a feeding tube is used in a technique called 'gavage'. In dermal toxicity studies, skin exposures are generally continuous for 24 hours. In inhalation toxicity studies, there is typically up to 8 hours of continuous exposure.

In a well-conducted study, 3–6 dose levels are tested, depending upon the route of exposure, using 5–10 animals of each sex for each dose level. Exposed animals are observed for signs of disease or toxic effects, and the death of any animal is recorded. After a short time, typically 14 days, any surviving animals are sacrificed and all test animals and controls are examined for signs of disease or toxic effects.

The most common measure of acute toxicity is the 'median lethal dose' (LD_{50}), the dose level that is lethal to 50% of the test animals exposed to that dose: the lower the LD_{50}, the more potent the chemical or toxic substance.

Growing concern about the use of animals in laboratory research, combined with the sometimes poor reproducibility of LD_{50} results between laboratories and the increasing development and sophistication of other tests (see below), has resulted in efforts to substitute other tests for LD_{50} animal studies as a measure of acute toxicity.

Subchronic exposure tests

Properly conducted subchronic tests involve repeated exposure of two species of test animals for 5–90 days, by exposure routes corresponding to expected human exposures. Often, more than one exposure route is tested. At least 3 dose levels are used to help define the dose–response relationship and to identify what are called the no observed adverse effects level, or NOAEL, and the lowest observed adverse effects level, or LOAEL. As implied, the NOAEL is the dose at which no adverse effects are observed, and the LOAEL is the lowest dose at which adverse effects are observed. Another important level that may be estimated from subchronic tests is the maximum tolerated dose, or MTD. The MTD is the largest dose of the test chemical that a test animal can receive for the majority of its lifetime without demonstrating adverse effects other than carcinogenicity.

Subchronic tests provide useful information about the dose–response relationship of the test chemical or toxic substance. They also help to identify metabolic reactions and define appropriate dose levels for chronic toxicity tests (as described below).

Long-term chronic exposure tests

In studies of the chronic effects of a risk agent, test animals receive daily doses of the risk agent (e.g. a suspect chemical) for approximately 2 years. In well-conducted experiments, at least 3 dose levels are used, the highest being the MTD (for studies of carcinogenecity, however, the use of the MTD is controversial; see Issue Summary IV, below).

Because of the need to detect small effects, and because the doses in chronic studies are lower than in acute or subchronic studies, a larger number of test animals – usually about 50 of each sex for each dose level – must be used to detect statistically significant effects. Thus, two major drawbacks of chronic animal bioassays are the time they take to conduct and analyse (from 2 to 3 years) and their large cost owing to the number of animals required (several hundred, depending upon the number of species, sexes and doses tested).

Test animals are observed during the experiment and sacrificed at the end of the exposure period for examination of organs and tissues. Abnormal behaviour, physiological damage or other signs of adverse effects (such as differences in organ weights) in test animals are recorded and compared with control animals. Significant adverse effects are inferred from several pieces of data, including data indicating a statistically significant increase in the incidence of the effect between dosed animals and controls at each dose level; an increase in the severity of the adverse effects with increases in dose; an accelerated emergence of adverse effects with increases in dose; and an increase in the numbers (types) of adverse effects with increases in dose.

As predicators of acute and chronic adverse effects in other species, and in humans particularly, animal bioassays are limited and controversial. For example, long-term animal bioassays may not be completely reliable predictors of carcinogenicity in humans. In evaluating over 700 chemicals, groups of chemicals and industrial processes, the International Agency for Research on Cancer (IARC) concluded that the available data provide causal evidence of human carcinogenicity for only 30 chemicals. Of these 30 human carcinogens, only 19 chemicals exhibited significant evidence of carcinogenicity in animals; data on the remaining 11 were limited, inadequate or unavailable to determine animal carcinogenicity.

Not all chemicals that cause cancer in one animal species also cause cancer in other species. The National Cancer Institute and the National Toxicology Program, in the USA, tested 224 chemicals for carcinogenicity in rats and mice; of these 224 chemicals, 75 were carcinogenic in both rats and mice, 32 were carcinogenic only in rats and 33 were carcinogenic only in mice.

As well as producing varying effects in different species, many carcinogens affect different organs in different species. Thus, from test results in one or two animal species, it is not possible to predict which organs will be affected or which species most closely resemble human beings in their response to the chemical.

There are several reasons for the difficulties in estimating human responses to test chemicals on the basis of animal bioassay results. Physiology and metabolic pathways that affect the response to a test chemical differ considerably among species. Another limitation is the large differences between the doses of the test chemical used (per kilogram of body weight) in the animal bioassays and the doses to which humans are typically exposed (see Issue Summary IV, below). Doses used in animal bioassays are necessarily relatively high so as to increase the sensitivity of the experiments, whereas human exposures tend to be much lower (and, as discussed below, actual doses to human tissues may be lower still). Thus, extrapolation from high test doses used in animal studies to the generally lower concentrations found in human environments creates large uncertainties in the validity of such bioassays as a means of identifying potential hazards. (A fuller discussion of scientific aspects of extrapolation to low dose occurs later in this section.)

Despite these shortcomings of animal bioassays, they are widely viewed as the best available analogy for identifying potential adverse human health effects of exposure to risk agents in the absence of good human data. For a summary of several key issues associated with using the results of such tests in hazard identification, see Decision Points I, below.

Decision Points I: Animal bioassay data in hazard identification

Although most experts accept the validity of using animal bioassay data to infer adverse human health effects, many issues are unresolved. For example, the use of these data requires the use of assumptions or judgements on the part of the risk assessor. For example, using a positive result from an animal test to infer an adverse human health effect represents a more conservative pessimistic judgement, while using negative animal data to infer the absence of adverse human health effects represents a less conservative or optimistic judgement. Other scientific questions that are unresolved include:

● What degree of confirmation of positive results should be necessary? Is a positive result from a single animal study sufficient, or should positive results from two or more animal studies be required? Should negative results be disregarded or given less weight?

● Should a study be weighted according to its quality and statistical power?

● How should evidence of different metabolic pathways or vastly different metabolic rates between animals and humans be factored into the risk assessment?

● How should the occurrence of rare tumours be treated? Should the appearance of rare tumours in a treated group be considered evidence of carcinogenicity even if the finding is not statistically significant?

● How should data for experimental animals be used when the exposure routes in experimental animals and humans are different?

● Should a dose-related increase in tumours be discounted when the tumours in question have high or extremely variable spontaneous rates?

● What statistical significance should be required for results to be considered positive?

● Does an experiment have special characteristics (for example, the presence of carcinogenic contaminants in the test substance) that lead one to question the validity of its results?

● How should findings of tissue damage or other toxic effects be used in the interpretation of tumour data? Should evidence that tumours may have resulted from these effects be taken to mean that they would not be expected to occur at lower doses?

● Should benign and malignant lesions be counted equally?

● Into what categories should tumours be grouped for statistical purposes?

● Should only increases in the numbers of tumours be considered, or should a decrease in the latent period for tumour occurrence also be used as evidence of carcinogenicity?

Short-term in vitro cell and tissue culture tests

In the past decade there has been an explosive growth in the quantity, variety and quality of laboratory tests using short-term *in vitro* (literally, in glass) cell and tissue cultures to study the effects of chemicals and other risk agents on biological organisms. The low cost and relative speed with which cell and tissue tests can be conducted have earned them a popular role in screening potentially hazardous substances and in providing additional sources of evidence for carcinogenicity.

This popularity has resulted primarily from (1) an increased demand for quicker and less expensive techniques to screen chemicals and other risk agents for potentially adverse effects on a routine basis; (2) rapid and revolutionary advances in biological techniques for manipulating genetic material, monitoring cellular behaviour, and initiating tissue culture growth; and (3) increasing pressures from animal welfare activists and others to develop alternatives to live animal assays.

Much of the development of *in vitro* techniques has occurred in the area of genetic toxicity tests for identifying chemicals that may be human mutagens and carcinogens. *In vitro* tests for genetic toxicity can be organized into the following categories: assays for genetic mutation, assays for chromosome effects, assays for disruption of DNA repair or DNA synthesis mechanisms, and assays for cellular transformation.

The predictive value of *in vitro* genetic toxicity tests for carcinogenicity is controversial. Most of the debate has centred upon the predictive value of the Ames test, which is the most widely used mutagenicity assay. Early research investigating the relationship between carcinogenicity and mutagenicity in the Ames test has reported correlations exceeding 90%. More recent evidence, which includes testing of a larger number of non-carcinogens, indicates the correlation is not as great as originally suggested. In examining the animal bioassay and *in vitro* test results of 73 chemicals studied in the National Toxicology Program, one study reported that 83% of chemicals with positive Ames tests were also rodent carcinogens. However, only 51% of the chemicals with negative Ames test results were non-carcinogens. Similarly, in an evaluation of results for 224 chemicals studied by the National Cancer Institute and the National Toxicology Program,

69% of Ames test mutagens were also animal carcinogens, while only 43% of non-mutagens were non-carcinogens.

Other short-term tests do not appear to predict carcinogenicity better than the Ames test. In two tests for chromosome effects, approximately 70% of chemicals with positive results were carcinogens, and 50% of chemicals with negative results were non-carcinogens. As might be expected, results of short-term tests on known human carcinogens show mixed results.

In general, the accuracy of *in vitro* tests for carcinogenicity is compromised by several factors, including (1) the lack of direct correspondence between the mechanisms of genetic toxicity used in the assays and the current understanding of carcinogenesis; (2) the difficulty of extrapolating from simple cellular systems to complex, higher organisms; (3) the use of different protocols and different interpretive rules by different laboratories; (4) the limited number of chemicals tested (except for the Ames test) by the assays, making validation difficult; and (5) the limited number of non-carcinogens tested.

For a summary of several key questions associated with the use of data from short-term *in vitro* tests, see Decision Points II, below.

Decision Points II: Short-term *in vitro* test data in hazard identification

The usefulness of short-term test data in estimating human adverse health effects is controversial. Unresolved scientific questions include:

- How much weight should be placed on the results of various short-term tests?
- What degree of confidence do short-term tests add to the results of animal bioassays in the evaluation of carcinogenic risks for humans?
- Should *in vitro* transformation tests be accorded more weight than bacterial mutagenicity tests in seeking evidence of a possible carcinogenic effect?
- What statistical significance should be required for results to be considered positive?
- How should different results of comparable tests be weighted? Should positive results be accorded greater weight than negative results?

The use of *in vitro* tests for adverse effects other than carcinogenicity has been much less widely examined. *In vitro* toxicity tests have been used mainly to study mechanisms of toxicity, but they are increasingly being developed as complements or alternatives to existing animal bioassays for estimating toxic effects. Scientists conduct *in vitro* toxicity tests on cell and tissue types ranging from microorganisms to tissue cultures from human organs. The choice depends partly upon the specific site and nature of the toxic effects of concern. For example, liver cells are used extensively, especially in hepatotoxicity tests, because the liver plays such an important role in the removal of toxic substances. Similarly, some tests with nerve tissue have been used to correlate neurotoxic effects with the presence of chemicals around the tissue. Measures of toxic damage in *in vitro* tests include changes in rates of cell reproduction, rates of synthesis of certain substances, changes in membrane permeability, and damage to some part of the cell structure.

Environmental epidemiological studies

Environmental epidemiological studies are concerned with the patterns of disease in human populations and the factors that influence these patterns. In general, scientists view well-conducted environmental epidemiological studies as the most valuable information from which to draw inferences about environmental health risks. A positive finding in a well-conducted environmental epidemiological study is generally viewed as strong evidence that a chemical or other risk agent poses a health risk to humans.

Unlike the other analytical approaches described in this section, risk assessors can use epidemiological methods to study the direct effects of chemicals and other risk agents on human beings. Also, epidemiological studies help identify actual hazards to human health without prior knowledge of disease causation. They also can complement and validate information about hazards generated by animal laboratory studies.

Compared to other techniques used in environmental health risk assessment, epidemiology is relatively well suited to situations in which exposure to the risk agent in question is high (such as in some occupational settings) or in which health effects are unusual (such as rare forms of cancer).

However, very few substances currently subject to regulatory and societal concern fall into these two categories. As a result, epidemiological studies used in risk assessment have important limitations that constrain their usefulness. These limitations arise not from epidemiology *per se*, but rather from the nature of the specific risk assessment needs to which epidemiology is sometimes applied.

A second limitation of environmental epidemiological studies is that they have poor sensitivity and are generally unable to detect small increases in health risk unless very large populations are studied. At low exposure levels, adverse effects may be very difficult to detect. For example, to identify any change in the number of genetic defects that could be caused by extremely small amounts of a chemical, a study would need to observe a large population of people for several generations. Moreover, even a positive result would not prove 100% certainty of harm, and a negative effect would not prove certainty of zero risk. Even if a carefully conducted study of 1000 exposed and unexposed people showed no excess cancer in the exposed population, it would be inappropriate to infer that the risk is non-existent.

These points underline the importance of the concept of statistical power in environmental epidemiological studies. The concept of statistical power is used by epidemiologists to decide whether statistical techniques are sufficient to reveal the effect under investigation. It also provides information relevant to the decision of whether the investigation should proceed.

After an epidemiological study is completed, its statistical value is determined by its confidence limits. Its epidemiological significance is also determined by:

- the consistency of association
- the strength of association
- the temporal relationship of association
- the specificity of association
- the biological plausibility of association.

In general, statistical significance and statistical power are not by themselves sufficient for results to be considered positive.

A third limitation of environmental epidemiological studies is that they can be conducted only for chemicals or other risk agents to which people already have been exposed.

A fourth limitation is the difficulty of establishing experimental controls. For obvious moral and ethical reasons, as well as pragmatic ones, researchers can neither control nor account completely for the behaviour of study subjects that may affect their health and therefore influence the study results.

A fifth limitation is the difficulty of describing and evaluating the effects of exposure to multiple sources of risk. This is particularly true in community health studies (see Issue Summary III, below). If both exposed and unexposed groups in a study are exposed to other risk agents, the study results may be difficult to interpret.

Epidemiological studies are often described as being either descriptive or observational. Furthermore, different types of observational studies exist, including case-control studies and cohort studies. Although other types of epidemiological studies exist, such studies are infrequently undertaken. For example, experimental epidemiological studies are sometimes conducted, but they require the deliberate application or withholding of a possible disease factor and observing the appearance or lack of appearance of any effect. For obvious ethical reasons, such studies are rare.

Descriptive and observational epidemiological studies are described below.

Descriptive epidemiology

Descriptive epidemiological studies examine the distribution and extent of disease in populations according to such basic characteristics as age, gender and race. The primary goal of a descriptive epidemiological study is to generate clues about the causes of disease. Descriptive epidemiological studies often provide data for more detailed follow-up epidemiological and toxicological studies.

Data for descriptive epidemiological studies come from several sources, including summaries of self-reported symptoms in exposed populations, case reports prepared by medical personnel, and studies that demonstrate a correlation between occurrences of health problems and the presence of a hazardous environmental or occupational condition.

Observational epidemiology

Data for observational epidemiological studies come from observations of individuals or relatively small groups of people. These studies are analysed using statistical methods to determine if an association exists between exposure to a risk agent and a disease outcome and, if so, the strength of the association. Often the hypothesis to be investigated is generated by a descriptive epidemiological study.

Two of the most common types of observational epidemiological studies are cohort studies and case-control studies. Cohort studies compare groups exposed to different levels of a chemical or other risk agent. They permit a direct estimate of the risk of disease associated with a particular exposure. Case-control studies compare the exposure histories of two matched groups: a group of individuals who exhibit symptoms of a particular disease, called cases, and a group of otherwise similar individuals who do not exhibit disease symptoms, called controls. A well-conducted case-control study requires a control group that is as similar as possible to the case group in all other ways except the presence of disease symptoms. Eligibility criteria are used to eliminate confounding factors such as age, race, gender and smoking. An additional confounding factor in case-control studies is that individuals in both groups may differ systematically in their recollection of past events.

For a summary of key questions associated with using data from case-control, cohort and other types of epidemiological studies, see Decision Points III, below (see also Case Study I, below, which examines the ways in which such studies have been used in assessing the health effects of dioxins).

Issue Summary III: Community health studies

Community health studies are a relatively common type of environmental epidemiological study that have received increased attention in recent years. The discovery of industrial chemicals in the water supply of a community, for example, may spark local concerns about the degree to which cancer cases, miscarriages and other health problems in the community may have been caused by exposure to industrial chemicals through food, water, air or soil. This concern may prompt officials, or citizens themselves, to conduct a community health study.

Community health studies are frequently used by researchers or public groups to draw attention to environmental health problems. In a typical community health study

---

of a chemical, the rate of occurrence of disease for people exposed to the chemical is compared with the average rate for that disease in other communities or in the country as a whole. The investigators survey people who have been exposed and collect information on the age, gender and disease history during a defined period of time. If the rate of occurrence of disease is greater than the average rate used for comparison, and if the difference is greater than would be expected owing to chance variation, then further, more detailed epidemiological investigation is typically undertaken.

One difference between experts and laypersons is that community residents often see a positive correlation in a community health study as evidence of a cause-and-effect relationship. However, correlation is not the same as cause-and-effect. For experts, a positive correlation is only suggestive and is used to develop hypotheses for further analytical studies. Being a type of correlational study, a community health study is usually not sufficient by itself to prove that the exposure of concern is associated with adverse health effects, unless the adverse health effects are rare or specific to the chemical of concern.

A significant difficulty with many community health studies and other such correlational studies is that the exposure history of individuals with and without disease is unknown. Also, the occurrence of disease can be affected by such factors as smoking, diet, exercise, access to health care facilities, and genetic influences. These factors, which are difficult to account for even in analytical epidemiology studies, are not usually considered in correlational studies. Thus, except for rare health problems that have well-understood causes, observations from community health studies are often too difficult to isolate from multiple confounding causes (such as smoking or diet). Consequently, they cannot provide definitive evidence of a risk. On the other hand, community health studies can be useful in identifying unusual patterns of disease occurrence and in indicating potential links between exposures to risk agents and disease.

Decision Points III: Epidemiological data in hazard identification

Although epidemiological data can be useful in assessing environmental health risks, many issues are unresolved. For example, experts often differ in answers they give to the following questions:

● What relative weights should be given to studies with differing results? For example, should positive results outweigh negative results if the studies that yield them are comparable? Should a study be weighted in accordance with its statistical power?
● What relative weights should be given to results of different types of epidemiological studies? For example, should the findings of a prospective study supersede those of a case-control study, or should those of a case-control study supersede those of a descriptive study?
● What statistical significance should be required for results to be considered positive?
● Does a study have special characteristics (such as the questionable appropriateness of the control group) that lead one to question the validity of its results?
● What is the significance of a positive finding in a study in which the route of exposure (e.g. inhalation, dermal exposure or ingestion) is different from the route of exposure for population at risk?
● Should evidence on different types of responses be weighted or combined (for example, data on different tumour sites and data on benign versus malignant tumours)?

Structure–activity relationship analysis

The simplest first step in any assessment of a potentially hazardous chemical is to compare it with similar chemicals for which the presence or absence of a hazard is known. One such approach is known as structure–activity relationship (SAR) assessment. EPA, for example, frequently uses this technique to determine whether more data (for example, from *in vitro* or laboratory animal tests) may be required.

SAR assessment involves comparing the molecular structure and chemical and physical properties of a chemical having unknown hazards with the molecular structures and properties of other, similar chemicals having known toxic or carcinogenic effects. Knowledge of the relationship between a particular structural feature or property and the physiological or molecular mechanisms by which the feature or property induces adverse effects strengthens the usefulness of SAR assessment.

The predictive value of SAR data is, however, often uncertain. Seemingly insignificant differences in chemical structures or properties may in fact obscure significant differences in hazardous characteristics. For example, the chemical relatives of several well-documented carcinogens are themselves not carcinogenic.

SAR assessment is potentially the most widely applicable and usable technique for assessing chemical hazards because molecular structures are readily identifiable and, in theory, any adverse effect can be assessed. In practice, however, predicting an adverse effect from a substance may not always be possible because of the lack of data about the particular adverse effect in structurally comparable substances.

Exposure assessment

Exposure assessment techniques estimate or directly measure the quantities or concentrations of a risk agent (or break down by-products) received by individuals or populations. Exposure assessments address the following multiple part question: What individuals or populations are, or may be, exposed to how much, of what, in what way, for how long, and under what circumstances.

Exposure assessments, as defined above, typically estimate concentrations of a risk agent (or its by-products) at a particular point of contact with a human being. Contact may occur as a result of inhalation, ingestion, or skin contact.

Some exposure assessments rely on data derived from analysis of body fluids or tissue samples to identify exposed populations and to determine exposure levels. Analyses of these types are needed to estimate doses, that is, concentrations or quantities of a given risk agent reaching body tissues, organs or cells where damage may occur.

Most exposure assessments are complicated by the fact that humans move from place to place and engage in a variety of activities that affect how much, when and for how long they are exposed to a given risk agent through the air, water, land or food. Some exposure assessments attempt to control for this variability by assuming or tracking – by using daily logs or surveys, for instance – the activity patterns of the target population.

Gathering the data necessary to account for such time–activity patterns is difficult and costly. Thus, many risk assessments use average exposures when better information is not available. This is analytically equivalent to assuming that all members of an exposed population are exposed to the same amount or concentration of the risk agent. In addition, constant or average exposure levels over time may be assumed. Whether these assumptions are reasonable depends upon the specific risk agent being assessed and the purpose of the risk assessment.

The specific methods or techniques used in exposure assessments vary depending upon the nature of the risk agent, knowledge about the source or sources, and knowledge about the activity patterns of exposed populations. For environmentally mobile risk agents, exposure assessments typically employ three kinds of approaches, which are discussed below:

● analogies
● monitoring
● exposure modelling.

Analogies with other risk agents

Information about the transport and fate of a particular risk agent in the environment can, in some cases, be inferred by comparison with what is known about the transport and fate of similar risk agents. The use of analogies to predict the environmental behaviour of risk agents is similar in concept to the use of structure–activity relationships to identify hazards. For example, some classes of chemicals, owing to their physical and chemical characteristics, are known to disperse and react with other chemicals in relatively predictable ways under given environmental conditions.

Analogies with other risk agents generally do not predict environmental transport and fate as accurately as actual measurements of environmental concentrations. However, such analogies may identify general characteristics of the risk agent that support specific judgements or assumptions used in exposure models.

Monitoring

The most accurate information about exposure comes from monitoring data. Moreover, monitoring data provide an accuracy benchmark for exposure models.

Monitoring data are typically collected in close proximity to the populations or environments of concern. There are two basic kinds of exposure monitoring: personal monitoring and ambient (or site or location) monitoring.

Personal monitoring involves using one or more techniques to measure the actual concentrations of a given risk agent to which individual humans are exposed, regardless of the location. Personal monitoring may include sampling of the food people eat, the air they breathe or the water they drink.

Personal monitoring may also involve the sampling of human body fluids (for example, blood or urine). This type of monitoring is often referred to as biological monitoring.

Ambient (or site or location) monitoring, in contrast to personal monitoring, involves collecting samples from the air, water, soil or food at fixed locations and then analysing the samples to determine environmental concentrations at that location. Ambient monitoring is clearly a more practical technique than personal monitoring when large geographical areas or human populations are exposed.

There are several potential sources of error in monitoring techniques. One of the most important is a poorly designed sample. For example, an important variable in sample design is the time period during which a sample reading is taken. Readings taken during different time periods may show different patterns and levels. For example, in a study of chemical air emissions at an industrial facility, levels may be high for 8 hours during intensive daytime industrial activity and low for the next 16 hours. Similarly, monitoring results can be biased by the selection and location of monitoring sites, such as at busy traffic intersections.

In addition to these problems, monitoring studies can be costly, time-consuming and difficult to generalize to other environmental situations. Furthermore, monitoring data may not be representative of the full range of exposure situations, since such data are collected under a defined set of conditions. For example, air monitoring systems for chemicals are typically designed to measure outdoor concentrations of chemicals. However, many people spend a substantial amount of their time indoors.

Despite these limitations, the main advantage of monitoring techniques over other methods is that they provide actual measured data from locations that are close to the exposed populations and environments of concern. For the same reason, monitoring data are typically more accurate than model predictions (see below). Monitoring data can be erroneous, however, and need to be periodically checked and questioned. This is especially true if monitoring data differ substantially and inexplicably from expected amounts. In some cases, the monitoring data will be found to be in error. In most cases, however, the model data are in error and the monitoring data can be used to improve the model's accuracy.

Exposure modelling

When monitoring data are either inadequate or inappropriate for estimating exposure, risk assessors frequently use models to simulate the behaviour of the risk agent in the environment. In most of the literature on risk assessment, such models are generally known as exposure models. Many such models exist, and many are highly specialized. For example, models exist that are specific to particular sources, toxic substances and environmental settings (such as watersheds and lakes).

All environmental models are limited by two types of uncertainty. First, there is uncertainty in the data used in the models. Secondly, models are only mathematical representations of environmental conditions. As such, they are necessarily imperfect predictors of the behaviour of the risk agent in the real environment. There is a complex relationship between the degree of simplification of a model and the amount of uncertainty in the model. Although complicated models may represent more characteristics of the real environment, their generally greater demand for data means that many factors must be estimated. Also, uncertainty can multiply with the number of factors estimated, sometimes creating greater aggregate uncertainty than is generated in a simpler, less data-intensive model.

The predictive capabilities of a model are ideally validated and improved through field testing. However, the data required for such testing are difficult to collect and interpret. Although some models have been validated in specific cases, procedures for validating models are not universally accepted. Moreover, validation of a model under one set of environmental conditions does not necessarily support its applicability to a different set of conditions.

Although a detailed discussion of exposure models is beyond the scope of this chapter, five general types of models are briefly described below: (1) atmospheric models, (2) surface-water models, (3) groundwater models, (4) multimedia models, and (5) food chain models.

1 *Atmospheric models.* The atmospheric transport of a chemical or other risk agent may be estimated by applying known laws of physics and chemistry to data from monitoring systems. However, in many cases, monitoring data are not available. Attempts to predict the transport and fate of chemicals and other risk agents have led to the development of many sophisticated models that simulate the transport and transformation of chemicals and other risk agents in the atmosphere.

Many atmospheric models incorporate equations that account for the rates of transformation, degradation, or deposition, that is, through settling or precipitation, of a risk agent released in the atmosphere. These phenomena are especially important when the transformation products of a risk agent pose a significantly greater or lesser hazard than the risk agent emitted from the source.

2 *Surface-water models.* Risk assessments often incorporate surface-water models in exposure assessments when it is believed that the risk agent may affect drinking water, food supplies or recreational resources derived from streams, rivers, lakes or other surface-water bodies.

Many surface-water models divide surface-water bodies into compartments or boxes. The transport of the risk agent is traced by mathematical equations that assume conservation of energy and mass going into and out of each box. Refinements to the compartmental model concept attempt to account for complex flow conditions (for example, tidal forces), sedimentary deposition, biological degradation and uptake, and chemical transformation and decay.

3 *Groundwater models.* Chemicals and other risk agents released or deposited on or in the ground can move through soil and rocks into groundwater, thereby threatening drinking-water supplies and possibly discharging into surface-water bodies.

Groundwater models estimate the vertical movement of water containing specific risk agents into the soil and between the ground surface and the groundwater zone. Traditional soil models rely on mathematical equations to describe statistically the behaviour of the risk agent moving with water through the soil.

Although compartmental models may provide more sophisticated treatment than traditional models, no single model yet exists that simulates all physical, chemical and biological processes associated with the behaviour of all risk agents in soils.

The simplest groundwater transport models calculate the movement of a chemical or other risk agent as a function of the linear velocity of the groundwater (known as advection); and the spreading or mixing of the chemical or other risk agent in the groundwater (known as dispersion). More complex groundwater models account for differences in density, adsorption on soil or rock particles, chemical and biological transformations, and the flow of water through fractured geological media.

4 *Multimedia models.* Although some air and water models account for deposition of chemicals and other risk agents into another medium (such as air, water, soil or groundwater), most of the models in the categories described above are limited to the assessment of a single environmental medium or exposure pathway. However, the movement of a chemical or other risk agent among different media is a critical factor in exposure assessment. For example, one study estimated that 50–85% of all chemicals released to a single medium will eventually have at least 5% of their mass in another medium.

Because of this, risk assessors have devoted increasing attention to multimedia pollutant behaviour. For example, risk assessors have begun to develop and use multimedia models to account for transfers of chemicals and other risk agents among different media and exposures from multiple environmental pathways. Most of these models consist of linked, single-medium models, which may simulate the physical and chemical processes that drive the transport of chemicals and other risk agents, such as between air and water, water and soil, and water and crops. However, the data requirements for such models are substantial, and scientific understanding of intermedia transport processes is still embryonic.

5 *Food chain models.* Food chain models simulate the transport, transformation and accumulation of risk agents in the environment as they are deposited (for example, in sediments) and ingested by different species representing the various parts of the food chain.

As with other models, the data requirements for food chain models are substantial. Moreover, large uncertainties exist on such critical subjects as the uptake, behaviour and retention of specific risk agents in plants and animals later consumed as food.

For a summary of several key questions associated with exposure assessment as a whole, see Decision Points IV, below.

Decision Points IV: Exposure assessment

Many unresolved issues exist in exposure assessment. For example, experts often differ in answers they give to the following questions:

- How should one extrapolate exposure measurements from a small segment of a population to the entire population?
- How should one predict dispersion of specific risk agents into the atmosphere attributable to convection and wind currents or predict seepage rates of risk agents into soils and groundwater?
- How should dietary habits and other variations in lifestyle, hobbies and other human activity patterns be taken into account?
- Should point estimates or a distribution be used?
- How should differences in timing, duration, and age at first exposure be estimated?
- What is the proper unit of dose?
- How should one estimate the size and nature of the populations likely to be exposed?
- How should exposures of special risk groups, such as pregnant women and young children, be estimated?

Dose–response assessment

Dose–response assessment, the third step in a risk assessment, involves (1) determining the dose of the risk agent received by exposed populations, and (2) estimating the relationship between different doses and the magnitude of their adverse effects. In essence, dose–response assessment involves efforts to quantify or describe statistically the qualitative relationship identified in the hazard-identification stage between a risk agent and any adverse effects.

It should be noted that the determination of 'delivered dose,' that is, the amount of a risk agent that is received by exposed populations, is sometimes discussed in the risk assessment literature under the heading 'exposure assessment' rather than under the heading 'dose–response assessment'. Many such inconsistencies can be found in the risk assessment literature and illustrate the embryonic state of the field.

Determining dose

Some risk assessments assume that the concentration of a risk agent that reaches the immediate vicinity or the body surfaces of the target population represents the dose to which the target population is exposed. The difficulty with this simple assumption is that the physiological and metabolic systems of organisms can act on risk agents and potentially increase, decrease or modify the amounts received by relevant parts of the human body. In response to this problem, increasing numbers of scientists have focused their attention on developing improved methods for estimating the amount of a chemical or other risk agent that is actually taken into the human body and how the chemical or risk agent interacts with particular tissues or organs.

To distinguish between ambient exposures and actual doses, analysts frequently use two measures of dose. One is the absorbed dose – the amount of a risk agent that is absorbed by:

- the lungs (for inhalation exposures)
- the gastrointestinal tract (for ingestion exposures)
- the skin (for dermal exposures).

The other measure is the internal, or effective, dose – the amount of a risk agent reaching a tissue or an organ where it inflicts damage.

Determining the absorbed dose usually is performed by applying a number of standard adjustment factors to environmental concentrations of a risk agent. Such factors may include, where appropriate, the number of adults and children in the exposed population; the amounts of drinking water consumed by members of the population; the amounts of air inhaled by exposed individuals, adjusted for age and level of physical activity; the amount of the chemical or other risk agent at the site of absorption in the respiratory or intestinal tract; and the absorption rates of skin, lung tissue, bronchial tissue and intestinal tissue. Generally, the data needed to determine the values of these adjustment factors are not available for the specific populations exposed to the risk agent. Standard values or statistical distributions are typically used, but these values may introduce some error into estimations of dose for actual exposed populations.

Determining the effective dose of a chemical or other risk agent is more difficult than calculating the absorbed dose. For example, the chemical of concern may be a metabolite, i.e. it poses a health risk only after it has been metabolized by the body. Moreover, the human body has complex mechanisms for responding to chemicals and other risk agents. For example, some toxic chemicals can be metabolized and excreted, whereas others may accumulate in certain tissues or organs. Some risk assessments use models of chemical and metabolic activity to determine the fate of a chemical or other risk agent from the time it enters the bloodstream and/or fluids to the time it interacts with tissues or organs. Such models are often called *pharmacokinetic models*.

Pharmacokinetic models often require enormous amounts of data on anatomy, physiology, rates of decay and metabolism, and biochemical interactions. Such data are becoming increasingly available. When such data are available, they are often derived from experiments on laboratory animals (usually rats or mice). As such, the data must be carefully weighed in light of the poorly understood biological differences between animals and humans, as well as the differences between relatively homogeneous, inbred laboratory animals and more heterogeneous human populations.

Given these difficulties and problems, the typical risk assessment equates effective dose with absorbed dose (or even environmental concentrations).

Dose–response estimation

To estimate the responses of humans to a given dose of a chemical or other risk agent, risk assessors conduct mathematical extrapolations. In rare instances, epidemiological data are available that demonstrate the magnitudes of adverse effects across a range of exposures (doses) that are comparable to the doses of concern. Most epidemiological data, though, are available only for doses significantly higher than the doses of concern. Analysts extrapolate the effects resulting from high doses to the lower doses to which the populations at risk are exposed. For most risk agents, adequate epidemiological data do not exist, and data from laboratory animal studies (similar to those described for hazard identification) are used.

As discussed above, animals used in toxicity studies receive high doses of the chemical or other risk agent in question to compensate for the low sensitivity of such studies. Toxicologists generally make two assumptions about the effects of exposure at low doses. The first is that thresholds exist in a population for most biological effects. That is, for non-carcinogenic, non-genetic, toxic effects, doses of the chemical exist below which no adverse effects are observable in a population of exposed individuals. The second assumption is that no thresholds exist for genetic damage or carcinogenic effects.

The first assumption is widely accepted by the scientific community and is supported by empirical evidence. The threshold for a chemical is, as mentioned earlier, often called the no observed effects level (NOEL) or the no observed adverse effects level (NOAEL). The difference between the NOEL and the NOAEL hinges upon the definition of adverse effects. As discussed above (see section on hazard identification), toxicologists usually estimate NOELs or NOAELs from toxicity studies.

The second assumption, regarding no thresholds, is more controversial but is adopted by all US federal regulatory agencies as a precautionary measure (see Issue Summary VI, below).

Extrapolations from high experimental doses to low doses require the use of mathematical models, which are often represented graphically as dose–response curves.

Dose–response extrapolation

Choosing an appropriate dose–response curve or extrapolation model for carcinogens is difficult because relatively little is known about the biological mechanisms involved in carcinogenesis, especially the latency period between exposure and effects. Different extrapolation models are based on different approaches to characterize carcino-genic activity. The following is a brief discussion of some of these models.

One category of models are termed mechanistic models. These models derive from particular theories about the biological steps involved in the formation of cancerous tumours. Mechanistic models include one-hit and multihit models, which are based on informed judgements about the number of 'hits' (or interactions between a chemical and a cell) required to make a cell become cancerous. Another mechanistic model, the multistage model, is the most frequently used extrapolation model. It derives from the theory that developing tumours go through several stages before they become clinically detectable.

Another category of models are termed threshold distribution models. These models are not based on mechanistic theories of carcinogenesis. Rather, they assume that different individuals have different tolerances and that this variability in tolerance in an exposed population can be described as a probability distribution. Within this category, the probit, logit and Weibull extrapolation models each adopt different probability distributions for the tolerance levels of individuals in the exposed population.

A third category of models are termed time-to-tumour models. These models attempt to describe the relationships among dose, tumour latency and cancer risk. Several models of this type have been developed, but none seems to have significantly improved the precision of estimates of risk.

In general, there is little scientific basis for deciding which of the many low-dose extrapolation models most accurately simulates the true dose–response relationship. Furthermore, no single model has gained universal acceptance within the scientific community. In some cases, risk assessors estimate dose–response using several extrapolation models as an indication of the uncertainties in extrapolating to low doses.

For non-carcinogenic health effects, extrapolation from high to low doses involves identifying the NOEL or the NOAEL and describing the dose–response relationship that best fits the observed data from animal bioassay, *in vitro* or epidemiological studies.

Species extrapolation

Differences in size, metabolism, anatomy, physiology and population heterogeneity make dose extrapolation among species a highly uncertain activity. For example, because of size differences, risk assessors frequently standardize the experimental dose of a chemical or other risk agent on the basis of body weight or body surface area. In such cases, the dose may be measured in terms of milligrams per kilogram of body weight or in terms of milligrams per square metre of body surface area. There is no clear consensus as to which extrapolation principle – body weight or body surface – is more appropriate; substantial variability results in risk estimates derived from the two methods.

Differences in genetic variability or heterogeneity between the populations are difficult to adjust for due to a lack of accepted principles. Laboratory species are generally inbred, and so they are thought to have a relatively homogeneous response to chemicals and other risk agents in comparison to highly variable human populations. Assuming that the exposed human population will respond identically to groups of inbred laboratory animals introduces considerable uncertainty into risk estimates.

Metabolic, physiological and anatomical differences among species also complicate interspecies extrapolation. Where differences are known – for example, in enzyme activity – such information is clearly useful. Often, however, data on these differences are insufficient to make reliable quantitative adjustments to dose–response estimates.

For a summary of questions associated with dose–response assessment, see Decision Points VI, below).

Decision Points V: Epidemiological data in dose–response assessment

Estimating the relationship between the dose of a risk agent and the response by a human requires many assumptions and judgements on the part of the risk assessor. Unresolved scientific questions include:

● What dose–response models should be used to extrapolate from observed doses to relevant doses?
● Should dose–response relations be extrapolated according to best estimates or according to upper confidence limits?
● How should risk estimates be adjusted to account for a comparatively short follow-up period in an epidemiological study?

● For what range of health effects should responses be tabulated? For example, should risk estimates be made only for specific types of cancer that are unequivocally related to exposure, or should they be made for all types of cancers?
● How should exposures to other carcinogens, such as cigarette smoke, be taken into consideration?
● How should one deal with different temporal exposure patterns in the study population and in the population for which risk estimates are required? For example, should one assume that lifetime risk is only a function of total dose, irrespective of whether the dose was received in early childhood or in old age? Should recent doses be weighted less than earlier doses?
● How should physiological characteristics be factored into the dose–response relation? For example, is there something about the study group that distinguishes its response from that of the general population?

Decision Points VI: Animal bioassay data in dose–response assessment

Many scientific uncertainties confront the risk assessor in attempting to extrapolate results of studies using laboratory animals to expected effects on humans. Unresolved scientific questions include:

● What mathematical models should be used to extrapolate from experimental doses to human exposures?
● Should dose–response relations be extrapolated according to best estimates or according to upper confidence limits? If the latter, what confidence limits should be used?
● What factor should be used for interspecies conversion of dose from animals to humans?
● How should information on comparative metabolic processes and rates in experimental animals and humans be used?
● If data are available on more than one non-human species or genetic strain, how should they be used? Should only data on the most sensitive species or strain be used to derive a dose–response function, or should data be

combined? If data on different species and strains are to be combined, how should this be accomplished?

- How should data on different types of tumours in a single study be combined? Should the assessment be based on the tumour type that was affected the most (in some sense) by the exposure? Should data on all tumour types that exhibit a statistically significant dose-related increase be used? If so, how? What interpretation should be given to statistically significant decreases in tumour incidence at specific sites?

Risk characterization

Risk characterization is the fourth and final step of the risk-assessment process. It is designed to integrate the results of all parts of the risk assessment process to generate several types of risk estimates. These include estimates of the types and magnitudes of adverse effects that the risk agent may cause and estimates of the probabilities that each effect will occur. Ideally, these estimates are accompanied by a description and discussion of uncertainties and analytical assumptions, since characterizing risk includes characterizing uncertainty and assumptions.

As described above, risk assessments typically focus on one or two adverse human health effects. Since these effects do not reflect the full range of adverse effects that a risk agent may cause, the risk statement ideally includes a discussion of adverse effects that were not assessed and why they were excluded from the assessment.

For a summary of some of the key questions associated with this fourth step of the risk-assessment process, see Decision Points VII, below.

The form of the numerical risk estimates depends upon the measure of risk chosen. One of the most common risk measures used in risk assessments is individual lifetime risk. This risk measure states the excess, or increase in, probability that an individual will experience a specific adverse effect as a result of exposure to the risk agent of concern. Individual lifetime risks are often presented as very small probabilities, such as 1×10^{-6}, or a one-in-a-million chance that an individual will develop the adverse effect. Unless otherwise indicated, individual lifetime risk means

the likelihood of experiencing an effect owing to a continuous lifetime exposure. Individual lifetime risk is calculated by multiplying the potency of a substance by the dose an individual receives. For chemicals and other risk agents with a threshold for exposure, the potency of the chemical is zero for dose levels below the threshold. For carcinogenic chemicals, which are assumed to have no threshold, a linear dose–response relationship is assumed. The risk at a high dose level is divided by that dose to determine potency (also known as unit cancer risk).

Population risk – also called societal risk – is another frequently used measure of risk. Population risk may be expressed as the number of cases of illness or disease resulting from 1 year of exposure, or as the number of cases occurring in 1 year. It is usually calculated as individual risk times the number of people exposed. This calculation assumes a linear dose–response relationship, which may or may not be appropriate.

Another common measure of risk is the 'relative risk'. Relative risk is a comparison of rates of disease occurrence between those exposed to the chemical or other risk agent and those not exposed. Thus, relative risk is the risk in the exposed population compared to the risk in the unexposed population.

Loss of life expectancy is yet another measure of risk. It is expressed as days or years of life expected to be lost owing to exposure to a particular chemical or other risk agent.

The choice of risk measures, as noted above, is often a reflection of the way in which the analyst collects and organizes data. The choice of a particular measure is not value-neutral, however, and should be considered as only one possible way of characterizing risk.

Decision Points VII: Risk characterization

The expressions of risk developed during the risk-characterization stage require combining information from the previous steps. Unresolved questions include:

- What are the statistical uncertainties in estimating the extent of health effects? How are these uncertainties to be computed and presented?
- What are the biological uncertainties in estimating the extent of health effects? What is

their origin? How will they be estimated? What effect do they have on quantitative estimates? How will the uncertainties be described to decision-makers?

● Which dose–response assessments and exposure assessments should be used?

● Which population groups should be the primary targets for protection, and which provide the most meaningful expression of the health risk?

Identifying and evaluating errors and uncertainties in risk assessments

By definition, error and uncertainty are inherent in all risk assessments. Frequently the source and magnitude of the errors or the uncertainties are not clearly or adequately described. One critical aspect of evaluating risk assessments or other risk information, therefore, is to identify and evaluate the assessment and expression of error and uncertainty.

Error and uncertainty arise from three kinds of sources. First, they occur as a result of natural variability over time and space in the environment. For example, rainfall, wind velocity, temperature and other environmental conditions vary from location to location and from time period to time period. These variations make statistical descriptions of the behaviour of risk agents in the environment inherently uncertain. Only in rare instances are sufficient data available to accurately estimate and characterize probabilities.

Secondly, error and uncertainty arise in the measurement or estimation of variables used to characterize the risk agent, the environment and the exposed populations.

Thirdly, error and uncertainty arise from models that do not accurately reflect the real environments or exposed populations of concern. Examples include uncertainties arising from untested assumptions in animal studies or the use of an exposure model that fails to account for the biodegradation of a chemical.

Analysis of uncertainty

A critical issue in risk assessment is to determine how much different sources of uncertainty contribute to the overall variability of the final risk estimates. The kinds of error and uncertainty described above affect all stages of the risk-assessment process: hazard identification, exposure assessments and dose–response assessments. Analysing the sources and magnitudes of uncertainties helps focus debate and identify areas of missing scientific information.

One means for expressing uncertainty is to conduct a worst-case/best-case risk assessment. In worst-case/best-case risk assessment, the lowest and highest extreme values are calculated to determine the upper and lower bounds of risk estimates. The upper bound, or highest risk, represents the worst possible, or most pessimistic, case, while the lower bound, or lowest risk, represents the best possible, or most optimistic, case. The range of final risk estimates obtained with this method of assessment is likely to be extremely large for most risk assessments.

Confidence intervals are a relatively common method of limiting the problems with extreme upper- and lower-bound estimates. Risk assessors may refer to the '95th percent confidence interval' to indicate that they are 95% sure that the true value lies within that interval. Such intervals are still likely to be large, however, and there is an implicit policy judgement in selecting 95% as a measure of confidence.

In many risk assessments, analysts simply acknowledge the existence of uncertainty but make no efforts to analyse or quantify it. Many final reports contain only a point estimate of the risk. If this approach is taken, the best point estimate is usually the mean or median (based on sample data or expert judgement).

Point estimates are easy to understand – especially for people with little or no statistical training. However, such simplicity comes at a high price. Point estimates obscure important elements of the analysis and mislead by hiding the existence of uncertainty and variability.

Issue Summary IV: Use of the maximum tolerated dose in animal bioassays for carcinogens

Considerable controversy exists concerning the use of large doses of chemicals in laboratory tests for carcinogenicity. In most animal bioassays, high doses of chemicals are administered to compensate for the insensitivity of the bioassays. Cancer occurs at very low rates; for example, lung cancer affects fewer than 8 in 10 000 people in the USA every year, an incidence rate of less than 0.08%. Such low incidence rates are virtually impossible to detect in animal studies.

To explore this issue in greater detail, scientists have conducted studies using large numbers of animals. Among these studies, perhaps the best known is the 'Megamouse Study'. In this study, 24 192 mice were subjected to seven different dose levels of a potent liver and bladder carcinogen. Even with that many test animals, the lowest incidence of observed tumours was about 1%.

Practical considerations prohibit using such large numbers of animals in most studies; typical animal tests may use 50 or 60 animals of each species and sex at each dose level. Very high doses of substances are often necessary to ensure that chemicals that are carcinogens do not yield negative results.

The highest dose used in carcinogenicity tests is the maximum tolerated dose (MTD), which is the dose an animal species can tolerate for a major portion of its lifetime without significant impairment of growth or observable toxic effect other than carcinogenicity. The importance of the MTD in carcinogenicity testing is demonstrated by results of long-term animal tests conducted for the National Toxicology Program. Of 52 chemicals judged as carcinogens, two-thirds would not have been found carcinogenic if the high dose selected had been one-half the MTD actually used.

One problem with doses as high as the MTD is that an organism's normal mechanisms of self-dence may be overwhelmed, allowing cancer to be induced or promoted. Additionally, very high doses of a chemical may have a qualitatively different impact on the organism than the same substance at a low dose: the distribution of a chemical in the body may be altered, or processes that detoxify or eliminate the chemical may be affected. A carcinogenic response at high dose levels may not be indicative of effects at low exposure levels. This issue is at the heart of many debates about the effects of chemicals on humans. For example, in the debate about the growth hormone Alar, the apple industry pointed out that a child receiving the same MTD used in the laboratory animal studies would have to eat 28 000 apples a day.

In response to this problem, researchers have concentrated their attention on the mechanisms that lead to cancer and how the mechanisms may change as the dose changes. The goal of such studies is to be able to incorporate information on the distribution of the substance within the organism and metabolism of chemicals in selecting the MTD.

Issue Summary V: Carcinogenicity characterization

What is a carcinogen? The mechanisms by which cancerous tumours form are still poorly understood. Currently accepted theories of carcinogenesis characterize the formation of tumours as a multistage process. Carcinogenic chemicals may 'cause' cancer by initiating the process by which tumours form ('initiators') or by promoting the unrestrained growth of cells once a cell has been transformed to a precancerous state ('promoters'). In addition, some carcinogenic chemicals may not initiate or promote cancerous growth but may cause other metabolic changes that in turn lead to cancer.

For many carcinogens, the exact mechanism by which they cause the cancer is not well understood. In the absence of scientific data on the mechanisms by which a given chemical causes cancer, regulatory agencies typically infer that the chemical has carcinogenic properties by weighing the evidence from both human and animal studies. Several different agencies and international institutions have developed various weight-of-evidence criteria for determining whether a chemical should be considered carcinogenic. These criteria are shown below.

US Environmental Protection Agency

Category	Criterion
A	Human carcinogen, with sufficient evidence from epidemiological studies
B1	Probable human carcinogen, with limited evidence from epidemiological studies

B2	Probable human carcinogen, with sufficient evidence from animal studies and inadequate evidence or no data from epidemiological studies
C	Possible human carcinogen, with limited evidence from animal studies in the absence of human data
D	Not classifiable as to human carcinogenicity, owing to inadequate human and animal evidence
E	Evidence of non-carcinogenicity for humans, with no evidence of carcinogenicity in at least two adequate animal tests in different species, or in both adequate animal and epidemiological studies

International Agency for Research on Cancer

Category	Criterion
1	Carcinogenic to humans, with sufficient epidemiological evidence
2A	Probably carcinogenic to humans, with (usually) at least limited human evidence
2B	Probably carcinogenic to humans, but having (usually) no human evidence
3	Sufficient evidence of carcinogenicity in experimental animals

National Toxicology Program

Category	Criterion
a	Known to be carcinogenic, with evidence from human studies
b	Reasonably anticipated to be a carcinogen, with limited evidence in humans or sufficient evidence in experimental animals

American Conference of Governmental Industrial Hygienists

Category	Criterion
A1	Confirmed human carcinogen, recognized to have carcinogenic or cocarcinogenic potential
A2	Suspected human carcinogen, based on either limited epidemiological evidence or

demonstration of carcinogenicity in experimental animals
Indirect carcinogenic activity occurs primarily as secondary effects of some other toxic or physiological action by the substance or its metabolites

Issue Summary VI: Threshold doses for chemical carcinogens?

Chemicals that do not cause cancer can generally be tolerated in small amounts and detoxified within the body with no adverse effects. However, there is a strong ongoing debate among scientists over whether carcinogenic chemicals in small doses can be detoxified, or whether even a minute amount of the chemical leads to the development of cancer. If a carcinogenic chemical can be tolerated in small amounts, then a threshold dose can be assumed below which a person is not affected by the chemical. If very small doses can cause an adverse reaction, then no threshold dose exists for that chemical.

Some individuals appear to have thresholds even for chemical carcinogens. One reason for differing thresholds among individuals is physiological and genetic variation.

The threshold/no-threshold argument refers to a population threshold. If a population threshold exists, then there are doses of a carcinogenic chemical for which no cases of cancer will result, no matter how many individuals are exposed. The population threshold is defined to be the lowest of the individual thresholds of all members of the population.

Currently, it is not agreed whether population thresholds exist for carcinogens. Proponents of the no-threshold view argue that irreversible, self-replicating lesions may result from a mutation in a single cell. Those arguing against the no-threshold hypothesis cite the existence of metabolic detoxification, DNA repair, and other mechanisms that may act to overcome the effects of potential carcinogens at low doses. In addition, some carcinogens are suspected of promoting cancer by acting on transformed cells at the later stages of the carcinogenic process. Such carcinogens may not cause cancer by genetic mutation and may exhibit threshold effects. In any case, scientific evidence has not yet proven the existence or non-existence of threshold doses for carcinogens.

In the interest of protecting public health, federal agencies generally assume that there are no thresholds for cancer-causing chemicals. For example, the Environmental Protection Agency, as a matter of prudence, typically assumes that there are no thresholds in setting exposure standards for cancer-causing chemicals.

Case Study I: Dioxins and the use of epidemiological studies

Dioxins are a family of chemical compounds that have inspired considerable scientific and public controversy. Dioxins are formed as a result of several processes, including as by-products in the manufacture of 2,4,5-T, a herbicide used on crops and in the Vietnam War as a defoliant known as Agent Orange.

The controversy over the uses and health effects of dioxins, as discussed here, illustrates the challenges that scientists face in interpreting the results of epidemiological studies.

Most of what is known about dioxins is based upon studies of one particular dioxin: 2,3,7,8-tetra-chlorodibenzo-*p*-dioxin, or TCDD. As shown in animal tests, TCDD is one of the most acutely toxic man-made compounds known. However, the animal species used in these tests differed widely in their susceptibility. For example, guinea pigs proved to be 5000 times more susceptible than hamsters. The results of LD_{50} experiments on various species are shown below.

Species	LD_{50}	mg/kg body weight
Guinea pig		1
Male rat	22	
Female rat		45
Monkey	70	
Mouse	114	
Rabbit	115	
Dog		300
Bullfrog	500	
Hamster	5000	

Humans have been exposed to high concentrations of dioxin through industrial accidents and occupational exposures. Studies of exposed populations after these high dose incidents have shown an association between TCDD and acute adverse

health effects, including liver disorders, loss of appetite and weight, loss of sex drive, nerve damage, severe fatigue, and – most commonly – a severe skin condition called chloracne. All of these effects, except chloracne, diminished after exposure stopped.

Most of the controversy over TCDD relates to the presence or absence of chronic – as opposed to acute – adverse health effects in humans. Epidemiological studies have yielded ambiguous results and these results have been used to support conflicting interpretations. The first known dioxin accident occurred in Nitro, West Virginia, in 1949, when a vat contaminated with TCDD exploded. Twenty years later, according to one study, the death and cancer rates of 122 workers were no higher than normal. The highly publicized explosion at Seveso, Italy, in 1976, resulted in TCDD contamination of a large residential area; although acute adverse health effects on the population were observed, no long-term effects have yet been documented.

Factory workers, farmers and Vietnam veterans exposed to TCDD have also been studied. According to some scientists, no long-term adverse human health effects have been clearly demonstrated. However, others have argued that the weight of evidence from the epidemiological studies supports the conclusion that TCDD has adverse effects on the human immune system and causes birth defects and damage to fetuses.

Several epidemiological studies have also produced conflicting results regarding the carcinogenic effects of TCDD. Some of this uncertainty may be the result of population study groups that were too small, doses that were too low, or exposures that were too short in duration to detect adverse health effects. Some epidemiological studies attempting to link TCDD to specific cancers have been complicated by the fact that the exposed groups were exposed to mixtures of chemicals.

In 1982, the National Toxicology Program rated the evidence from carcinogenicity assays in mice as 'inadequate'. However, other federal agencies, including the Environmental Protection Agency (EPA), used results from animal tests to make a weight-of-evidence determination that TCDD is probably carcinogenic.

In vitro cell culture tests of TCDD have been less ambiguous. Researchers have demonstrated that TCDD is a potent promoter of cell transformation. Studies also suggest that it may initiate genetic damage as well. TCDD has also been shown in some studies to suppress cell-mediated immunity, suggesting that such immune effects could make exposed individuals more susceptible to cancer from other sources.

Given these uncertainties, it is clear that the debate and research on TCDD will continue. This debate was heightened by the downgrading of the risk of dioxin by the EPA in 1991. However, given that TCDD is extremely persistent in the environment, and given the suggestive evidence of its health effects, concern about TCDD and other dioxins is unlikely to diminish until the uncertainties are substantially reduced.

Appendix A: Questions to ask about risk-assessment studies

Below is a list of questions that can be asked of any risk assessment. In interpreting answers to these questions, expert help may be needed.

1   *Questions relating to the objective of the study*
- What is the nature of the problem that stimulated this study? Why was the study done? What motivated the study?
- What were the original objectives of the study? what questions or hypotheses did the study initially intend to answer? Did the objectives and/or questions change during the course of the study?
- What was the original population to which the study applied? Did this population change during the course of the study? Are the results being extrapolated to populations other than the original population?

2   *Questions relating to the design of the study*
- Was the study an experiment, an analysis of records, or other type of study?
- Was sampling involved? Is the population and sampling description available? If sampling was involved, how was the sample selected? Are there possible sources of selection bias which would make the sample atypical or non-representative? If so, what provisions were made to deal with this bias?
- If control groups or benchmarks were used, what is the nature of the control group or standard of comparison? Is the control group or standard of comparison adequate to the task and unbiased?
- Was the study original research or simply a review of existing literature?

3   *Questions relating to the methods used in the study*
- Were the methods used in analysing the data the most appropriate, effective and efficient for the purpose of the study? Were the methods applied correctly? Is a clear and detailed description of the methods available?
- Were the instruments used in the study (questionnaires, laboratory tests, testing equipment) properly designed for their purpose?
- If training of investigative staff was required (for example, interviewers or coders), were they adequately trained? Was there significant variation in the results obtained by different investigators? If so, how were these differences interpreted and handled?
- Were the methods or approaches used in the study new or novel? If new or novel, how were they validated?

4   *Questions relating to the observations*
- Are there clear definitions of the terms used to record observations, including criteria for health outcomes?
- Was the method of classification or measurement consistent for all the subjects and relevant to the objectives of the study? Are there possible biases in measurement, and, if so, what was done to deal with them?
- Are the observations reliable and reproducible?

5   *Questions relating to the presentation of findings*
- Are the study findings presented clearly, objectively and in sufficient detail to enable the reader to judge them?
- Are the findings internally consistent? Do the numbers add up properly or are there missing cases? Are the tables based on different populations? If so, why?

6   *Questions relating to the analysis*
- Are the data worthy of statistical analysis? If so, are the methods of statistical analysis appropriate to the source and nature of the data? Is the analysis correctly performed and interpreted?
- Is there sufficient analysis to determine whether 'statistical differences' exist and whether they may in fact be due to lack of comparability of the groups in sex, age distribution or other characteristics of the study population?
- Have the study results or claims been successfully repeated? Do different studies of different populations at different times show much the same results?

- Have the study results or claims been successfully tested using more than one method? Have the results or claims been re-evaluated using different measurement or statistical techniques.
- Do the study results or claims test high for statistical significance? Is the probability small that the same effect could have occurred by chance alone?
- What is the statistical strength of the study result or claim? How substantial is the strength of association? Are the claims of a strong or clear effect supported by a strong strength of association?
- Are the study results or claims specific as to health effects of the risk agent or are they general in nature?
- Can the study results or claims be explained by confounding factors or other relationships?
- What is the amount of detail in describing data and possible weaknesses in the study? What types of data are missing? How much data are missing? What variables are missing? How significant is the missing data or variables?

- What are the greatest sources of uncertainty in the results? What does the investigator feel is known well and what is not known?

7 *Questions relating to the conclusions*
- Are the conclusions clearly stated?
- Are the conclusions of the study justified by the findings and substantiated by the evidence presented? Which ones are? Which ones are not? Are the conclusions linked to the original objectives of the study?
- Are the generalizations confined to the populations from which the sample was drawn? If not, why not?
- What are the implications of the study? What action does it suggest? What additional studies are needed?
- Could this study be replicated? If not, why not?
- Has the study been peer-reviewed by qualified professionals?
- Has the study been published or accepted for publication in a scientific journal? If not, why not? If not, will it be submitted for publication in a scientific journal?

Chapter 6

Risk communication

VT Covello

Introduction

Risk communication can be defined as the exchange of information among interested parties about the nature, magnitude, significance or control of a risk. Interested parties include government agencies, corporations or industry groups, unions, the media, scientists, professional organizations, special interest groups, communities and individual citizens. Information about risks can be communicated through a variety of channels, ranging from media reports and warning labels to public meetings or hearings.

In recent years, the literature on risk communication has grown rapidly. Hundreds of articles and books have been published on the topic, most of which focus on the challenges of communicating information during crisis and non-crisis situations about risks of exposures to environmental and occupational risk agents – particularly the risks of exposure to chemicals, heavy metals, and radiation in the air, water, land and food.

Why the sudden interest in risk communication? One explanation is the increased number of hazard communication and right-to-know laws relating to exposures to environmental risk agents. Another stems from increased public fear and concern about exposures to environmental and occupational risk agents and the corresponding demand for risk information. A third explanation is the expansion of media interest in environmental and occupational risk issues, which in turn reflects greater public interest in such issues. A fourth explanation is the increasing political nature of

risk debates and the advantages that accrue to those with effective risk communication skills.

The purpose of this chapter is to review the literature on risk communication. The specific aim is to provide the reader with a general outline of the field and to relate this work to the practical needs of those with risk communication responsibilities.

Science and perception

A significant part of the risk communication literature focuses on problems and difficulties in communicating risk information effectively. These problems and difficulties revolve around issues of science and perception and can be organized into four categories: (1) characteristics and limitations of scientific data about risks; (2) characteristics and limitations of spokespersons in communicating information about risks; (3) characteristics and limitations of the media in reporting information about risks; and (4) characteristics and limitations of the public in evaluating and interpreting risk information. Each is described below.

Characteristics and limitations of scientific data about risks

One source of difficulty in communicating information about risks is the uncertainty and complexity of data on health, safety and environmental risks. Risk assessments, despite their strengths, seldom provide exact answers. Due to limitations in scientific understanding, data, models and methods, the results of most risk assessments are at best approximations. Moreover, the resources needed to resolve these uncertainties are seldom adequate to the task.

These uncertainties invariably affect communication with the public in the hostile climate that surrounds many environmental issues. For example, uncertainties in environmental risk assessments often lead to radically different estimates of risk. An important factor underlying many debates about risks are the different assessments of risk produced by government agencies, industry and public interest groups.

Characteristics and limitations of spokespersons in communicating information about risks

A central question addressed by the literature on risk communication is why some individuals and organizations are trusted as credible sources of risk information and others are not. For example, numerous studies have found that scientists and officials in industry and government – two of the most prominent sources of risk information – often lack trust and credibility. These same studies have found that public distrust of government and industry is grounded in several beliefs: that they have been insensitive to public concerns and fears about environmental and occupational risks, unwilling to acknowledge problems, unwilling to share information, unwilling to allow meaningful public participation, and negligent in fulfilling their responsibilities to protect the health and safety of workers and the public. Compounding the problem are beliefs that environmental laws are too weak and that government and industry have done a poor job in protecting the environment.

Several factors compound these perceptions and problems. First, many scientists and officials have engaged in highly visible debates and disagreements about the reliability, validity and meaning of the results of environmental and occupational health risk assessments. In many cases, equally prominent experts have taken diametrically opposed positions on issues as diverse as the safety of nuclear power plants, hazardous waste sites,

asbestos, electric and magnetic fields, lead, radon, PCBs, arsenic and dioxin. While such debates can be constructive for the development of scientific knowledge, they often undermine public trust and confidence.

Secondly, resources for risk assessment and management are seldom adequate to meet demands by citizens and public interest groups for definitive findings and rapid action. Explanations by scientists and officials that the generation of valid and reliable toxicological or epidemiological data is expensive and time consuming – or that risk assessment and management activities are constrained by resource, technical, statutory, legal, or other limitations – are seldom perceived to be satisfactory. Individuals facing what they believe is a new and significant risk are especially reluctant to accept such claims.

Thirdly, coordination among responsible authorities is seldom adequate. In many debates about risks, for example, lack of coordination has severely undermined public faith and confidence. Compounding such problems is the lack of consistency in approaches to risk assessment and management by authorities at the local, regional, national and international levels. For example, few requirements exist for regulatory agencies to develop coherent, coordinated, consistent and interrelated plans, programmes and guidelines for managing risks. As a result, regulatory systems tend to be highly fragmented. This fragmentation often leads to jurisdictional conflicts about which agency and which level of government has the ultimate responsibility for assessing and managing a particular risk. Lack of coordination, different mandates and confusion about responsibility and authority also lead, in many cases, to the production of multiple and competing estimates of risk. A commonly observed result of such confusion is the erosion of public trust, confidence and acceptance.

Fourthly, many scientists and officials lack the skills needed to communicate effectively information about risk. For example, many scientists and officials use complex and difficult technical language and jargon in communicating information about risks to the media and the public. The use of technical language or jargon is not only difficult to comprehend but can also create a perception that the official or expert is being unresponsive, dishonest or evasive.

Finally, scientists and officials have often been insensitive to the information needs of the public and the differences between expert and lay perceptions of risk. Scientists and officials often operate on the assumption that they and their audience share a common framework for evaluating and interpreting risk information. However, this is often not the case. One of the most important findings to emerge from risk perception and communication studies is that people take into consideration a complex array of qualitative and quantitative factors in defining, evaluating and acting on risk information.

One of the costs of this heritage of mistrust and loss of confidence is the public's reluctance to believe risk information provided by government and industry. Programmes for overcoming this distrust have focused on improvements in risk assessment, risk management and risk communication. In the risk communication arena, two areas have received the greatest attention: (1) skills enhancement, and (2) credibility enhancement.

Skills enhancement is based on three fundamental risk communication principles: that perceptions are realities; that the primary goal of risk communication is to establish trust and credibility; and that risk communication is a skill (*Table 6.1*). The verbal and non-verbal skills listed in *Tables 6.2* and *6.3* represent a sampling of the practical tools and techniques identified in the applied risk communication literature.

Credibility enhancement is based on research indicating that trust and credibility are built on a foundation of perceived caring and empathy; perceived competence and expertise; perceived honesty and openness; and perceived dedication and commitment (*Table 6.4*). Activities that enhance credibility include outreach efforts aimed at improving coordination and collaboration with organizations and individuals perceived to be credible. Surveys indicate that organizations and

individuals perceived to be relatively high to medium in credibility on environmental and occupational risk issues include health and safety professionals, educators, scientific organizations, professional organizations, the media, non-management employees, non-profit voluntary health organizations, environmental groups, and citizen or employee advisory groups (*Table 6.5*).

Characteristics and limitations of the media in reporting information about risks

The mass media play a critical role in transmitting risk information. Given this importance, researchers have focused their attention on the role of the mass media and on characteristics and limitations

Table 6.1   Key formulae underlying effective risk communication

$P = R$

[Perceptions (P) equal realities (R): what is perceived as real will be real in its consequences]

$G = T + C$

[The primary goal (G) of risk communication is to establish high levels of trust (T) and credibility (C); the secondary goal is to convey facts and figures]

$C = S$

[Effective risk communication (C) is a complex skill (S): as with any complex skill, it requires significant amounts of knowledge, training and practice]

Table 6.2   Verbal risk communication skills

Jargon. Avoid jargon; define all technical terms

Organizational identity. Use personal pronouns; avoid using the organization's name

Attacks. Attack issues; avoid attacking those with higher credibility

Humour. Avoid humour (jokes, cartoons, sarcasm, etc.)

Risk/benefit comparisons. Discuss risks and benefits in separate communications

Risk comparisons. Use risk comparisons for perspective; not acceptability

Negative allegations. Don't repeat negative allegations

Speculation. Don't speculate about worst cases or 'what if' situations

Key messages. Stress performance, trend lines and achievements

Technical details and debates. Avoid providing excessive amounts of technical detail

Quantitative health risk numbers. Avoid risk statements stated as quantitative probabilities

Guarantees. Talk about achievements, not about the lack of guarantees

Zero risk. Emphasize the value of zero risk as a goal

Comparisons with others. Avoid comparing your organization with other organizations

Length of answers to questions. Limit answers to 2 minutes or less

Length of presentations. Limit presentations to 15–20 minutes or less

Visuals. Use visuals and graphics as much as possible

Abstractions. Use examples, analogies and stories to establish meaning

Testing. Test and practise all answers and presentations

Table 6.3 Non-verbal risk communication skills

Poor eye contact. Messages: dishonest, closed, unconcerned, nervous

Excellent eye contact. Messages: honest, open, competent, sincere, dedicated, confident, knowledgeable, interested

Frequent blinking. Messages: nervous, deceitful, inattentive

Sitting back in chair. Messages: uninterested, unenthusiastic, unconcerned, uncooperative

Sitting forward in chair. Messages: interested, enthusiastic, concerned, cooperative

Arms crossed on chest. Messages: uninterested, unconcerned, defiant, not listening, arrogant, impatient, defensive, stubborn

Frequent hand-to-face contact. Messages: dishonest, deceitful, nervous

Hidden hands. Messages: deceptive, guilty, insincere

Open hands. Messages: open, sincere

Speaking from behind barriers. Messages: dishonest, deceitful, formality, unconcerned, uninterested, superior

Speaking from an elevated position. Messages: superiority, dominance, judgemental

Clenched hands. Messages: anger, hostility, determination, uncooperative

Table 6.4 Indicators of trust and credibility

Perceived caring/empathy (50%) – e.g. perceived sincerity, ability to listen, ability to see issues from the perspective of the other

Perceived competence/expertise (15–20%) – e.g. perceived intelligence, training, authoritativeness, experience, educational level, and professional attainment, knowledge, command of information

Perceived openness/honesty (15–20%) – e.g. perceived truthfulness, candidness, justness, objectivity, sincerity, disinterestedness

Perceived dedication/commitment (15–20%) – e.g. perceived altruism, diligence, self-identification, involvement, hard work

Table 6.5 Trust and credibility of sources of environmental information based on 1996 sample survey of the US population

Top third
● Local citizens that are perceived to be neutral, respected and well informed about the issue
● Health and safety professionals
● Educators (especially those from respected local schools)
● Non-profit voluntary health organizations
● Non-management employees
● Professional societies

Middle third
● Media
● Environmental groups

Bottom third
● Industry officials
● Federal government officials
● Environmental consultants from for-profit firms

Changes from previous years
Environmental groups: 10–15% loss of credibility
Media: 5–10% gain in credibility
Government and industry: 10% loss in credibility

of the media that contribute to problems in risk communication.

One of the major conclusions to emerge from risk communication research is that journalists are often biased toward stories that contain drama, conflict, expert disagreements and uncertainties. The media are especially biased toward stories that contain dramatic or sensational material, such as a minor or major accident at a chemical manufacturing facility or a nuclear power plant. Much less attention is given to daily occurrences that kill or injure far more people each year but take only one life at a time. In reporting about risks, journalists often focus on the same concerns as the public; for example, potentially catastrophic effects, lack of familiarity and understanding, involuntariness, scientific uncertainty, risks to future generations, unclear benefits, inequitable distribution of risks and benefits, and potentially irreversible effects.

Media coverage of risks is frequently deficient in that many stories contain oversimplifications, distortions and inaccuracies in reporting risk information. Media coverage is also deficient not only in what is contained in the story but in what is left out. For example, analyses of media reports on cancer risks show that these reports are often deficient in providing few statistics on general cancer rates for purposes of comparison; providing little information on common forms of cancer; not addressing known sources of public ignorance about cancer; and providing little information about detection, treatments and other protective measures.

Many of these problems stem from characteristics of the media and the constraints under which reporters work. First, most reporters work under extremely tight deadlines that limit the amount of time for research and for the pursuit of valid and reliable information. Secondly, with few exceptions, reporters do not have adequate time or space to deal with the complexities and uncertainties surrounding many risk issues. Thirdly, journalists achieve objectivity in a story by balancing opposing views. Truth in journalism is different from truth in science. In journalism, there are only different or conflicting views and claims, to be covered as fairly as possible. Fourthly, journalists are source dependent. Under the pressure of deadlines and other constraints, reporters tend to rely heavily on sources that are easily accessible and willing to speak out. Sources that are difficult to contact, hard to draw out or reluctant to provide interesting and non-qualified statements are often left out. Finally, few reporters have the scientific background or expertise needed to evaluate the complex scientific data and disagreements that surround many debates about risks. Given these limitations, effectiveness in communicating with the media about risks depends in part on understanding the constraints and needs of the media and adapting one's behaviour and information to meet these needs.

Characteristics and limitations of the public in evaluating and interpreting risk information

Much of the risk communication literature focuses on characteristics and limitations of the public in evaluating and interpreting risk information. These include: (1) inaccurate perceptions of levels of risk, (2) difficulties in understanding probabilistic information related to unfamiliar activities or technologies, (3) strong emotional responses to risk information, (4) desires and demands for scientific certainty, (5) strong beliefs and opinions that are resistant to change, (6) weak beliefs and opinions that are easily manipulated by the way information is presented, (7) ignoring or dismissing risk information because of its perceived lack of personal relevance, (8) perceiving accidents and mishaps as signals, (9) using health, environmental or occupational risks as proxies or surrogates for other concerns, and (10) distinguishing between perceptions of risk and judgements of risk acceptability. Each of these characteristics is described below.

Inaccurate perceptions of risk

People often overestimate some risks and underestimate others. For example, people tend to overestimate the risks of dramatic or sensational causes of death, such as accidents at manufactur-

ing plants or waste disposal facilities, and underestimate the risks of undramatic causes, such as asthma, emphysema and diabetes. This bias is caused in part by the tendency for risk judgements to be influenced by the memorability of past events and by the imaginability of future events. A recent disaster, intense media coverage or a vivid film can heighten the perception of risk. Conversely, risks that are not memorable, obvious, palpable, tangible or immediate tend to be underestimated.

Difficulties understanding probabilistic information related to unfamiliar activities or technologies

A variety of cognitive biases and related factors hamper people's understanding of probabilities. This difficulty, in turn, hampers discussions of risk probabilities between experts and non-experts. For example, risk experts are often confused by the public's rejection of the argument that a cancer risk from a new activity is acceptable if it is smaller than 1 in 1 million. This is especially frustrating given that a one-in-a-million risk is an extremely small number and that the background chance of cancer is approximately 1 in 4. In rejecting this argument, people respond with one or more objections. First, they personalize the risk (For example: What if that one is me or my child?). Secondly, they raise questions of trust (For example: Why should I believe you – didn't you and your colleagues do the calculations?). Thirdly, they raise concerns about cumulative risks (For example: I am already exposed to enough risks in life – why do I need one more?). Fourthly, they question whether the risks are worth the benefits (For example: Is the activity that generates the risk really worth losing one life?). Finally, they raise ethical questions (For example: Who gave government and industry the right to play God and choose who will live or die?). Exacerbating the problem is the difficulty people have understanding, appreciating and interpreting small probabilities, such as the difference between 1 chance in a 100 000 and 1 chance in 1 million.

Given these difficulties, the risk communication literature contains explicit cautions about the use of probabilistic information in explaining risk decisions. This is especially the case when there is little time available for discussion. A more effective strategy is to focus the risk communication on

(1) the degree to which activity meets health, safety or environmental standards, as set or reviewed by trusted and credible authorities; (2) the relationship between the risk of activity in question and other risks; and (3) the degree to which the risk estimate is based on worst-case or pessimistic assumptions that are biased toward public health and safety.

These same problems hamper discussions between experts and non-experts on low probability/high consequences events and 'worst case scenarios'. In many such cases, the imaginability of the worst case makes it difficult for people to distinguish between what is remotely possible and what is probable.

Strong emotional responses to risk information

Strong feelings of fear, hostility, anger, outrage, panic and helplessness are often evoked by exposure to unwanted or dreaded risks. These emotions often make it difficult to engage in rational discourse about risk in public settings. Emotions tend to be most intense when people perceive the risk to be involuntary, unfair, not under their personal control and low in benefits. More extreme emotional reactions often occur when the risk affects children, when the adverse consequences are particularly dreaded – e.g. cancer and birth defects – and when worst-case scenarios are presented.

Desires and demands for scientific certainty

People often display a marked aversion to uncertainty and use a variety of coping mechanisms to reduce the anxiety generated by uncertainty. This aversion often translates into a marked preference for statements of fact over statements of probability – the language of risk assessment. People often demand to be told exactly what *will* happen, not what *might* happen.

Strong beliefs and opinions that are resistant to change

People tend to ignore evidence that contradicts their current beliefs. Strong beliefs about risks, once formed, change very slowly and are extra-

ordinarily persistent in the face of contrary evidence. Initial beliefs about risks tend to structure the way that subsequent evidence is interpreted. New evidence – e.g. data provided by a government or industry official – appears reliable and informative only if it is consistent with the initial belief; contrary evidence is dismissed as unreliable, erroneous, irrelevant or unrepresentative.

Weak beliefs and opinions that are easily manipulated by the way information is presented

When people lack strong prior beliefs or opinions, subtle changes in the way that risks are expressed can have a major impact. To test this hypothesis, one group of researchers asked two groups of physicians to choose between two therapies – surgery or radiation. Each group received the same information but with one major difference – probabilities were expressed either in terms of dying or in terms of surviving. Even though these two numbers are the same, the difference resulted in dramatic differences in the choice of therapy. Virtually the same results were observed for other test populations.

A variety of studies have demonstrated the powerful influence of such presentation or 'framing' effects. The experimental demonstration of these effects suggests that risk communicators can, under some circumstances, easily manipulate risk perceptions.

Ignoring or dismissing risk information because of its perceived lack of personal relevance

Most risk data relate to society as a whole. These data are usually of little interest or concern to individuals, who are more likely to be concerned about risks to themselves than about risks to society.

Perceiving accidents and mishaps as signals

The significance of an accident is determined only in part by its health, safety or environmental consequences, e.g. the number of deaths or injuries that occur. Of equal if not greater importance is what the accident or mishap signifies or portends.

A major accident with many deaths and injuries, for example, may have only minor social significance (beyond that to the victims' families and friends) if it occurs as part of a familiar and well-understood system (e.g. a train wreck). However, a minor accident in an unfamiliar or poorly understood system – such as a leak at a radioactive waste disposal site – can have major social significance as a harbinger of future, possibly catastrophic events.

Using health, environmental or occupational risks as proxies or surrogates for other concerns

The specific risks that people focus on reflect their beliefs about values, social insitutions, nature and moral behaviour. Risks are exaggerated or minimized accordingly. Debates about risks often are a proxy or surrogate for debates about other, more general social, economic or political concerns. The debate about nuclear power, for example, has often been interpreted as less a debate about the specific risks of nuclear power than about other concerns, including the proliferation of nuclear weapons, the adverse effects of nuclear waste disposal, the value of large-scale technological progress and growth, and the centralization of political and economic power in the hands of a technological elite.

One conclusion that can be drawn from these observations is that risk is not an objective phenomenon perceived in the same way by all interested parties. Instead, it is a social construct with its roots deeply embedded in specific social contexts. A variety of scientific, psychological, social and cultural factors determine which risks will ultimately be selected for societal attention and concern. Scientific evidence about the magnitude of possible adverse consequences is only one of these factors.

Distinguishing between perceptions of risk and judgements of risk acceptability

Even though the level of risk is related to risk acceptability, it is not a perfect correlation. Two factors affect the way people assess risk and evaluate acceptability; these factors modify the correlation.

First, the level of risk is only one among several variables that determines acceptability (*Table 6.6*). Some of the most important variables that matter to people in evaluating and interpreting risk information are described below.

1 Catastrophic potential, i.e. people are more concerned about fatalities and injuries that are grouped in time and space (e.g. fatalities and injuries resulting from a major accidental release of toxic chemicals or radiation) than about fatalities and injuries that are scattered or random in time and space (e.g. automobile accidents).
2 Familiarity, i.e. people are more concerned about risks that are unfamiliar (e.g. leaks of chemicals or radiation from waste disposal facilities) than about risks that are familiar (e.g. household accidents).
3 Understanding, i.e. people are more concerned about activities characterized by poorly understood exposure mechanisms or processes (e.g. long-term exposure to low doses of toxic chemicals or radiation) than about activities characterized by apparently well-understood exposure mechanisms or processes (e.g. pedestrian accidents or slipping on ice).
4 Uncertainty, i.e. people are more concerned about risks that are scientifically unknown or uncertain (e.g. risks from a radioactive waste facility designed to last 20 000 years) than about risks that are relatively known to science (e.g. actuarial data on automobile accidents).
5 Controllability, i.e. people are more concerned about risks that they perceive to be not under their personal control (e.g. accidental releases of toxic chemicals or radiation from a waste disposal facility) than about risks that they perceive to be under their personal control (e.g. driving an automobile or riding a bicycle).
6 Voluntariness, i.e. people are more concerned about risks that they perceive to be involuntary (e.g. exposure to chemicals or radiation from a waste or industrial facility) than about risks that they perceive to be voluntary (e.g. smoking, sunbathing or mountain climbing).
7 Effects on children, i.e. people are more concerned about activities that put children specifically at risk (e.g. milk contaminated with radiation or toxic chemicals; pregnant women exposed to radiation or toxic chemicals) than about activities that do not put children specifically at risk (e.g. adult smoking).

Table 6.6 Factors important in risk perception and evaluation

Factor	Conditions associated with increased public concern	Conditions associated with decreased public concern
Catastrophic potential	Fatalities and injuries grouped in time and space	Fatalities and injuries scattered and random
Familiarity	Unfamiliar	Familiar
Understanding	Mechanisms or process not understood	Mechanisms or process understood
Uncertainty	Risks scientifically unknown or uncertain	Risks known to science
Controllability (personal)	Uncontrollable	Controllable
Voluntariness of exposure	Involuntary	Voluntary
Effects on children	Children specifically at risk	Children not specifically at risk
Effects manifestation	Delayed effects	Immediate effects
Effects on future generations	Risk to future generations	No risk to future generations
Victim identity	Identifiable victims	Statistical victims
Dread	Effects dreaded	Effects not dreaded
Trust in institutions	Lack of trust in responsible institutions	Trust in responsible institutions
Media attention	Much media attention	Little media attention
Accident history	Major and sometimes minor accidents	No major or minor accidents
Equity	Inequitable distribution of risks and benefits	Equitable distribution of risks and benefits
Benefits	Unclear benefits	Clear benefits
Reversibility	Effects irreversible	Effects reversible
Personal stake	Individual personally at risk	Individual not personally at risk
Origin	Caused by human actions or failures	Caused by acts of nature or God

8 Effects manifestation, i.e. people are more concerned about risks that have delayed effects (e.g. the development of cancer after exposure to low doses of chemicals or radiation) than about risks that have immediate effects (e.g. poisonings).

9 Effects on future generations, i.e. people are more concerned about activities that pose risks to future generations (e.g. genetic effects due to exposure to toxic chemicals or radiation) than to risks that pose no special risks to future generations (e.g. skiing accidents).

10 Victim identity, i.e. people are more concerned about risks to identifiable victims (e.g. a worker exposed to high levels of toxic chemicals or radiation) than about risks to statistical victims (e.g. statistical profiles of automobile accident victims).

11 Dread, i.e. people are more concerned about risks that are dreaded and evoke a response of fear, terror or anxiety (e.g. exposure to radiation or carcinogens) than to risks that are not especially dreaded and do not evoke a special response of fear, terror or anxiety (e.g. common colds and household accidents).

12 Trust in institutions, e.g. people are more concerned about situations where the responsible risk management institution is perceived to lack trust and credibility (e.g. lack of trust in certain government agencies for their perceived close ties to industry) than they are about situations where the responsible risk management institution is perceived to be trustworthy and credible (e.g. trust in the management of recombinant DNA risks by universities and by the National Institutes of Health).

13 Media attention, i.e. people are more concerned about risks that receive much media attention (e.g. accidents, leaks and other problems at waste disposal facilities) than about risks that receive little media attention (e.g. on-the-job accidents).

14 Accident history, i.e. people are more concerned about activities that have a history of major and sometimes minor accidents (e.g. leaks at waste disposal facilities) than about activities that have little or no history of

major or minor accidents (e.g. recombinant DNA experimentation).

15 Equity and fairness, i.e. people are more concerned about activities that are characterized by a perceived inequitable or unfair distribution of risks and benefits (e.g. inequities related to the siting of waste disposal facilities) than about activities characterized by a perceived equitable or fair distribution or risks and benefits (e.g. vaccination).

16 Benefits, i.e. people are more concerned about hazardous activities that are perceived to have unclear, questionable or diffused benefits (e.g. waste disposal facilities) than about hazardous activities that are perceived to have clear benefits (automobile driving).

17 Reversibility, i.e. people are more concerned about activities characterized by potentially irreversible adverse effects (e.g. nuclear war) than about activities characterized by reversible adverse effects (e.g. injuries from sports or household accidents).

18 Personal stake, i.e. people are more concerned about activities that they believe place them (or their families) personally and directly at risk (e.g. living near a waste disposal site) than about activities that do not place them (or their families) personally and directly at risk (e.g. disposal of hazardous waste in remote sites or in other nations).

19 Nature of evidence, i.e. people are more concerned about risks that are based on evidence from human studies (e.g. risk assessments based on adequate epidemiological data) than about risks based on animal studies (e.g. laboratory studies of the effects of radiation using animals).

20 Human vs. natural origin, i.e. people are more concerned about risks caused by human actions and failures (e.g. accidents at waste disposal sites caused by negligence, inadequate safeguards or operator error) than about risks caused by acts of nature or God (e.g. exposure to geological radon or cosmic rays).

These factors explain, in large part, the aversion of parts of the public toward activities and technologies such as nuclear power. They also help to explain phenomena such as the 'not in my back yard' (NIMBY) response to chemical, nuclear and related facilities. For example, many residents in communities where unwanted industrial facilities exist or are planned believe that government and industry officials: (1) have excluded them from meaningful participation in the decision-making process; (2) have denied them the resources needed to evaluate or monitor independently the associated health, safety or environmental risks; (3) have denied them the opportunity to give their 'informed consent' to management decisions that affect their lives and property; (4) have imposed or want to impose upon them facilities that provide few local economic benefits; (5) have imposed or want to impose upon them facilities that entail high costs to the community (e.g. adverse impacts on health, safety, wildlife, recreation, tourism, property values, traffic, noise, visual aesthetics, community image and quality of life); (6) have imposed or want to impose on them facilities that provide most of the benefits to other parties or to society as a whole; and (7) have dismissed their opinions, fears and concerns as irrational and irrelevant.

Critical to resolving NIMBY and related risk controversies is recognition that a fairly distributed risk is more acceptable than an unfairly distributed one. A risk entailing significant benefits to the parties at risk is more acceptable than a risk with no such benefits. A risk for which there are no alternatives is more acceptable than a risk that could be eliminated by using an alternative technology. A risk that the parties at risk have control over is more acceptable than a risk that is beyond their control. A risk that the parties at risk assess and decide voluntarily to accept is more acceptable than a risk that is imposed on them. These statements are true in exactly the same sense in which it is true that a small risk is more acceptable than a large risk. Risk is multidimensional; size is only one of the relevant dimensions.

If the validity of these points is accepted, then a whole range of risk communication and management options present themselves. Because factors such as fairness, familiarity and voluntariness are as relevant as size in judging the acceptability of a risk, efforts to make a risk fairer, more familiar and more voluntary are as appropriate as efforts to make the risk smaller. Similarly, because control is important in determining the acceptability of a risk, efforts to share power, such as establishing and assisting advisory committees or supporting third-party research, audits, inspections and monitoring, can be effective in making a risk more acceptable.

Secondly, deciding what level of risk ought to be acceptable is not a technical question but a value question. People vary in how they assess risk acceptability. They weigh the various factors according to their own values, sense of risk and stake in the outcome. Because acceptability is a matter of values and opinions, and because values and opinions differ, debates about risk are often debates about values, accountability and control.

Risk comparisons

A significant part of the risk communication literature focuses on risk comparisons. Interest in risk comparisons derives in part from the perceived difficulties in communicating complex, quantitative risk information to laypersons and the need to put risk information in perspective. Several authors have argued that comparisons provide this perspective.

In a typical risk comparison, the risk in question is compared with the risks of other substances or activities. Because comparisons are perceived to be more intuitively meaningful than absolute probabilities, it is widely believed that they can be used effectively for communicating risk information. A basic assumption of the approach is that risk comparisons provide a conceptual yardstick for measuring the relative size of a risk, especially when the risk is new and unfamiliar.

Risk comparisons have several strengths that address important facets of this problem. They present issues in a mode that appears compatible with intuitive, natural thought processes, such as the use of analogies to improve understanding; they avoid the difficult and controversial task of converting diverse risks into a common unit, such as dollars per life lost or per day of pain and suffering; and they avoid direct numerical reference to small probabilities, which can be difficult to comprehend and evaluate in the abstract.

Many risk comparisons are advanced not only for gaining perspective and understanding, but also for setting priorities and determining which risks are acceptable. More specifically, risk comparisons have been advocated as a means for determining which risks to ignore, which risks to be concerned about, and how much risk reduction to seek. A common argument in many risk comparisons, for example, is that risks that are small or comparable to already accepted risks should themselves be accepted.

The risk comparison literature contains two basic types of risk comparisons: (1) comparisons of the risks of diverse activities; and (2) comparisons of the risks of similar or related activities. Each type is described below.

Comparisons of the risks of diverse substances, activities and technologies

The basic strategy in this type of comparison is to compare – along a common scale or metric – the risk of a new or existing substance, activity or technology to the risks of a diverse set of substances, activities or technologies. For example, the health risks of new pesticide might be compared to the risks of sunbathing, smoking and driving. An underlying but untested assumption is that the health risks of the new or existing substance, activity or technology can be more easily appreciated by people if placed in comparative perspective.

Approaches

A variety of different scales have been used by researchers for comparing risks, including scales based on the annual probability of death, the risk per hour of exposure, and the overall loss in life expectancy. Data for constructing such scales are typically drawn from diverse sources, including public health and accident data collected by various government agencies.

One of the most commonly used scales for comparing risks is the annual death rate. Using such a measure, it can be shown, for example, that citizens in the USA face, on average, a 2 in 1000 risk of dying from cancer, a 5 in 10 000 risk of dying in an accident, a 2.5 in 10 000 risk of dying in a motor vehicle accident, a 1 in 10 000 risk of being murdered, and a 5 in 10 million risk of being killed by a lightning bolt. These risks can be contrasted with other risks. For example, the average smoker faces a 3 in 1000 risk of dying each year from smoking, the average mountain climber faces a 6 in 10 000 risk of being killed in a climbing accident, and the average hang glider faces a 4 in 10 000 annual risk of being killed in a hang gliding accident. On an annual basis, the risk of smoking is substantially greater than the risk of hang gliding, mountaineering, boxing and working in a mine; somewhat greater than the risk of military service during the Vietnam era; and nearly as great as the risk of stunt flying.

One deficiency in these risk comparisons is their lack of sensitivity to age differences. For example, at age 5 the risk of dying from all causes is less than 1 in 1000; at age 40 it is about 2 in 1000; and at age 80 it is about 83 in 1000. Given the large effect that age can have on risk estimates, an alternative procedure that takes this factor into account is to calculate the expected loss in life expectancy due to various causes. Several authors have taken this approach and have shown that the risk of dying from cigarette smoking is twice as great as the risk of being a coal miner; and that the risk of dying in a motor vehicle accident is twice as great as the risk of dying in an accident at home.

Other formats for comparing risks have also been developed. For example, one format is to compare a set of activities with approximately equal risks, such as the risk of activities estimated to increase a person's chance of death (during any year) by 1 in 1 million. Using this measure, researchers have found that each of the following activities presents the same risk: smoking 1.4 cigarettes, riding 10 miles by bicycle, eating 40 tablespoons of peanut butter, drinking 30 12-ounce cans of diet soda containing saccharin, and living within 5 miles of a nuclear reactor for 50 years.

Adopting a somewhat different approach, researchers have calculated the time needed to accumulate a one-in-a-million risk of death from a variety of activities. Using this measure, it can be shown that the risk of dying in a motor vehicle accident is approximately equivalent to the risk of dying from being on police duty; and that the risk of dying from employment in trade or manufacturing is approximately equivalent to the risk of dying from a fall.

Many of the risk comparisons described above have been advanced not only for gaining perspective and understanding but also for setting priorities and determining which risks are acceptable. More specifically, they have been advocated as a means for determining which risks to ignore, which risks to be concerned about, and how much risk reduction to seek.

Based on such arguments, researchers have constructed scales ranking risks from acceptable to unacceptable. In one such study, activities falling in the upper zone, representing risks of death per year of exposure of less than 1 in 1 million, were deemed acceptable. The basic argument was that the risks of these activities were insignificant – insignificance being defined as the level of risk

that individuals routinely accept in their personal and daily activities. For example, since individuals routinely accept the risk of being struck by lightning – which poses a risk of death of 1 in 1 million per year of exposure – risks of this size can be regarded as acceptable. Following the same logic, it was argued that activities representing risks of death that are greater than 1 in 1000 per year of exposure can be regarded as unacceptable. Activities falling in the middle zone of the scale were identified as the most problematic: the acceptability of these could not be determined *a priori*. Instead, they must be closely scrutinized and subjected to analysis and societal debate.

Numerous authors have criticized studies that use this type of approach for determining which risks are acceptable. The basic criticism is that such efforts fail to recognize the importance and legitimacy of basing decisions about the acceptability of a risk on factors other than the size of the risk.

Comparisons of the risks of similar or related substances, activities or technologies

Some researchers have adopted a narrower approach to risk comparison, limiting their comparisons to risks that are similar or closely related. Several examples are described below.

Foods, food products and food additives

To gain perceptive and improved understanding, a large number of studies have compared the risks posed by different foods, food products and food additives. One of the best known comparative analyses of the risks of different foods and food products are the studies on food risks, diet and cancer by Professor Bruce Ames and his colleagues at the University of California, Berkeley. These studies compared the cancer risks of foods that contain synthetic chemicals (e.g. food additives and pesticide residues) with the risks of natural foods. An important conclusion is that synthetic chemicals represent only a very small fraction of the total carcinogens in foods. The basic argument underlying this conclusion is that natural foods are not benign. Large numbers of potent carcinogens (e.g. aflatoxin in peanuts) and other toxins are present in foods that contain no synthetic chemicals. Many of these natural carcinogens are produced by plants as part of their natural defence mechanisms. Analysis shows that human dietary intake of these natural carcinogens in food is likely to be at least 10 000 times greater than the intake of potentially carcinogenic synthetic chemicals in food (although partial protection against the effects of natural carcinogens is provided by the many natural anti-carcinogens that also appear in food).

Some of Ames's critics have argued that his risk estimates are inflated. The same critics have argued against an implicit, and sometimes explicit, risk comparison argument that natural carcinogens in foods deserve greater societal and regulatory attention and concern than synthetic chemicals.

Energy production technologies

In the last two decades, a large number of studies have attempted to compare the risks of alternative energy production technologies. Perhaps the best known comparison of risks from alternative energy production technologies was an analysis conducted by Dr Herbert Inhaber for the Atomic Energy Control Board of Canada. The study compared the total occupational and public health risks of different energy sources for the complete energy production cycle – from the extraction of raw materials to energy end-use. The study examined the risks of 11 methods of generating electricity – coal, oil, nuclear, natural gas, hydroelectricity, wind, methanol, solar space heating, solar thermal, solar photovoltaic and ocean thermal. Two types of risk data were analysed: (1) data on public health risks from industrial sources or pollutant effects, and (2) data on occupational risks derived from statistics on injury, death and disease rates for workers. Total risk for the energy source was calculated by summing the risks for the seven components of complete energy production cycle: (a) materials acquisition and construction, (b) emissions from materials acquisition and energy production, (c) operation and maintenance, (d) energy back-up system, (e) energy storage system, (f) transportation, and (g) waste management.

The report concluded (a) that most of the risk from coal and oil energy sources is due to toxic air emissions arising from energy production, operation and maintenance; (b) that most of the risk from natural gas and ocean thermal energy sources is due to materials acquisition; (c) that most of the risk from nuclear energy sources is due to materials acquisitions and waste disposal; and (d) that most of the risk from wind, solar thermal and solar photovoltaic energy sources is due to the energy back-up system required (assumed to be coal). Alternative sources were compared on the basis of the calculated number of man-days that would be lost per megawatt year of electricity produced.

The most controversial aspect of the report was the conclusion that nuclear power carries only slightly greater risk than natural gas and less risk than all other energy technologies considered. Inhaber reported, for example, that coal has a 50-fold larger mortality rate than nuclear power. The report also argued (a) that, contrary to popular opinion, non-conventional energy sources, such as solar power and wind, pose substantial risks; and (b) that the risks of nuclear power are significantly lower than those of non-conventional energy sources. The relatively high risk levels associated with non-conventional energy sources were traced by Inhaber, in part, to the large volume of construction materials required for these technologies and to the risks associated with energy back-up systems and energy storage systems.

Following publication of the report, its methodology was severely criticized. Critics claimed (a) that the study mixed risks of different types, (b) that it used risk estimators of dubious validity, (c) that it made questionable assumptions to cover data gaps, (d) that it failed to consider future technological developments, (e) that it made arithmetic errors, (f) that it double-counted labour and back-up energy requirements, and (g) that it introduced arbitrary correction factors. Perhaps the most damaging criticism was that the study was inconsistent in applying its methodology to the various energy technologies. For example, while the study considered materials acquisition, component fabrication and plant construction in the analysis of unconventional energy sources and of hydropower, critics have claimed that the study did not follow the same approach for coal, nuclear power, oil and gas. Furthermore, the labour figures for coal, oil, gas and nuclear power included only on-site construction, while those for the renewable energy sources included on-site construction, materials acquisition and component manufacture.

Despite these criticisms, Inhaber's study represented a landmark effort in the literature on risk comparisons. It made a significant conceptual contribution by attempting to compare, in a systematic and rigorous way, the risks of alternative technologies intended to serve the same purpose. Also important were Inhaber's observations (a) that risks occur at each stage in product development (e.g. raw material extraction, manufacturing, use and disposal), and (b) that risks from each stage need to be added together to obtain an accurate estimate of the total risk.

Cancer

A variety of studies have used risk comparisons to put cancer risks in perspective. In perhaps the best known such study, Sir Richard Doll and his colleagues analysed data for a variety of causes of cancer, including industrial products, pollution, food additives, tobacco, alcohol and diet. Results of the study provided an important comparative perspective on cancer risks. The study found, for example, that the combined effect of food additives, occupational exposures to toxic agents, air and water pollution and industrial products account for only about 7% of US cancer deaths. These results suggest that removing all pollutants and additives in the air, water, food and workplace would result in only a small decrease in cancer mortality (although even this small percentage represents a substantial number of lives). By contrast, the combined effects of alcohol, diet and smoking are related to 70% of US cancer deaths. Consequently, even a modest change in personal habits would result in a significant decrease in cancer mortality.

Other authors have adopted a different approach for comparing the risks of cancer. For example, researchers have compared data on the annual risks of cancer from various common or everyday activities. Smoking clearly poses the largest risk of cancer, with an annual risk of 1.2 in 1000. Drinking 1 beer per day, receiving an average number of diagnostic X-rays and background radiation at sea level all pose about the same annual risk of cancer – 2 in 100 000.

Other types of comparisons

A large number of other studies have also compared the risks of similar or diverse activities and technologies. Because of their policy significance, two types of risk comparisons have received special attention in the risk communication literature: (1) comparisons of different occupations or indus-

tries; and (b) comparisons of different sources of radiation. In the occupational arena, one study found that the annual job-related risk of death experienced by timber workers, miners and pilots – the most risky occupations – is several orders of magnitude greater than for school teachers, dentists and librarians – among the least risky occupations. Occupational risks of death range from 1 chance in 1000 per year to 1 chance in 1 million per year. In the radiation field, one study compared different sources of radiation exposure (e.g. natural, medical and occupational) and found that the single largest source of radiation exposure is radon emanating from the ground or construction materials and accumulating in closed buildings. Such a finding is, of course, only as useful as it is accurate. Only a few years ago, diagnostic X-rays were identified as the largest source of radiation exposure. Radon was not even listed in most tables as a source of radiation exposure.

One of the most ambitious attempts to compare risks was a 1987 study by the EPA, entitled *Unfinished Business: A Comparative Assessment of Environmental Problems*. A critical part of the study is a comparative ranking of 31 health and environmental risks. The ranking was performed by EPA experts and covered nearly every environmental problem addressed by EPA programmes, including air pollution, water pollution and hazardous waste. Risks were ranked in four major categories: cancer effects; non-cancer causing human health effects; ecological effects; and welfare effects (e.g. damage to materials). Factors not included in ranking environmental problems were benefits to society; qualitative aspects, such as whether the risk is voluntary or equitable; and economic or technical controllability.

An important finding of the study was that the EPA's ranking of health and environmental risks did not correlate well with the public's ranking of health and environmental risks. For example, risks associated with hazardous waste sites were in the middle of the EPA ranking for cancer effects and at the lower end of the EPA ranking for non-cancer-causing health effects. By comparison, risks associated with hazardous waste sites were at the top of the public's rankings. Risks associated with radon were at the top of EPA's ranking, while the same risks were ranked at the bottom of the public's ranking. The report notes that the EPA risk rankings also do not correspond well with the agency's programme priorities. Agency priorities appear to be more closely aligned with public opinion than with estimated risks.

Another type of comparison that attempts to put risk information in perspective are 'concentration' comparisons. In such comparisons, the concentration of a toxic substance in the environment is compared to other measurement units such as length or time (*Table 6.7*). For example, 1 part per billion of a toxic chemical in drinking water is equivalent to 1 inch (25 mm) in 16 000 miles (26 000 km) and 1 second in 32 years. Although some insight is provided by such comparisons, the data often lack relevance and meaning unless coupled with data on the toxic potency of a particular chemical.

In addition to these comparisons, several studies have attempted to compare the costs of different risk reduction programmes. For example, one study compared the cost per fatality averted implied by various activities aimed at reducing risks. Researchers have also compared the cost per year of life saved of different various investments, and the cost per life saved of various risk-reduction regulations.

One general conclusion from these studies is that different health, safety and environmental programmes and investments vary enormously in their costs per lives saved. Disproportionate amounts of money are spent to reduce risks in some areas, while other areas are relatively neglected. One study found, for instance, that the cost-per-fatality-averted for different risk reduction programmes ranges between $10 000 and $1 billion; another study found that the cost-per-life-saved for various health investments ranges between $540 and $6.6 million per year; and a third study showed that the cost-per-life-saved of various proposed, rejected and final regulations ranges between $100 000 and $72 billion (for final regulations only, the range is $100 000 to $132 million, with an average and median of $23 million and $2 million, respectively).

Limitations of risk comparisons

As indicated in the examples cited above, critics have noted significant limitations of the risk comparison approach. The most important are (1) failing to identify and emphasize uncertainties involved in the calculation of comparative risk estimates; (2) failing to consider the broad set of quantitative dimensions that define and measure risk; and (3) failing to consider the broad set of qualitative dimensions that underlie people's concerns about the acceptability of risks and technologies. Each is described below.

Table 6.7 **Some US examples of concentration comparisons organized by unit categories**

Unit	*1 part per million*	*1 part per billion*	*1 part per trillion*
Length	1 in./16 miles	1 in./16 000 miles	1 in./16 000 000 miles (a 6-in. leap on a journey to the sun)
Time	1 min/2 years	1 sec/32 years	1 sec/320 centuries (or 0.06 sec since the birth of Jesus Christ)
Money	1 cent/$10 000	1 cent/$10 000 000	1 cent/$10 000 000 000
Weight	1 oz/31 tons	1 pinch salt/10 tons of potato chips	1 pinch salt/10 000 tons of potato chips
Volume	1 drop vermouth/80 'fifths' of gin	1 drop vermouth/500 barrels of gin	1 drop of vermouth in a pool of gin covering the area of a football field 43 ft deep
Area	1 ft^2/23 acres	1 in./160-acre farm	1 ft^2/the state of Indiana; or 1 large grain of sand on the surface of Daytona Beach
Action	1 lob/1200 tennis matches	1 lob/1 200 000 tennis matches	1 lob/1 200 000 000 tennis matches
Quality	1 bad apple/2000 barrels	1 bad apple/2 000 000 barrels	1 bad apple/2 000 000 000 barrels

Failing to identify and emphasize uncertainties involved in the calculation of comparative risk estimates

A critical flaw in many risk comparisons is the failure to provide information on the assumptions underlying the calculation of comparative risk estimates. Since risk estimates are typically drawn from a variety of different data sources, tables of comparative risks may contain risk estimates based on one set of assumptions, together with non-comparable estimates based on another set of assumptions. Similarly, tables of comparative risks may contain risk estimates based on actuarial statistics (e.g. deaths from motor vehicle accidents) together with estimates based on controversial models, assumptions and judgements (cancer deaths from chronic exposure to pesticides or air pollutants).

A related flaw in many risk comparisons is the failure to describe and characterize uncertainties. This flaw can seriously undermine the value and potential usefulness of risk comparisons for risk communication purposes. Tables of risks that report only single values for adverse health, safety or environmental consequences, for example, ignore the range of possibilities and may provide an inaccurate picture of the risk problem to the public. Given the various biases, errors and other sources of uncertainty that can undermine the validity and reliability of a risk assessment, it is critical that tables of comparative risks provide the fullest possible information on potential errors and inaccuracies in each computed risk value – including qualifiers, ranges of uncertainty, confidence intervals and standard errors. To date, it is more the exception than the rule for results of comparative risk studies to be presented with full disclosure of the strengths and limitations of the assessment and with full disclosure of the degree to which assessment results are based on controversial data and judgements. Risk comparisons that do not include such information can produce a false sense of certainty.

Failing to consider the broad set of quantitative dimensions that define and measure risk

Most lists of comparative risks are unidimensional. They present statistics for only one dimension of risk, such as expected annual mortality rates or reductions in life expectancy. The use of such narrow quantitative measures of risk can, however, obscure the importance of other significant quantitative dimensions, such as expected annual probability of injury or disability, spatial extent, concentration, persistence, recurrence, population at risk, delay, maximum expected fatalities, transgenerational effects, expected environmental damage (e.g. ecological damage or adverse effects on endangered species), and maximum expected environmental damage.

Significant distortions and misunderstandings also result from comparative analyses that fail to provide the full range of relevant quantitative risk information. Consider some of the problems involved in comparing the risks of aircraft travel to the risks of travelling by automobile or train. Using a measure of risk to an individual based on the number of deaths per hundred million passenger miles, travelling as an aircraft passenger appears to pose slightly less risk to an individual (0.38 deaths per hundred million passenger miles) than being an automobile passenger (0.55 deaths per hundred million passenger miles); and slightly more risk than travelling as a train passenger (0.23 deaths per hundred million passenger miles). However, for aircraft travel, the landing and take-off phase represents the period of highest risk; thus it can be argued that a better estimate of individual risk is the number of passenger journeys rather than the number of miles travelled. Using this measure, travelling as an aircraft passenger (1.8 deaths per million passenger journeys) poses slightly greater risk than travelling as an automobile passenger (0.027 deaths per million passenger journeys) or as a train passenger (0.59 deaths per million passenger journeys). As a result, if distance travelled is the selected measurement criterion, then aircraft travel is marginally safer than automobile travel and marginally less safe than train travel; but if number of journeys is the selected measurement criterion, then aircraft travel is marginally less safe than both automobile travel and train travel.

A related deficiency is the failure in most risk comparisons to estimate the total quantitative risk of technologies and activities included in the risk comparison. Technological activities encompass a variety of different components; stages of development (e.g. extraction of raw materials, production, consumption and disposal); and relationships (direct and indirect) with other technological and societal activities. Detailed examination of the risks of these different components, stages of development and relationships may significantly alter the overall ranking of a technology or activity. Consequently, any risk comparison that claims to be comprehensive must either present risk data for each of these aspects, or explicitly acknowledge those aspects of the analysis that have been excluded.

Even when the analyst provides data on the total quantitative risk of an activity or technology, the comparison can nevertheless be misleading if it fails to provide risk data for sensitive, susceptible or high-risk groups. These include children, pregnant women, the elderly, and individuals who are particularly vulnerable or susceptible because of illness or disease. Most lists of comparative risks present population averages. However, population averages often mask important subpopulation variations in susceptibility.

Important distinctions also can be masked in other ways. For example, it is not always clear from risk comparison tables what is included in the specific risk entries. For example, do deaths from smoking include cardiovascular disease and emphysema as well as lung cancers? Are the risk estimates based on the entire population or only the population that is exposed?

Even if the analyst carefully and accurately reports risk data, misunderstandings can develop if important situational qualifiers are left out. For example, the risk calculation for driving includes many different driving situations. Yet speeding home from a party just before dawn is two orders of magnitude more dangerous than driving to the supermarket. Similarly, the risk of being hit by lightning for people who remain on a golf course during a thunderstorm is much higher than the average risk for the US population.

A related deficiency stems from the failure to recognize the importance of framing effects on risk comparisons. Different impressions are created by different presentation formats. Each format for presenting or expressing risk information, such as deaths per million people, deaths per unit of concentration or deaths per activity, is likely to have a different impact on the audience. Context can be equally important. For example, an individual lifetime risk of 1 in 1 million in the US is mathematically equivalent to approximately 0.008 deaths per day, 3 deaths per year or 200 deaths over a 70-year lifetime. Many people will view the first two numbers as small and insignificant, whereas the latter two statistics are likely to be perceived as sufficiently large to warrant societal or regulatory attention.

A final deficiency is the failure in most risk comparisons to acknowledge deficiencies in the quality of the data. Most risk comparisons draw on diverse data sources that vary considerably in quality. Because of the high cost and difficulty of collecting original data, researchers seldom have access to data developed exclusively for the comparison. Instead, a variety of existing data sources are used, each varying in quality. As a result, comparative risks often contain data of high quality together with data of questionable scientific validity and reliability.

Failing to consider the broad set of qualitative dimensions that underlie people's concerns about the acceptability of risks and technologies

Risk comparison is often advocated as a means for setting priorities or for determining which risks are acceptable. A common argument is that risks that are small, or that are comparable to risks that are already being accepted, should themselves be accepted. A number of critics have argued, however, that such claims cannot be defended. Although carefully prepared lists of comparative risk statistics can provide insight and perspective, they provide only a small part of the information needed for setting priorities or for determining which risks are acceptable.

Judgements of acceptability are related not only to annual mortality rates – the focus of most risk comparisons – but also to a multiplicity of qualitative dimensions or factors. These factors were discussed earlier in the section on risk perceptions and include voluntariness, controllability, fairness, effects on children, familiarity and benefits.

Because of the importance of these factors, comparisons showing that the risk of a new or existing activity or technology is higher (or lower) than the risks of other activities or technologies may have no effect on public perceptions and attitudes. For example, comparing the risk of living near a nuclear power or chemical manufacturing plant with the risk of driving x number of hours, eating x tablespoons of peanut butter, smoking x number of cigarettes a day or sunbathing x number of hours may provide perspective but may also be highly inappropriate. Since such risks differ on a variety of qualitative dimensions – e.g. perceived benefits, extent of personal control, voluntariness, catastrophic potential, familiarity, fairness, origin and scientific uncertainty – it is likely that people will perceive the comparison to be meaningless.

For example, it is often tempting for risk communicators to use the following argument during a meeting: the risk of *a* (e.g. emissions from an incinerator or facility) is lower than the risk of *b* (driving to the meeting or smoking during breaks). Since you (the audience) find *b* acceptable, you are obliged to find *a* acceptable.

This argument has a basic flaw in logic; its use can severely damage trust and credibility. Some listeners will analyse the argument this way: 'I do not have to accept the (small) added risk of living near an incinerator just because I accept the (perhaps larger, but voluntary and personally beneficial) risk of sunbathing, bicycling, smoking or driving my car. In deciding about the acceptability of risks, I consider many factors, only one of them being the size of the risk – and I prefer to do my own evaluation. Your job is not to tell me about what I should accept but to tell me about the size of the risk and what you are doing about it.'

The fundamental argument against the use of risk comparisons is that it is seldom relevant or appropriate to compare risks with different qualities for risk acceptability purposes, even if the comparison is technically accurate. Several reasons underlie the argument. First, there are important psychological and social differences among risks with different qualities. Risks that are voluntary and result from lifestyle choices, for example, are more likely to be accepted than involuntary and imposed risks.

Secondly, people recognize that risks are cumulative; that each additional risk adds to their overall risk burden. The fact that a person is exposed to risks resulting from voluntary lifestyle choices does not lessen the impact of risks that are perceived to be involuntary and imposed.

Finally, people perceive many types of risk in an absolute sense. An involuntary increased risk of cancer or birth defects is a physical and moral insult regardless of whether the increase is small or whether the increase is smaller than risks from other exposures.

Aggravating the problem is the lack of attention given in most risk comparisons to how people actually make decisions about the acceptability and tolerability of a risk. Judgements about risks are seldom separated from judgements about the risk decision process. Public responses to risk are shaped both by the characteristics of the activity or technology and by the perceived adequacy of the decision-making process. Risk comparisons play only a limited role in such determinations.

Guidelines for improving the effectiveness of risk comparisons

Despite the limitations reviewed above, researchers have found that a well-constructed and well-documented risk comparison can be useful in communicating risk information. It can, for example, provide (1) a benchmark and yardstick against which the magnitude of new or unfamiliar risks can be calibrated and compared; (2) a means for determining and communicating the relative numerical significance and seriousness of a new or existing risk; and (3) a means for informing and educating people about the range and magnitude of risks to which they are exposed.

For a risk comparison to achieve these goals and purposes, however, the limitations and deficiencies of the approach must specifically be addressed. Results from experimental studies and case studies suggest the following guidelines: (1) the risks that are compared should be as similar as possible; (2) dissimilarities between the compared risks should be identified; (3) sources of data on risk levels should be credible and should be identified; (4) limitations of the comparison should be described; (5) the comparison should have only one purpose – numerical perspective; and (6) all comparisons should be pilot tested.

In summary, the risk comparison approach can be a powerful tool in risk communication. However, the simplicity and intuitive appeal of the method is often deceptive. Many factors play a role in determining the legitimacy and effectiveness of a risk comparison. The success of the comparison as a risk communication will depend on the degree to which these factors have been adequately recognized, considered and addressed.

Conclusions

Given the passage of increasing numbers of right-to-know laws, and given increasing demands by workers and the public for risk information, risk communication will be the focus of increasing attention in years to come. The findings reported in this chapter are only a sampling of results from the emerging area of risk communication research. However, several general principles and guidelines for communicating information about risks can be extrapolated from this literature (see below). Although many of these principles and guidelines may seem obvious, they are so often violated in practice that a useful question is why are they so frequently not followed.

Principle 1. Accept and involve the public as a legitimate partner.

Discussion: Two basic tenets of risk communication in a democracy are generally understood and accepted. First, people and communities have a right to participate in decisions that affect their lives, their property and the things they value. Secondly, the goal of risk communication should not be to diffuse public concerns or avoid action. The goal should be to produce an informed public that is involved, interested, reasonable, thoughtful, solution-oriented and collaborative.

Guidelines:
- Demonstrate your respect for the public and your sincerity by involving the community early, before important decisions are made.
- Make it clear that you understand the appropriateness of basing decisions about risks on factors other than the magnitude of the risk.
- Involve all parties that have an interest or a stake in the particular risk in question.

Principle 2. Plan carefully and evaluate performance.

Discussion: Different goals, audiences and media require different risk communication strategies. Risk communication will be successful only if carefully planned.

Guidelines:
- Begin with clear, explicit objectives, such as providing information to the public, motivating individuals to act, stimulating emergency response, or contributing to conflict or dispute resolution.
- Evaluate the information you have about risks and know its strengths and weaknesses.
- Classify the different subgroups among your audience.
- Aim your communications at specific subgroups in your audience.
- Recruit spokespersons who are good at presentation and interaction.

- Train your staff – including technical staff – in communication skills and reward outstanding performance.
- Whenever possible, pretest your messages.
- Carefully evaluate your efforts and learn from your mistakes.

Principle 3. Listen to your audience.

Discussion: People in the community are often more concerned about issues such as trust, credibility, control, competence, voluntariness, fairness, caring and compassion than about mortality statistics and the details of quantitative risk assessment. If you do not listen to people, you cannot expect them to listen to you. Communication is a two-way activity.

Guidelines:
- Do not make assumptions about what people know, think or want done about risks.
- Take the time to find out what people are thinking: use techniques such as interviews, focus groups and surveys.
- Let all parties that have an interest or a stake in the issue be heard.
- Recognize people's emotions.
- Let people know that you understand what they said, addressing their concerns as well as yours.
- Recognize the 'hidden agendas', symbolic meanings and broader economic or political considerations that often underlie and complicate the task of risk communication.

Principle 4. Be honest, frank, and open.

Discussion: In communicating risk information, trust and credibility are your most precious assets. Trust and credibility are difficult to obtain. Once lost they are almost impossible to regain.

Guidelines:
- State your credentials; but do not ask or expect to be trusted by the public.
- Disclose risk information as soon as possible (emphasizing any appropriate reservations about reliability).
- Do not minimize or exaggerate the level of risk.
- Speculate only with great caution.
- If in doubt, lean toward sharing more information, not less – or people may think you are hiding something.
- Discuss data uncertainties, strengths and weaknesses – including the ones identified by other credible sources. Identify worst-

case estimates as such, and cite ranges of risk estimates when appropriate.

Principle 5. Coordinate and collaborate with other credible sources.

Discussion: Allies can be effective in helping you communicate risk information. Few things make risk communication more difficult than conflicts or public disagreements with other credible sources.
Guidelines:
- Take time to coordinate all inter-organizational and intra-organizational communications.
- Devote effort and resources to the slow, hard work of building bridges with other organizations.
- Use credible and authoritative intermediaries.
- Consult with others to determine who is best able to answer questions about risk.
- Try to issue communications jointly with other trustworthy sources such as credible university scientists, physicians, trusted local officials and opinion leaders.

Principle 6. Meet the needs of the media.

Discussion: The media are a prime transmitter of information on risks. They play a critical role in setting agendas and in determining outcomes. The media are generally more interested in politics than in risk; more interested in simplicity than in complexity; and more interested in danger than in safety.
Guidelines:
- Be open with and accessible to reporters.
- Respect their deadlines.
- Provide information tailored to the needs of each type of media, such as graphics and other visual aids for television.
- Prepare in advance and provide background material on complex risk issues.
- Follow up on stories with praise or criticism, as warranted.

- Try to establish long-term relationships of trust with specific editors and reporters.

Principle 7. Speak clearly and with compassion.

Discussion: Technical language and jargon are useful as professional shorthand. But they are barriers to successful communication with the public.
Guidelines:
- Use language appropriate to the audience.
- Use vivid, concrete images that communicate on a personal level.
- Use stories, examples and anecdotes that make technical risk data come alive.
- Avoid distant, abstract, unfeeling language about deaths, injuries and illnesses.
- Acknowledge and respond (both in words and with actions) to emotions that people express – anxiety, fear, anger, outrage, helplessness.
- Acknowledge and respond to the distinctions that the public views as important in evaluating risks.
- Use risk comparisons to help put risks in perspective; but avoid comparisons that ignore distinctions that people consider important.
- Always try to include a discussion of actions that are under way or can be taken.
- Promise only what you can do, and be sure to do what you promise.
- Never let your efforts to inform people about risks prevent you from acknowledging – and saying – that any illness, injury or death is a tragedy.

Analyses of case studies suggest that these principles and guidelines can form the basic building blocks for effective risk communication. Each principle recognizes, in a different way, that effective risk communication is an interactive process based on mutual trust, cooperation and respect among all parties. Each principle also recognizes that effective risk communication is a complex art and skill that requires substantial knowledge, training and practice.

Chapter 7

Survey design

KM Venables

Introduction: the scope of occupational epidemiology

Epidemiological surveys have an important place in occupational health and much of our present knowledge of the effects of occupational exposures on man has come from epidemiological research. Despite the relevance of epidemiology to their work, occupational physicians and hygienists are often reluctant to carry out their own surveys. This chapter aims to encourage the diffident by describing the necessary steps in planning and undertaking surveys. It concentrates on studies of morbidity, rather than mortality. The general concepts underlying epidemiological surveys are discussed in Chapter 4.

A survey may be *descriptive*, performed perhaps to aid planning about resource allocation in an occupational health service. It may be *analytical*, testing hypotheses about the relationship between occupational exposure and its effects. It may form part of the *evaluation* of a control measure which reduces exposure or aims to limit its effects. These three ways of using epidemiology are complementary and a single study may have descriptive, analytical and evaluative components. For example, describing the accident rates in different areas in a factory would give information which is useful in itself, may confirm theories about the causes of certain types of accident and also could form the first phase of an evaluation of accident prevention measures. Although even the simplest survey goes through several stages (*Figure 7.1*) they can be accomplished quickly if necessary. Few surveys are so urgent that speed takes priority over preparation and a poorly planned and executed survey could produce actively misleading results. Preparations for a study, and the analysis of results, always take longer than collecting the data, sometimes considerably longer.

Questions

The first step is the recognition of a question or questions which should be answered by an epidemiological survey. This may seem an obvious point, but occasionally surveys are proposed from a wish to 'do something' about an occupational health problem. Further thought may suggest that action, rather than research, is needed or that clinical or toxicological research would be more appropriate than epidemiology. The availability of an exposed population, set of records or series of patients may prompt the collection of data before questions have been formulated adequately. Although such opportunities should not be neglected, careful consideration of the questions to be answered can only improve a study's quality.

There is no shortage of questions to be answered by occupational epidemiology. They are constantly generated by the results of toxicological research, and by drawing analogies with the results of research in fields other than occupational health. Of greater concern is that many ideas for surveys are raised, but, like the elephant's question in *Figure 7.2*, remain only ideas and are

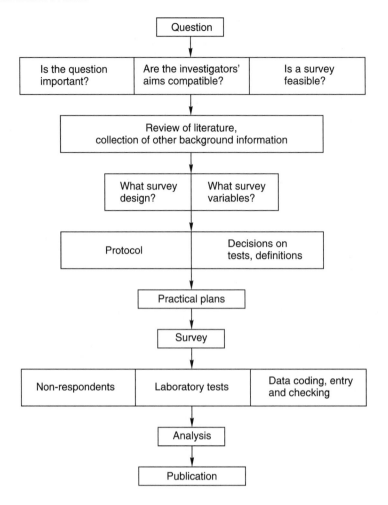

Figure 7.1 Stages in survey

never translated into practical planning and execution. The important steps in translating ideas into action are consideration of the question's importance, discussing the idea with potential collaborators and assessing the survey's feasibility.

How important is the question?

Medawar writes lucidly and wittily on scientists' thought-processes and activities and has commented that anyone '*who wants to make important discoveries must study important problems*. It is not enough that a problem should be interesting – almost any problem is interesting if it is studied

in sufficient depth' and again, 'the problem must be such that it *matters* what the answer is' [1]. Occupational medicine and hygiene are essentially problem-solving disciplines which identify and quantify problems and recommend, execute and evaluate measures to control them. It is thus often easier to follow Medawar's advice than in the fields of basic research about which he wrote.

What is the likely result of the study? Will it lead directly to action to improve workers' health, perhaps by providing information useful in setting environmental standards or in deciding an occupational health service's priorities? There may be no immediate practical result, but the survey will help in understanding the causes or natural history of disease, leading ultimately to prevention. If the

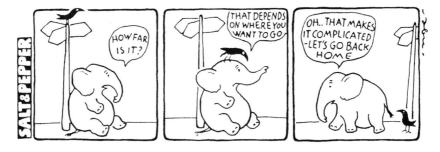

Figure 7.2 A survey in search of a question. Included by kind permission of the artist Abu Abraham (First printed in *The Guardian*, 1981, and reproduced by permission)

survey's prospects for disease prevention and improved working conditions seem remote, one must question the value of doing it. Burr [2] has made similar points about medical research in general and also commented that little is gained by confirming what everybody believes, or by refuting something which nobody believes. Research investigates issues between these two extremes, in the area of genuine doubt.

Plans for studies are sometimes made prematurely, when reviewing the literature or talking to others with similar interests would show that the questions have already been answered. Conversely, the potential investigator may find that his ideas are fresh and will make a worthwhile contribution. Sometimes 'facts', accepted as common knowledge, are revealed as untested assumptions.

Collaboration

Few surveys can be done single-handed and at least one formal meeting of all potential collaborators should be held. It is very difficult to plan surveys by telephone, letter or in casual conversation. The purposes of the meeting are clarification of the survey's aims and a decision about its feasibility. Talking to other interested persons brings more factual information and a range of perspectives to bear on the problem and always helps to refine questions. Quite disparate aims may be compatible, as long as they are positive and clearly defined. For example, a company physician who wishes to know the prevalence of a particular disease in a factory can work easily with a research department whose primary objective is, say, the validation of a new survey technique. A vague wish to 'do research' will accomplish little.

Feasibility

Discussion may reveal that, at present, the survey is not feasible. It will require access to a population of workers or to a set of records. A population cannot be assumed accessible if the views of management and unions are not known. The adequacy and completeness of records must be assessed and confirmation sought that they can be used for research purposes. A study will not be immediately feasible if it appears to require technical expertise not available to the current collaborators. The plan can be discussed further after talks with management and unions, custodians of records or with further collaborators.

To ensure the study gets done, one person must be appointed to write a protocol and be responsible for planning and, probably, analysis. He need not have initiated the survey, but must be able to devote time to the project and be sufficiently knowledgeable to take day-to-day decisions about the study. His first practical step in a survey of an occupational population is identifying one person in the company (assuming a survey at a single company) of sufficient seniority to take decisions without lengthy consultation. Such a person is invaluable even when an occupational health service performs an in-house investigation. He should liaise between the investigators and the company, ensure the survey does not disrupt production, make practical arrangements on-site, provide information about the worksite and workforce and keep the company and unions informed about progress. Frequently the personnel officer or safety officer assumes this role, but whoever does must be committed to the success of the survey and prepared to spend time on it.

Protocol

Much information is needed to perform a survey, which is collated in a protocol, or series of increasingly detailed protocols, under headings such as in *Table 7.1*. A protocol is simply a 'road map' for the survey, a written document containing the survey's aims and methods and discussing other important issues. Even simple surveys require a protocol. Its preparation clarifies ideas about the study: it acts as an *aide-mémoire* during analysis, or if planning must be halted for a time; it is circulated to collaborators and other interested parties, thus avoiding misunderstandings; and it forms the basis for a submission for funding if additional personnel or equipment are needed.

The literature pertaining to the problem must be reviewed. If the problem is well known, with a large literature, it is wise to consult experts. Reviewing the literature may lead to changes in the way questions are framed. The protocol should contain a succinct account of publication in the field, focusing on the particular questions the survey asks. The review should include the methodology proposed for measuring the variables in the study, and the current legislation may also be relevant.

Information about the process, materials handled, ventilation, other protective measures and past environmental measurements is collected. The investigators must arrange to see the process for themselves. For a population survey, a person-

nel list must be obtained of all workers to be studied. Groups such as cleaners, security, managerial, clerical and occupational health staff, and contract, part-time and night workers, are easily forgotten in preparing these lists, which must be carefully scrutinized for completeness. Meetings must be arranged with management and unions, so that queries are answered and concerns voiced. Helpful practical suggestions and information arise from these meetings.

Information about the proposed methodology should also be collected. Manufacturers of equipment may have extensive technical literature and some may keep bibliographies of publications about their equipment or supply names of other people using it.

Survey objectives

The aims, or objectives, of the survey evolve from general, broad ideas into specific aims which are achievable. For example (and hypothetically), let us assume that clinical observation suggests that chemical industry workers may be at risk of skin rashes. The question 'do chemicals cause skin rashes?' is too general. A list of likely chemicals must be drawn up and the type of skin condition defined. Let us say it is decided to focus on acetic acid and urticaria. The question 'does acetic acid cause urticaria?' is specific, but not framed in epidemiological terms. It could, for example, be answered by studying experimental animals. Epidemiology notes associations and seeks, by the design of the study and by comparison with other evidence, to establish if an association is causal. Bradford Hill [3] has discussed the features of an association which suggest causality. 'Is urticaria associated with exposure to acetic acid?' is the right phrasing for an epidemiological study but still does not suggest a specific design. 'Is the incidence rate of new cases of urticaria higher in workers exposed to acetic acid than in unexposed workers?' would be asked in a longitudinal study. 'Do persons with urticaria report exposure to acetic acid more frequently than persons without urticaria?' would be asked in a case-referent study.

Tests of statistical significance will ultimately be applied to the data. These assume a 'null hypothesis' of no association, a concept discussed in standard textbooks of statistics. Some find it helpful to phrase questions as null hypotheses. In the

Table 7.1 Headings for a protocol

General objectives
Review of the literature
Other background information
Specific objectives
Design: including sampling, controls, non-respondents
Methods: including equipment, techniques
Observations: including record forms, definitions
Analysis
Timetable
Ethical and 'political' issues
Cost

example above, assuming a cross-sectional survey, this would be 'workers exposed to acetic acid have a similar prevalence rate of urticaria to unexposed workers'.

Design

Type of study

Discussion of survey methodology starts with design and the reasons for choosing a particular study type should be stated in the protocol. Epidemiological surveys are *cross-sectional, longitudinal* or *case-referent* in design. Cross-sectional surveys measure disease prevalence, longitudinal surveys measure incidence or follow changes over time and case-referent studies compare the proportion exposed in cases and referents. The *prevalence rate* expresses the number of cases with disease as a proportion of the population studied at a defined point in time (or sometimes, over a period of time). Prevalence is an appropriate measurement for chronic diseases with no clearly defined starting point. Acute events, such as accidents or acute illnesses, are best described using the *incidence rate*, the number of new cases arising in the population over a period, with both population and time in the denominator.

One of several advantages of longitudinal studies is that they follow events from exposure prospectively. Cross-sectional and most case-referent studies have no true time dimension, although they can make retrospective enquiries of their subjects. The cross-sectional and case-referent designs have a practical advantage in that studies can be undertaken quickly, whereas longitudinal surveys, particularly morbidity surveys, may take some time to set up and carry out. Case-referent studies are carried out increasingly frequently, often to study potential associations between occupational exposures and rare diseases. Schlesselman [4] discusses this design in detail. Cross-sectional surveys may produce biased results if the disease affects 'survival' in a job. However, cross-sectional surveys are common in occupational medicine, and almost all occupational hygiene surveys are cross-sectional. Because of this, this chapter's emphasis is on cross-sectional studies, but the issues discussed are relevant to any type of survey.

Sampling and choice of referents

Other design issues are sampling and the choice of referents (controls). If the workforce is large, it may be more economical of effort to sample, usually by stratified random sampling in order to focus on groups most likely to show the effect under investigation. Statistical advice may be needed on the size of the sample. Usually, surveys look at the effects of a specific exposure and unexposed referents are available from within the workforce, but it may be desirable to include a referent group from another workforce, or perhaps from the general population. Referent groups are often difficult to find, rarely entirely satisfactory, and the advantages and disadvantages of the group chosen should be discussed.

Surveys aim to see all of the population, or of the sample. Response rates of 85% or more are acceptable, but anything less will throw considerable doubt on the results. The survey planning must encourage response, with explanatory letters and meetings for workers, physical siting of investigations close to the place of work and repeated assurances that no pay will be lost and that results will be confidential. Although all surveys are voluntary, it is reasonable to stress that the results will be important, perhaps for workers worldwide on similar processes, and will be meaningless if participation is low. Plans should be made to see as many non-respondents as possible, perhaps with only some of the main survey's tests, and for comparing them to respondents using available information from personnel and occupational health service records.

Variables

There are three types of variable: *exposure, response* and *potential modifiers*. Occupational exposure has two components, duration and intensity. Duration is obtained from company records or from an occupational history. There are various ways of estimating intensity. None is accurate, in the sense of measuring the concentration of a toxic agent at its target organ. The best estimates are environmental measurements made specially for the survey by, or with the advice of, a hygienist familiar with both technical considerations and the biological mechanism through which the agent exerts toxicity. The biological model may be that accumulated exposure is important, expressed as the product of duration and some measure of average intensity summed over jobs with different exposure intensities. This model is often assumed when there is little information on an agent's toxicology in man. There may be evidence for other modes of action. For example, short peaks of high exposure may be more toxic than the equivalent 'dose' as a long-term, low-intensity stimulus. The survey may make use of past environmental measurements made by the company. Sometimes, no measured values for exposure are available and intensity is estimated qualitatively, for example by ranking job titles into 'high', 'medium' and 'low' exposure categories.

That survey variables are only indirect estimators of the 'true' quality we wish to measure is emphasized when we consider response variables. For example, 'asthma' is notoriously difficult to define [5]. Because it cannot be 'measured' directly, surveys of asthma usually include several variables known to be associated with the condition, such as various respiratory symptoms and measures of lung function.

The other variables included are those thought to modify exposure, for example, respiratory protection, or modify response, for example sex, age, prescribed medication or alcohol consumption. It is particularly important to note effect-modifiers which are unevenly distributed through exposure categories and confound the relationship between the two. Smoking is often a confounding variable in studies of respiratory and cardiac disease and of cancer because smoking may, itself, cause the disease under investigation and also be a more common habit in people with high exposure than people with little exposure. This is often the case if exposure relates to socioeconomic class, and *Table 7.2* gives a hypothetical example of confounding by smoking.

Tests, records and definitions

The choice of tests may be aided by consultation with experts. For example, there are several components of lung function which are measurable. For each there are several methods and for each method, equipment from different manufacturers. The protocol should justify the choice of test and new and untried procedures should be described in detail. In protocols which will be discussed with lay managers and union officials, an outline of routine procedures should also be provided. This readership will, rightly, wish to know exactly how each test is carried out and if any might be uncomfortable or unpleasant for individual subjects.

Method criteria

Survey methods must be safe (for example, electrically, if a factory environment contains combustible material), acceptable to essentially healthy people (a requirement which disqualifies many hospital tests used on patients) and also simple and robust enough for repetitive use during the investigation. Methods must be valid, that is provide a meaningful estimate of the quality or quantity they are measuring. It is sometimes assumed that the newest, most complex equipment must give the most valid results, but this is not so. Technological sophistication may have considerable disadvantages. Measurements should also be reproducible, and the protocol should refer to calibration, standardization and quality control procedures and discuss other unwanted variation, such as caused by the timing of biological tests where there is a chronological rhythm, or observer bias if subjective judgements are to be made. Where possible, standard methods should be used, with known validity and reproducibility

Table 7.2   An apparent effect of exposure because of confounding by smoking

	Total		Case		Prevalence of disease (%)
	Smokers	*Non-smokers*	*Smokers*	*Non-smokers*	
Exposed (manual) workers ($n = 100$)	80	20	40	5	45
Unexposed (clerical) workers ($n = 100$)	20	80	10	20	30

This hypothetical example assumes no effect of exposure, but half of smokers have the disease, compared with a quarter of non-smokers. More exposed workers smoke than in the unexposed group chosen as their referents. This leads to a 1.5-fold excess of the disease in the exposed group.

characteristics, which allows comparison of the results with those from other surveys using the same methods. If this is not possible, it is desirable to incorporate formal measurement of these qualities, during the main survey or in a pilot study. The principles of these assessments are discussed by Barker and Rose [6].

Record forms

The proposed record forms should be included in the protocol, such as questionnaires or forms for recording the results of biological measurements. To keep data collection and analysis simple, the number of questions, and of tests, must be rigorously pruned until only the essentials remain. But once the tests (or questions) are decided upon, as much information as they can reasonably provide should be recorded. Some variables are continuous, for example height or blood pressure. It makes sense to record continuous variables with as much precision as the instrumentation allows, for example height to the nearest ½ cm, or blood pressure to the nearest millimetre of mercury (mmHg). The record forms should state the precision required and include enough space, or recording boxes, for the number of digits expected. Other variables are categorical: dichotomous such as 'Yes' and 'No' answers in a questionnaire, ordinal scales, such as of the severity of a symptom, or implying no order, such as categories of marital status. For categorical scales, decisions must be made on whether multiple answers are permissible and whether 'unsure' or 'unknown' answers are allowed, or if the worker (or investigator) must make a choice between the options suggested. The forms must indicate this clearly. All record forms should be tested by the investigators before the survey for clarity and ease of completion. Design is particularly important for questionnaires, both interviewer-administered and self-completed types. The reader is referred to books which discuss questionnaire design [7,8].

Records storage

If the survey is a large one, the storage of records may be a major practical issue. Even small surveys require some thought about record storage and retrieval. A numbering system which gives each subject a unique number and which is carried across all record forms is essential. Names, addresses and dates of birth are not unique identifiers and should not be used. Every page of a multipage form should contain the identity number, as staples and paperclips have a limited life, and personal environmental samples and biological samples should share the same numbering system as other information.

Specifying definitions

Many definitions can be specified before the survey. For example, one may specify how long a subject should have stopped smoking to be classified as an ex-smoker. Others can only be stated precisely when the results are known, but the approach to definition can be specified. For example, it may be known from the expected survey numbers that grouping by, say, quartiles of measured environmental exposure will give reasonable numbers for comparison between groups.

Planning the analysis

If the survey's questions have been well formulated, the basic lines of analysis will be clear and should be presented in the protocol. 'Fishing expeditions' through large numbers of variables may give statistically significant associations by chance. Unexpected findings may, of course, be important, but the temptation to 'fish', which is greatly facilitated by the power of available computer packages, should be curbed by specifying the major analyses in advance. In a survey which examines only a limited number of variables, it may be possible to draw up a complete set of 'dummy' tables in advance.

Thinking about the analysis at an early stage has two other benefits. First, it will highlight questions or definitions which are not yet sufficiently concrete. Secondly, it will suggest ways of improving record forms. Answers to questionnaires, for example, can be precoded, which increases accuracy in transferring data to computer. *Figure 7.3* shows different ways of recording information from a questionnaire used in surveys of occupational asthma. The person who will be responsible for data entry, either by first transferring it to a coding form or entering directly from the survey forms, should review the survey forms. Attention to their layout will increase the accuracy of transcription.

(1)   What happens to your   Better ☐   Same ☐   Worse ☐
       wheezing on holiday?

(2)   What happens to your   (for 'better' enter 1,
       wheezing on holiday?   'same' 2, 'worse' 3)

(3)   What happens to your   Better ☐ 1   Same ☐ 2   Worse ☐ 3
       wheezing on holiday?

Figure 7.3 Recording answers in a questionnaire. The answers (better, same, worse) do not follow any obvious numbering and mistakes could be made in data entry to a computer file without precoding. The second option is not uncommon in interviewer-administered questionnaires and requires the interviewer to enter the correct code in a box. The third option is preferable as the interviewer (or subject) has to think only about the reply to the question and not about coding it.

Timetables

There are two types of timetable which should be prepared and included in the protocol. One is an overall timetable, including health and environmental measurements, any subsequent laboratory tests and data analysis. Protocols for surveys involving interviews and tests on individual workers also should include a timetable for the survey participant. *Table 7.3* illustrates the considerations which may apply when deciding on the individual's timetable. Tests whose results may be influenced by other tests must always be separated. For example, an interviewer recording symptoms may be influenced by the subject's occupational history, so different investigators should administer symptoms and occupational questionnaires. As a general rule , it is always wise to take a blood sample as the last test, and to arrange some privacy. Very occasionally people faint when donating blood and fear of needles is not uncommon.

Ethical and 'political' issues

Strictly ethical issues, such as the use of invasive medical procedures, rarely arise in epidemiological surveys, but it is a sensible practice to submit protocols to the appropriate Ethical Committee. More commonly, surveys present problems with an 'ethico-political' component concerning the confidentiality of results, provision of medical advice to individual workers, provision of advice to the firm or publication of results. In general, all the environmental measurements and the group results of biological measurements should be freely available to management and unions but the individual's results are confidential. A few subjects may need further investigation because of clinically abnormal results, such as raised blood pressure or low lung function. They must be offered advice and if the company employs a doctor, he could readily provide it. However, transmission of results to the company doctor may not be acceptable to unions, or to individual workers. The general practitioner is an alternative to whom abnormal findings may be referred. Each worker with abnormal findings must be asked individually if his results may be passed on and the reason for this explained to him. The potential conflict between confidentiality and the provision of medical advice needs sensitive handling and an agreed procedure. Although not strictly part of the survey, it may take almost as much time to perform, and to the individual worker is probably more important.

The provision of advice to the firm, on environmental control or medical surveillance, may be the proper concern of the investigators, if they have expertise in these areas. Otherwise advice may be given by the occupational health service or perhaps by the Health and Safety Executive (HSE) if the company does not have its own occupational health professionals.

Most surveys produce results of general interest which should be published. This may be an alarming prospect for management, who will be concerned that commercial secrets may be revealed or the company may receive adverse publicity.

Table 7.3 Two hypothetical timetables for survey tests

Accumulated time (min)	Time table 1 Subjects				Timetable 2 Subjects			
	A	B	C	D	A	B	C	D
5	1				1			
10					2	1		
15	2	1			3a	2	1	
20					3a	3b	2	1
25	3	2	1			3b	3a	2
30	3						3a	3b
35		3	2	1				3b
40		3						
45			3	2				
50			3					
55				3				
60				3				

Tests 1 and 2 take 5 min, but test 3 takes 10 min and is the 'rate-limiting' test. Either the investigators carrying out tests 1 and 2 spend an equal amount of time doing nothing (timetable 1) or there are two investigators (3a and 3b) for test 3 (timetable 3). Timetable 2 sees subjects at a faster rate than timetable 1 (at intervals of 5 compared to 10 min) and individuals are away from work for a shorter time (20 compared to 30 min) but has the potential disadvantage that four (instead of three) workers are away from their posts at any one time.

The protocol should state that the company's name need not be used in publications or presentations, and the company may see drafts so any commercial secret may be deleted or obscured by appropriate rephrasing. However the protocol must state that the company has no right of veto over publication and will not hold the copyright of published material.

Costs

Protocols submitted to finding organizations must contain detailed costings to justify the total sum requested. Even if no additional funding is sought, the protocol should contain an approximate estimate of the survey costs, including that for staff time, the use of equipment, stationery, laboratory and computer time and the cost of any travelling and accommodation. In collaborative surveys, costings provide a crude method of estimating the input of each participant department, if this seems important. Costings also focuses the mind on whether the questions, and the likely answers, justify the effort and time involved in doing the survey.

Practical plans

Detailed planning proceeds when the protocol has been drafted. Administrative and technical details must be arranged, such as rooms booked at the site, forms duplicated, equipment serviced and calibrated, supplies purchased and arrangements made for the transport of equipment and supplies. It is rare for industrial sites to have facilities for disposal of contaminated waste such as used needles, so appropriate containers must be supplied which must be taken away for incineration.

The investigators need not be the originators of the study, although greater continuity is achieved if they take part. The ideal field-worker is neutral, consistent and meticulous in following his instructions. Procedures will require training, but often do not require special technical qualifications or experience. Indeed, the well-qualified field-worker, such as a doctor, may be a liability, as he may have his own theories about the cause of the disease studied which may unconsciously bias his behaviour.

It is helpful to list every activity, however trivial, which each investigator must perform and to do a 'dry run' for several hypothetical subjects on paper or with colleagues acting as subjects. This is often revealing, suggesting that more rooms or more investigators are needed than was originally envisaged. A procedure initially assigned to one investigator may, on examination, break down into a series of tasks which contains clear switches from one mode of thought to another. It is better that he be bored doing repetitive tasks than hurried and liable to omit important items so the procedure might be better split into two or three and shared out among additional investigators. One field-worker should have enough time for liaison with the company about any problems arising at the survey.

Dates must be confirmed with all investigators and it is wise to have reserves in case of illness. Dates are then confirmed with the responsible person at the firm. Special arrangements may be necessary to cover night and weekend shifts. Some advance preparation may be necessary, such as the distribution of a questionnaire. Some firms prefer a fixed appointment system, which has advantages if many tests are to be performed or if the study group is scattered about a large site. A looser timetable, with groups arriving for survey at predefined intervals, will often suffice and is more flexible than individual appointments. Timetabling should ensure that environmental and biological measurements are made as closely together in time as practicable and all workers seen over the shortest possible time. Surveys involving several sites should also be close in time. This minimizes the effects of fluctuations in variables over time, such as changes in exposure across the week, or longer periods, or the effects of epidemic viral infections on biological measurements. This means a concentrated effort by the investigators.

The survey

The site team should arrive the night before or at least 1 h before the survey starts. Supplies should be checked and equipment, including any in reserve in case of breakdowns, checked and recalibrated if necessary. People handling blood (or other samples) should wear laboratory coats and any other protective clothing which they usually wear to prevent infection from blood-borne pathogens. No investigator wishes to be discourteous to subjects but pressures of time may mean he gives an unhelpful impression, which will reduce participation. All members of the team must be prepared to answer queries about the survey's aims and methods, though without revealing specific

hypotheses, which may influence the subject's answers to questionnaires. Name-badges for investigators, notices on doors and chairs where subjects will wait all make the survey easier for the subject. If the planning has been thorough, the survey should go smoothly. The investigators' performance should be checked regularly to ensure each understands his instructions and is carrying them out, and equipment needs regular calibration. Problems should be referred to one person and close liaison maintained with whoever at the firm is coordinating the timetable.

Towards the end of the survey an approximate response rate should be calculated and the coordinator from the firm asked to establish which workers not yet seen are at work, so they can be encouraged to participate while the team is present. If a second survey is necessary to see non-respondents, a provisional date can be arranged. A poor response rate would suggest that planning was inadequate and the survey may need to be repeated.

Sufficient crude data-processing should be performed immediately after the survey for a preliminary report including at least an assessment of the response rate. Workers with clinically abnormal findings may be referred for advice, if this was not done at the survey. Any second survey of non-respondents and any laboratory tests on environmental and biological samples will be performed at this stage.

Analysis

For computer data-processing, the results will be coded into a computer-readable form and entered into a computer file. The accuracy of coding and entering must be checked by comparison with the raw data or by repeat coding of all or a sample of the results. Special programs may have to be written and checked for some analyses and some variables may need special handling, such as transformation. The analysis proceeds by asking specific questions and meetings of collaborators are helpful as it progresses. Florey and Leeder [9] discuss the documentation required, which is important, for personnel may change during a lengthy analysis. Finally, the results are sufficiently processed for publication. The experience of the survey, discussion of results and comments from other people almost always stimulate further questions, and possibly further surveys.

Acknowledgements

I thank my teachers, especially Corbett McDonald, and all my students.

References

1. Medawar, P.B. *Advice to a Young Scientist*, p. 13. Harper and Row, New York (1979)
2. Burr, M.L. Medical memorandum: criteria for planning a research project. *Community Medicine*, **1**, 157–159 (1979)
3. Bradford Hill, A. *A Short Textbook on Medical Statistics*, 11th edn. Hodder and Stoughton, London (1984)
4. Schlesselman, J.J. *Case-Control Studies: Design, Conduct, Analysis.* Oxford University Press, New York (1982)
5. Porter, R. and Birch, J. (eds) *Ciba Foundation Study Group, no. 38. Identification of Asthma.* Churchill Livingstone, Edinburgh (1971)
6. Barker, D.J.P. and Rose, G. *Epidemiology in Medical Practice*, 3rd edn. Churchill Livingstone, Edinburgh (1984)
7. Bennett, A.E. and Ritchie, K. *Questionnaires in Medicine: A Guide to Their Design and Use.* Nuffield Provincial Hospitals Trust, Oxford University Press, London (1975)
8. Moser, C.A. and Kalton, G. *Survey Methods in Social Investigation*, 2nd edn. Gower, Aldershot (1971)
9. Florey, C. du V. and Leeder, S.R. *Methods for Cohort Studies of Chronic Airflow Limitation. WHO Regional Publications, European Series No. 12.* WHO Regional Office for Europe, Copenhagen (1982)

Further reading

Abramson, J.H. *Survey Methods in Community Medicine: An Introduction to Epidemiological and Evaluative Studies*, 3rd edn. Churchill Livingstone, Edinburgh (1984)

Checkoway, H., Pearce, N.E. and Crawford-Brown, D.J. *Research Methods in Occupational Epidemiology. Monograph in Epidemiology and Biostatistics*, Vol. 13. Oxford University Press, New York (1989)

McDonald, J.C. *Epidemiology of Work-Related Diseases.* BMJ Publishing Group, London (1995)

Chapter 8

Sickness absence

SJ Searle

Definitions and background

Sickness absence is defined as absence attributed by the employee to illness or injury and accepted as such by the employer. This definition emphasizes that the phenomenon concerns absence due to incapacity for work, as declared by the employee, the presence of a specific medical condition in the individual being only one of many factors which may precipitate the inception of a spell of absence. Absence due to normal pregnancy or confinement is not normally included as sickness absence. In order for the employer to accept the absence as 'sickness absence', some form of certification is necessary either by a doctor as a medical certificate or by the employee in the form of a self-certificate.

Medical certificates may or may not show the true underlying cause of the sickness absence and often doctors use broad terms such as debility to indicate psychological causes of absence. Evidence suggests that sickness absence due to major psychiatric disorders is substantially under-reported; studies concerning minor psychiatric morbidity (symptoms of anxiety and depression which fall short of major psychiatric illness) suggest that those suffering from such problems have a higher than average severity of absence due to all causes.

Self-certificates completed by individual employees should always be required to state a specific reason for the sickness absence and descriptions such as 'unwell' should not be accepted. As an individual pattern of sickness absence builds up, the reasons given for absence on self-certificates may give some indication as to whether there is an underlying medical problem.

Sickness absence is not synonymous with morbidity, but in large groups of employees it is possible to obtain an indication of the broad diagnostic groups which may be of concern to a company and which may indicate appropriate preventive initiatives. For instance, a large amount of sickness absence for low back pain may indicate an ergonomic problem with lifting and handling which requires appropriate risk assessment and management

The primary concern of the general practitioner or family practitioner is the maintenance of a good doctor–patient relationship rather than serving the needs of an employer to control absence. In order to assist in effective management of sickness absence the occupational health practitioner must be able to bridge this gap by providing good, clear information to the primary care physician about work task demands and possibilities and by interpreting the medical assessment of the problem in clear, functional and temporal terms which allow management to take appropriate action. The process of interactions which focuses on the central role of the occupational health practitioner as interpreter of medical information to management and of management information to the treating physician is illustrated in *Figure 8.1*.

There is also a feedback loop to this process in managing rehabilitation after ill-health, whereby the manager can report back to the occupational health practitioner on progress and performance prior to further advice concerning progression of work activities. Also the occupational health prac-

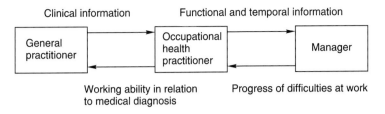

Figure 8.1 The occupational health practitioner as interpreter

titioner may then provide information about progress at work back to the primary care physician or medical specialist to inform them concerning decisions about the employee's future medical management.

Individual sickness absence behaviour

The presence of a medical condition in an individual is only one of many factors which will produce the inception of a spell of sickness absence. Individuals with the same medical condition may remain at work or take absence, depending on the interaction of many factors. The model of individual sickness absence behaviour [1] shown in *Figure 8.2* considers these factors at the level of the individual employee. Later in the chapter the interaction of organizational factors with these personal factors will be discussed as they can impact substantially on the management of the problem both at individual and organizational level.

The health status of the individual includes minor ailments, current symptoms, clinically diagnosed illness and psychological stress. The interaction between the individual's constitution, lifestyle factors and the range of health problems, which may range from minor ailments to serious disease, determines the health status. At an organizational level, the sickness tolerance threshold determines whether and when the individual decides to assume the sick role, with the associated expectations of obtaining diagnosis, treatment and restoration of health. In adopting the sick role the individual will aim to seek and receive treatment to restore health or stop the progression of disease. The absence tolerance threshold will determine whether the balance of work demands, social demands and the individual perception of the severity of illness leads to absence from work. An individual with a high absence tolerance threshold may continue in employment while attempting to resolve the problem, whereas those with low thresholds will commence a spell of absence from work. Ready access to occupational health advice at work may help an individual to

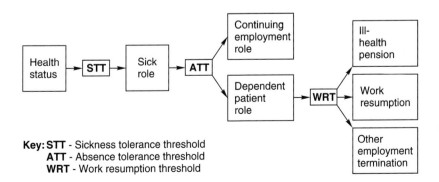

Figure 8.2 A model of individual sickness absence behaviour

stay at work by suitably modified work being arranged while the health problem is being managed.

The individual adopting the dependent patient role and commencing an absence from work will report sick, and for absences longer than a few days will seek medical certification of the absence. The majority of spells of sickness absence will end with resumption back to employment in some capacity. If this does not occur, the individual may be forced to substitute the dependent patient role for that of an unemployed, disabled or retired person.

Certification of sickness absence

In the UK self-certification of sickness absence was introduced in 1982, largely due to pressure from the representatives of general practitioners who were keen to reduce the burden of counter-signing the patient's statement about short term ill-health which could often not be well substantiated from a medical viewpoint. Those employees taking time off work for reasons attributed to ill-health have to complete a certificate of incapacity themselves to cover the first seven successive calendar days that they are away from work. Absence continuing after this has to be substantiated by a medical certificate issued by a doctor.

When self-certification was introduced many managers were concerned about the possibility that absence rates would increase with the removal of the doctor as gatekeeeper for sick pay in respect of short absences. Subsequently it became clear that this system increased the power of managers to control short-term absenteeism, as they could challenge individuals about adverse absence records more directly. An Industrial Society Survey reported in 1985 that many businesses have found the introduction of self-certification helpful in stimulating effective absence control procedures. Research in the British Post Office at that time showed no change for the worse in the pattern of sickness absence severity or frequency.

In the UK more medical certificates to refrain from work are issued on a Monday than other days of the week and the most likely day given for return to work is also a Monday. In Israel, however, where Sunday is the first day of the working week, more certificates are issued on that day. This supports the view that the patient rather than the doctor decides when a period of absence attributed to sickness will start and end, depending on the absence tolerance and work resumption thresholds referred to in *Figure 8.2*.

Costs and economic importance of sickness absence

In 1993 The Confederation of British Industry (CBI) reported that UK employers lose £13 billion annually as a result of sickness absence. This level of economic loss was confirmed by Davies and Teasdale [2] in a report for the Health and Safety Executive in the United Kingdom, and it was considered equivalent to 10% of the gross trading profits of UK industry. If the costs of litigation for work-related ill-health and injury are added, the economic impact of sickness absence is even greater.

Because of the costs involved and the disruption to work processes, whether in manufacturing or a service industry, the problems associated with sickness absence are of concern not only to doctors but also to employers, workers, trade unions, administrators of social insurance schemes and ultimately the taxpayer. Few organizations collect sufficient data to be able to estimate accurately their costs in this area. Regular surveys undertaken by the Industrial Society in the UK produce a response rate of only 30%, due to the lack of records on sickness absence even within relatively major companies.

Back pain is a common symptom, reported by about 60% of people at some time in their life. The Clinical Standards Advisory Group [3], in the UK, estimate that the major costs of back pain are in work loss and social security benefits. These costs amount to £480 million for diagnostic and treatment costs to the National Health Service, £3.8 billion for lost production in industry and £1.4 billion for social security benefits. Once back pain is established and the employee has adopted the dependent patient role, the prognosis is poor. Once patients are off work for more than 28 weeks, and particularly if loss of employment results, the chances of return to work are low irrespective of any health care intervention (see also Chapter 22). It is estimated that every 1% improvement in clinical services for back pain in the UK would save £38 million in lost production and £14 million in social security benefits.

Making appropriate early decisions about ill-health retirement can have a major impact on reducing employer costs of sickness absence. Malcolm [4] found that, in a local authority in the North-East of England, earlier and more consistent referral of employees with long-term sickness absence saved the authority £750 000 in one year.

Patterns of sickness absence

Sickness absence is broadly split into two types, long term and short term. Neither has a clear definition; long-term absence broadly includes absences of several weeks or more, whereas short-term absence relates to single day spells of absence or absences lasting less than a few weeks. Where organizational policies are in place it is essential that the difference between long- and short-term absence is defined in their terms in the policy, as referral and management actions will be triggered by the type of absence recorded and defined.

A local authority found that considerable savings were made by referring cases of long-term sickness absence to the occupational health service at 3 months' duration instead of after 6 months of absence. Most organizations would consider the 3-month definition rather long, as much illness may be well established by that time and, as in the example given earlier in relation to back pain, rehabilitation and eventual return to work may be more problematic. Usually 14 days or 28 days are taken as the threshold for initial referral to, or discussion with, the occupational health service. Obviously a balance has to be struck between excessive investigation and assessment of cases where the outcome is more easily forecast and the risk of missing a clinical problem where the likelihood of return to work can be improved by early clinical intervention and management flexibility in arranging appropriate work.

Generally long-term absence is more likely to be associated with significant medical problems than short-term absence which is more often due to self-limiting conditions, but the question of substance abuse may need to be considered (see Chapter 20). Frequent short-term absenteeism can be very disruptive to production or service delivery because of its unpredictable nature. It is generally regarded as being more amenable to management control than long-term absence. However, managers should always consider the possibility of significant medical problems in those taking frequent short-term absences and offers of help by referral to internal occupational health advice or encouragement to the employee to seek advice from the general practitioner should be given at interviews related to sickness absence of any sort.

Repeated short-term absences may also suggest a factor in the workplace which is triggering episodes of ill-health, such as exposure to a sensitizing agent resulting in occupational asthma, repeated absences due to workplace stress or musculoskeletal problems related to manual handling. Managers are increasingly responsible for assessing risks in the workplace and providing solutions to reduce those risks; they should be aware that information from sickness absence patterns may be of assistance to them in this and that the identification of underlying work factors may be more important in reducing sickness absence than a mechanistic and disciplinary approach to interviewing those with adverse attendance records. A partnership approach to managing these issues, involving the occupational health service and line managers with human resources managers taking a coordinating role, including the collection and collation of data, can be very constructive.

Measurement

Sickness absence is a repetitive event and requires measurement of both duration (number of days in a period) and frequency (number of spells in a period). Generally, absences with a greater medical basis have longer but fewer spells and absence patterns with a greater behavioural basis show shorter, more frequent spells. In any comparative study of sickness absence it is useful to have both these measures, as only then can conclusions be drawn as to how much absence is long term, and possibly more amenable to medical intervention, and how much is short term and perhaps more amenable to management control.

Spells of absence

A spell of absence is defined as an uninterrupted period of absence, irrespective of its duration. Short spells of sickness absence of 1 day or more should be included in calculations. When reviewing and comparing absence studies, care should be taken to consider whether all spells have been included in the calculations. Some American studies exclude absences of less than 1 week and thus appear to show low rates. When making annual analyses, a spell of absence commencing in one year and continuing into the next year contributes only to the spell rate in the first year, since rates are calculated for spells commencing during a period. Another term for the same calculation is spell inception rate.

The frequency rate (mean spells per person in the period) is calculated as follows:

$$\frac{\text{Total number of new spells of absence commencing in the period}}{\text{Average population at risk during the period}}$$

The period is usually 1 year, either a calendar or business year, but could be a shorter period.

Duration of absence

The duration of absence should preferably be counted in calendar days to enable comparison with other studies. However, some personnel or finance departments prefer to use actual working days or hours, as these reflect more closely the costs which are attributable to the company. Any published study which quotes absence rates should state the basis on which the duration of absence is calculated so that valid comparisons can be made. The first day, or substantial part of a day, that a person is absent is counted as the initial day. The final day of the absence is counted as the one preceding the day of return to work, or the day on which the employee is retired, dismissed or dies.

The severity rate (mean days per person in the period) is calculated as follows:

$$\frac{\text{Total days of absence attributed to sickness in the period}}{\text{Average population at risk during the period}}$$

Prevalence rates

Prevalence rates can be calculated for defined periods. They may be useful for monitoring the progress of epidemics or to identify days in the organization when absenteeism is particularly high or low. An example is the point prevalence rate which is calculated as follows:

$$\frac{\text{Number of persons absent on a day}}{\text{Population at risk on that day}}$$

Population at risk

For all the calculations described above it is necessary to determine the common denominator of the population at risk. This may be achieved in a number of ways, all of which provide an estimate of how many people are 'at risk' of being absent during the period considered in the study. Most sickness absence research considers annual rates and in that case person-years are used. This means the number of people at risk of taking absence in an organization throughout a defined year, which may be a calendar year or a business year. It is actually a head count and should include part-time staff as well as full-time staff. It allows for people leaving the organization or joining it during the year under consideration.

There are three ways of arriving at the estimate of population at risk:

1 Taking a mid-year census. This is satisfactory if the working population is stable during the period of study but would be very inaccurate if there was a major contraction, for instance a redundancy programme, during the year. Equally an expanding business would not reflect its population size accurately in a mid-year census.
2 Taking a mean of four quarterly population figures.
3 A mean annual population taken from a computerized payroll. This is derived from person-months or days, for salaried and weekly paid staff respectively, for every individual employed for some or all of the 12 months under study; it is the method of choice in terms of accuracy.

Where person-years are the appropriate denominator for mean frequency and severity rates the prevalence rate referred to above requires measurement of the total number of persons present for that period. Also, where frequency distributions are being used for comparing different factors, these distributions must relate to people present throughout the period of study; therefore, joiners and leavers during a period must be excluded in determining such distributions.

In studies of sickness absence it is advisable to obtain data covering at least 100 person-years in order to provide valid comparisons. Studies with smaller populations are unlikely to form the basis for any valid conclusions, beyond a descriptive approach to what has been found.

Frequency distributions

If duration and spells of absence during a period are plotted as frequency distributions, it can be seen that the distribution is highly skewed. The distribution never follows the normal distribution curve and is most similar to the negative binomial distribution of uneven risk which was first described earlier this century in relation to the concept of accident proneness. *Table 8.1* shows the distributions of days and spells of absence in a sample of postal staff. It can be seen that about a third of employees took no absence at all during the year and that three-quarters of employees took 5 days or less and no more than 2 spells of absence.

Considering this and other studies, it is a good rule of thumb that in any one year about one-third of the staff take no absence at all, about two-thirds will take a few short spells, usually self-certificated, and only one-third of employees in an organization will take longer medically certificated absence. As a result of the highly skewed distribution of absence, it is found in most organizations that about half the total absence is caused by less than one-tenth of the workforce.

Sickness absence policies should acknowledge that anyone can fall sick, and may have to take absence from work as a result, and should include a commitment to record information about absences so that the problem can be managed effectively without being excessively intrusive to the individual or time-consuming for the line manager or the human resources department. Using distributions to determine appropriate standards for attendance and trigger points for management interviews and referral for occupational health advice is one way to achieve this. *Table 8.2* shows the median number of days and spells and the number exceeded by the 5% of employees with the worst absence records. Similar tables could be constructed showing the days and spells taken by the worst 10% or 20%, in order to inform a decision about setting manageable trigger points for action.

Considering the information in *Table 8.2* it can be seen that if a trigger for management interviews for frequent absenteeism was set at 4 spells in one year then most staff, as seen from the median figure, will be well within this figure and all concerned in any control procedure can see that a fair system is in operation. Also there is no excessive use of management time in interviewing those who take an occasional spell of absence. Similarly, at least half of employees are seen to take no more than 7 days absence in a year, so a trigger of referral for occupational health advice could be

Table 8.1 Distribution of self-certificated absence: postal staff 1984–85

No. of days or spells	Percentage of days of absence	Cumulative percentage of days of absence	Percentage of spells of absence	Cumulative percentage of spells of absence
0	29.5	29.5	29.5	29.5
1	11.2	40.7	25.4	54.9
2	11	51.7	19.6	74.5
3	10	61.7	13.1	87.6
4	7.1	68.8	6.7	94.3
5	6.8	75.6	3	97.3
6	5.5	81.1	1.4	98.7
7	4.5	85.6	0.7	99.4
8	3.6	89.2	0.4	99.8
9	2.8	92.0	0.1	99.9
10	2.0	94.0	0.1	100
11	1.7	95.7	0	100
12	1.1	96.8	0	100
13	0.9	97.7	0	100
14	0.6	98.3	0	100
15–21	1.5	99.8	0	100
>21	0.2	100	0	100

Table 8.2   Absence criteria by grade, Post Office 1984–85: median and upper 5% values

Sex and grade	Median days	5% days	Median spells	5% spells
Men				
Managers	1.2	36	0.4	5
Clerks	2.3	29	0.7	4
Postmen	4.4	53	1.4	6
Other grades	1.9	35	0.7	4
Women				
Managers	2.5	33	0.8	4
Clerks	4.0	43	1.3	5
Postwomen	6.3	70	1.4	6
Other grades	5.3	76	1.2	5

set above this, say at 14 or 28 days. The figure also shows that more days and spells of absence are taken by the postmen and postwomen, the manual workers, than the clerical staff. This reflects the pattern shown in most organizations. It is clearly more difficult to attend work and perform a physically demanding task when suffering from acute respiratory symptoms or following an injury than it is to undertake more sedentary work. The type of work the individual is undertaking thus has an influence on the absence tolerance threshold shown in *Figure 8.2*.

If undertaking a study using sickness absence data it is wise to seek advice from a statistician at the outset. The highly skewed distribution of absence does cause some problems in statistical analysis when comparing different groups. It is not useful to use tests of statistical inference based on the normal distribution, such as t-tests. There can also be problems in using more sophisticated statistical models such as analysis of variance and multivariate analysis, as these rely on a normal distribution of the data.

While it is difficult to compare directly mean rates of duration and frequency of absence, it is possible to compare proportions of individuals with particular absence characteristics, such as high or low absence duration or frequency, using statistical tests for comparing qualitative data such as the chi-square (χ^2) test. It is also possible to use non-parametric statistical tests.

Percentage working time lost

Another common measure of absence, which is used in industry to monitor performance and set budgets for absence, is percentage working time lost. This is a point prevalence rate expressing the number of people absent on a single day as a percentage of the total population who should have attended for work on that day. It can also be calculated as the total scheduled hours lost, attributed to sickness, expressed as a percentage of total hours scheduled to be worked. The daily rates can be averaged over any period to give a picture of the trend in absence severity. Thus comparisons can be made week by week or month by month. Such data can be used to set targets for absence for use by line managers in controlling absence in their units and comparing their performance with others.

Percentage working time lost figures can be used to compare performance between different units within an organization, between organizations and between countries on a national basis. They are useful in budgeting for the costs of sickness absence and in setting management improvement targets. However, they do not give any indication of the proportion of absence which is short term or long term and are not helpful in defining the causes, either organizational or medical, behind the problem of sickness absence.

Measuring calendar days or working days lost

When setting up measurement systems of sickness absence in an organization, consideration should be given as to whether to measure calendar days lost or working days lost. Calendar days are mainly used in the medical and sociological literature on sickness absence and by some large organizations. This system tends to overestimate the amount of absence, including weekends when the individual may or may not be fit to attend work, and reflects incapacity for work rather than the true amount of absence from working duties. Sickness absence is very different from true morbidity, and where a new system of absence recording is being established there is good reason to use working days lost, as this reflects more truly the direct financial cost to the business as well as the potential impact on production or provision of a service.

When reviewing the literature and comparing studies of sickness absence in different settings, it is necessary to convert calendar days lost to working days lost or vice versa, to allow valid comparison. The conversion depends on the number of working days in the organization in question, but is computed by direct proportion as in the following example:

Calendar days per year = 365
Number of working days per year (organization with 5-day week) = 52 × 5 = 260
less average days holiday and bank holidays, say 25 = 260 − 25 = 235

If, for example, the mean duration of absence (calendar days) is 12 days per year, then the mean duration working days will be $12 \times \frac{235}{365} = 7.7$ working days per year.

Key variables

Three of the personal factors which affect sickness absence have a greater influence than any other. These three factors of age, gender and occupational status must therefore be controlled for in any comparative study. In comparing absence rates between groups of employees it is necessary to use stratification or standardization techniques to control for these factors which cause a lot of variation. From *Table 8.2* it can be seen that women have higher rates than men and that there can be up to a fourfold difference in absence rates between clerical staff and manual staff .

Age is the factor which has the greatest influence, with younger people taking more frequent spells of absence, perhaps reflecting an adjustment to work in relation to other lifestyle factors and social demands. Older people take fewer spells of absence, but have an increasing severity of sickness absence with age, showing a higher duration

of mean days lost due to sickness absence with increasing age. This is to be expected, as there is a greater likelihood of major ill-health due to degenerative disorders such as coronary heart disease and osteoarthritis, with advancing age. The vital importance of using age standardization is shown in a study by Sharp and Watt [5]. They studied the absence records of 2561 workers in two organizations where men and women had equal work status. Information was collected from personnel departments using a standardized form providing information on all absences of 1 or more calendar days, the length of absence and the location, age, gender and occupational status of the worker. Just under a quarter of the workforce were female. Female absence exceeded male absence for both spells and duration in days, being between 1.3 and 1.5 times greater in frequency (spells) and between 1.2 and 1.9 times greater in duration (days). When age standardization was applied, the differences disappeared, suggesting that there was little true difference in absence behaviour in respect of gender in this group of workers. This finding may reflect the equal work status between men and women in the study group, but it clearly demonstrates the value of using age standardization.

A number of studies from Sweden have considered the role of gender integration on sickness absence. These have shown that women working in extremely male-dominated occupations have high rates of sickness absence and also that men working in highly female-dominated occupations had the highest incidence of absence of all men in a particular Swedish county. Occupations with greater gender integration, or a more equal sex distribution, showed the lowest rates of sickness absence. These studies also showed that blue-collar, or manual, occupations had the highest sick leave rates.

Causes

Although days lost through absence attributed to sickness may be covered by a medical certificate, it does not follow that the cause is solely attributable to a medical condition or even medical factors.

The causes known to influence sickness absence can be divided into three levels. Geographical factors are those which cause variation between different countries and broad geographical regions and includes sociopolitical factors. Organizational factors may cause differences in rates between different organizations or subunits of organizations within the same geographical area. Personal factors are those which concern the individual worker and may include the presence of a specific medical condition. Analysis of geographical, organizational and personal factors in sickness absence sometimes refers to these broad categories as macro, meso and micro levels, focusing down from a broad socioeconomic viewpoint to a more personal view of individual behaviour. The factors affecting sickness absence at these three levels are summarized in *Table 8.3*.

Geographical factors

The strong influence of social factors on sickness absence rates can be seen by considering trends over the past 40 years. Between 1960 and 1980 sickness absence rates rose in most industrialized countries by up to 30%, with many more days lost through sickness absence than as a result of industrial action. During the 1980s the rate of increase fell off and a reduction was seen in some organizations and some countries, particularly the developing economies of the Pacific Rim where there appear to be lower absence rates associated with a strong work ethic. In the 1990s absence rates were seen to fall in the UK and a survey among European Community countries in 1994 showed the UK with the lowest absence rates at 3.2% working time lost, compared to 6.4% in The Netherlands, 5.5% in Germany and 4.4% in Belgium.

Social insurance may have a marked impact on when the individual decides to resume work. Generous provision, as in The Netherlands, tends to raise the work resumption threshold (see *Figure 8.2*), whereas more stringent controls applied to benefits will tend to lower the threshold, with an early return to work after illness becoming a greater economic necessity. The provision of Health Services will impact on the sickness tolerance threshold, with easy and early access to health care allowing the individual more opportunity to control health problems and remain at work in the continuing employment role. Unemployment and reduced job security as a result of the global recession in the 1980s may well have been a factor in the reductions in sickness absence seen in the late 1980s and early 1990s. There is increasing evidence that long-term unemployment can in itself have an adverse effect on health status. Social attitudes to work probably explain the low rates of absence seen in the Pacific Rim countries, where possible loss of face within the work group following withdrawal from work is a major factor stimulating the continuing employment role.

Organizational factors

This category includes the nature and function of the enterprise, its human resources strategy, operational methods and business processes. For instance, in the UK, engineering industries and the health service have twice the rates of absence found in the finance and education sectors of the economy. Operational methods that focus on teamwork, such as cellular production as opposed to a production line, allow individuals greater autonomy in how they do their job. Such working methods also require greater mutual support of and from individuals in the team, resulting in lower absence rates.

It was recognized many years ago that there was a relationship between the size of the organization and its absence rates, with larger organizations having higher absence rates. However, it is now clear that the relevant factor is the size of the working unit within the organization, rather than the size of the organization itself. Small working units have lower absence rates.

In large groups the worker may feel anonymous and lacking support, particularly if the supervision

Table 8.3 Some factors known to influence sickness absence

Geographical	Organizational	Personal
Climate	Nature	Age
Region	Size of unit	Gender
Social insurance	Industrial relations	Occupation
Health services	Sick pay	Job satisfaction
Epidemics	Supervisory quality	Personality
Unemployment	Working conditions	Life crises
Social attitudes	Personnel policies	Medical conditions
Pension age	Environmental hazards	Alcohol and other
Taxation	Occupational health	substance abuse
	service	Family
	Labour turnover	responsibilities
		Social activities
		Journey to work
		Length of service
		Gender integration

is poor. Absence of one or two people may easily be covered by others and management may give the impression that the absence has had little effect on the operations of the organization. Management interviews on return to work and continuing supportive contact during an absence can help to overcome such attitudes and substantially improve absence rates. Studies comparing Japanese-managed companies in the UK with traditionally British-managed firms show that the Japanese-run companies have lower absence rates. This may be associated with the greater adoption of total quality management, where workers feel more involved with the processes of the company and have a greater sense of worth and responsibility.

Good industrial relations and a high level of employee involvement in the organization help to reduce absence rates. Sickness absence rises where there is uncertainty about continuing employment, which is a worsening problem with companies increasingly reducing staff numbers as technology reduces the need for labour-intensive activities. Good communications about such changes, coupled with provision of suitable leaving packages and outplacement counselling, can help to reduce this adverse impact.

The level of company sick pay has an effect on sickness absence. Some companies do not provide sick pay to new entrants or for the first few days of an absence. Such firms have lower absence rates, probably as a result of raising the absence tolerance threshold, with absence being economically difficult when the individual is faced with a choice of pay or no pay. Firms who pay at full rates for the first 6 months of absence often find that long-term absences start to resolve around the time of reduction to half pay at the six-month stage.

Supervisory quality is a very important factor in controlling sickness absence. If people feel that their absence is not noticed, they are more likely to take repeated spells. Return to work interviews can have the effect of raising the awareness of the worker that his absence has been noticed and has had an adverse effect on his team or working unit as well as providing the opportunity to give information about access to occupational health advice and review any factors in the working environment that may have influenced the absence. A high level of supervisor training is required to achieve this end and a number of good video-based training aids are available commercially.

A number of studies have considered the effect of shift work on absence rates. Most show that shift workers have lower sickness absence rates than non-shift workers. This is despite some evidence of an increased incidence of gastrointestinal and stress-related disorders in shift workers.

Personnel policies may influence sickness absence. For instance, once it is established that an individual is unlikely to return to their normal job or modified work, dismissal on medical grounds may be considered. If pay is given in lieu of notice the recorded sick rate, which is heavily influenced by absence spells of long duration, may substantially reduce without any additional cost to the organization. Such a decision may also hasten decisions about appropriate replacement and training needs.

The presence of environmental hazards is a major factor, and common causes of adverse absence patterns are inappropriate manual handling methods, especially for repetitive tasks, and exposure to hazardous chemicals such as sensitizing agents which may result in occupational asthma or dermatitis. Managers should be increasingly aware of their responsibilities for identifying, controlling and monitoring such hazards, be they physical, chemical or biological. In the European Community countries legislation exists to require managers to undertake risk assessments and take appropriate action to control hazards. Giving support for such processes, for instance by providing health surveillance or environmental monitoring, introduces good opportunities for occupational health professionals to prove their worth to the organization as well as protecting individual workers.

Labour turnover is often directly correlated with rates of absence. Typically, turnover is highest in the first few months of employment, then short-term absenteeism becomes more pronounced as new employees learn the ropes, often having less autonomy in controlling and organizing their work than more established employees.

Personal factors

The three most important factors in this category are age, gender and occupational status, as discussed in the section on key variables. Age in particular must always be controlled for in comparative studies.

A number of large studies on sickness absence have suggested that the more autonomy a worker has in controlling working arrangements, the more support obtained from colleagues at work and from social relationships away from work, the lower the absence rates are. This applies to all diagnostic causes of absence including those considered to be stress related (see also Chapter 19).

Life crises such as marital breakdown, the sudden illness of a spouse or dependent relative and bereavement can result in increased sickness absence. Provision of counselling facilities either in-house or by using an external Employee Assistance Programme can help to reduce the impact of these events.

Rehabilitation programmes for alcohol misuse and other substance abuse have been shown in some studies to have a beneficial effect in reducing absenteeism and improving work performance. There is also some evidence that introducing smoking prohibition at work reduces sickness absence, particularly for spells of short-term respiratory illness.

Medical factors

Of over 30 factors identified in *Table 8.3* as influencing differences in sickness absence between groups only five are strictly medical as opposed to socioeconomic or organizational. These medical factors are the occurrence of epidemics, the availability of health services within an area, the effect of hazards in the working environment, the availability of occupational health services, and whether or not an individual suffers from a medical condition.

The occupational health practitioner advising a company can help to modify the effect of these factors. Advice on public health measures to control epidemics may be a large component of the work of an occupational health practitioner in developing countries and may contribute substantially towards the success of the enterprise. Advice to travellers overseas will also assist in controlling this factor. In developed countries, influenza epidemics are the main problem in this respect but influenza vaccination programmes are only cost effective if high take-up rates are achieved, which proves very difficult in practice.

When access to diagnosis and treatment for medical conditions is limited the company can be advised about medical insurance and the provision of private medical care where appropriate. Even in the UK, with the availability of a National Health Service, priorities for entry into the system may be different in terms of the test of clinical need as against the requirements of the earliest possible

return to effective work from the business perspective. Substantial savings can be made by selective use of early diagnostic and treatment facilities funded by the company where there are long waiting lists for access to diagnosis and treatment. This is particularly important in relation to back conditions as it has been made clear that people who are absent from work with back ache for longer than 6 months have a very poor prognosis for continued employment.

Some studies have shown that introducing an occupational health service, or an employee assistance programme providing counselling, can actually increase absence initially. This is probably by lowering the sickness tolerance threshold and stimulating the worker to assume the sick role and thence the dependent patient role (see *Figure 8.2*). Proving the effectiveness of occupational health interventions is a continuing challenge that demands close partnership in measuring outcomes between the organization and the occupational health service.

The identification and control of workplace hazards is of major importance and is dealt with in Chapter 5. More information on this topic can be gleaned from texts on occupational hygiene.

The occupational health practitioner has a major role in advising the individual and the organization on fitness to work, in relation to specific medical problems. This involves early diagnosis, good communications with the worker and treating physicians as well as with management to ensure that appropriate rehabilitation and resettlement measures are set in place. The central role of the occupational health practitioner is shown in *Figure 8.1*.

Comparative data

Comparative information about sickness absence in the UK is available from surveys undertaken by the Confederation of British Industry (CBI) and the Industrial Society. These surveys use estimates of percentage working time lost to compare differences between industrial sectors and regions.

The CBI conducted a survey in 1987 involving 431 companies with a total employee population of 1.2 million people. The results estimated an annual cost to UK industry of non-attendance at work to be £5 billion. Another survey in 1993, involving 300 companies representing 1.22 million employees, gave an estimate of current cost as

£13 billion. Taking all employees, the percentage working time lost was 3.5%, a fall of 0.5% from the previous 1987 estimate. The survey also emphasized the differential between manual workers, who took 10 days of sickness absence per year, and non-manual workers who took between 5 and 6 days per year as sickness absence.

Factors identified as reducing absence rates included management commitment, improved monitoring and the provision of absence statistics to line managers. Fear of redundancy among employees was considered to be less important. Organizations keeping only manual records for sickness absence had sickness absence levels 16% higher than those keeping computer-based records.

The Industrial Society has published three surveys, in 1985, 1990 and 1992. The last survey considered differences in managing attendance at work between Japanese-managed companies and traditionally British-managed companies [6]. They found a national mean absence rate of 3.97% compared to 5.05% in their 1990 survey. The rate for the public sector was 4.57%, the private sector 3.87% and for Japanese-owned and managed companies was only 2.35%. Japanese-owned companies had smaller working groups and gave more importance to communicating absence rates to their employees via team briefing groups and notice boards. Japanese respondents were more likely to ask about attendance records at recruitment interviews and tended to interview employees after each spell of absence, irrespective of its length. This approach appeared to result in an absence rate approaching half that in the UK public sector.

The economic sectors with the highest rates included the health services with 5.94% and engineering and vehicle manufacture with a rate of 5.46%. There were marked regional variations, with London showing an increase from 3.31% in 1990 to 4.97% in 1992 and the rates in Wales rising from 3.89% to 5.77%. The areas with the lowest absence rates were the Home Counties (South East England) at 2.98% and East Anglia at 3.37%.

Opinion was sought from respondents on the effect of the recession. Some felt it had reduced absence by highlighting the need for good attendance, where job security was perceived to be a problem. Other respondents felt that the recession had increased absence by adding to stress and pressure of work. Many companies had used individual absence records as one of the selection criteria in their redundancy policies.

Organizational management of sickness absence

The doctor working in an industrial or commercial environment is concerned with the health aspects of groups of individuals as well as individuals. This section considers this aspect of managing sickness absence.

Diagnosis

In this context the diagnosis of sickness absence relates to the identification of the real causes of sickness absence in groups of individuals. These factors may relate to the individual or the environment, both at work or away from work, but especially to the interaction between the two. Therefore medical, occupational, social and behavioural factors all need to be considered. Accurate diagnosis requires an understanding of the patient in their total environment. The occupational health practitioner needs to have a comprehensive working knowledge of the culture of the organization and the nature of the work carried out in the enterprise. This includes an understanding of expectations and behaviours which are prevalent and which could be deleterious to health, such as expectations to work excessive hours or tendencies to invade the privacy of individuals when they are away from work, such as contact while the employee is on leave.

Just as anonymized feedback can be given to management regarding the results of health surveillance in relation to physical environmental hazards in the workplace, so can summary information concerning psychological triggers and coping skills of groups of individuals be used to provide feedback to management. This can assist an organization in maintaining the mental health of employees in the current milieu of rapid organizational change.

Treatment

The organizational treatment of sickness absence refers to the role of the occupational health practitioner in preventing the inception of spells of sickness absence and reducing the duration of those that do occur. It also involves supporting the effective return to work of employees after illness or injury and helping those whose medical problems make them unfit to return to their previous occupation in terms of appropriate resettlement to alternative work or access to ill-health retirement where this is within the terms of the pension fund.

Examples of the prevention of inception of absence include health education initiatives that encourage healthy lifestyles and raise the sickness tolerance threshold referred to in *Figure 8.2*, thus preventing the employee from assuming the sick role as a precursor to taking absence from work. The increasing awareness of the adverse effects of smoking, alcohol and drugs in the workplace is an example. The occupational health practitioner can play a major role in establishing and reviewing policy in these areas, providing health education to employees and individual counselling and support to those who wish to change their lifestyle, for instance running smoking cessation programmes. There is also scope for input into food policies to promote healthy eating and ensure suitable provision for workers on shift systems. Occupational health input at the design stage of new plant, premises and work processes can help to prevent expensive ergonomic disasters at an early stage.

Close liaison with treating physicians, both general practitioners and specialists, is necessary in terms of ensuring an optimum return to effective work. Contact with other members of the primary care team, including mental health nurses and physiotherapists, is also essential. The normal constraints of professional confidentiality always apply and such contact must be with the properly informed consent of the employee. The occupational health practitioner can then interpret the medical information in the context of specialized knowledge about the limitations of the workplace and the organizational culture, as illustrated in *Figure 8.1*. Managers find that advice about likely dates for return to work, the prospective length of an absence or any modified work, and details about functional limitations, are of much greater help than medical jargon. Once an employee has returned to work the occupational health nurse is usually closer to the workplace, in terms of proximity and approachability, than the occupational physician and is best placed to undertake post-absence monitoring. If work problems are noticed in the recovery period, then suitable advice can be given to both the individual and the management

which may help to prevent the inception of a further spell of absence.

Prevention

Pre-employment health screening is little use as a predictor of future absence. The best criterion for assessing the risk of future absence is the past attendance record of an individual, a poor record probably reflecting a combination of low sickness tolerance threshold and a low absence tolerance threshold. It is worth encouraging recruitment officers to obtain and assess past attendance records in previous employment or during the school years for younger employees. The relatively good performance of Japanese-managed firms in the UK in sickness absence management is related in part to the fact that such firms are more likely to obtain detailed information about prospective employees' past work attendance and to discuss the topic at interview, compared to UK-managed firms.

Pre-employment assessment by the occupational health service of those who are known to have particular health problems may help to ensure appropriate work placement which will not adversely affect the employees' health status or work performance. It is important for the recruitment department to realize that this approach is much more effective than blanket rejection of all applicants declaring a particular medical problem. Legislation introduced in the UK on the treatment of people with disabilities has increased the importance of fair assessment of capability in relation to work demands in those people known to have a disability. Guidance on assessment of fitness to work, using a systematic approach and emphasizing the assessment of residual ability, is to be found in a publication from the Faculty of Occupational Medicine in the UK [7].

Effective management of sickness absence includes keeping good records on a group and an individual basis and feeding back information about absence and its effect on production or service at team briefings or meetings. This should be supported by the manager showing concern for the individual, acknowledging that anyone can fall ill, and also the effect of their absence on the job and the work team when an individual phones in to report sick.

Individual case management

The first essential step is to determine whether the absence is associated with a specific medical condition and to arrive at an accurate diagnosis. This may require contact with the individual's own medical advisers, in addition to a consultation with the occupational health practitioner. The individual must give written informed consent when the occupational health practitioner is seeking reports on health status in relation to work. This consent must be informed by a knowledge of the implications of the use of such information, such as work modification or consideration of long-term employment prospects. It is important for occupational health practitioners to have a clear idea of their ethical responsibilities in handling such information, given their position between the employee and the organization. It is clear that the primary responsibility of the occupational health practitioner is to each individual being assessed, while taking into account the needs of the organization. The occupational health service can be most effective if a climate is created in which many referrals are informal and at the request of the individual rather than mandatory referrals from management.

Consideration needs to be given to any possible work-related cause or aggravating factors, once a definitive diagnosis has been made. Problems such as alleged work-related upper limb disorder and work-related stress are becoming increasingly common and proving a burden to employers in terms of actual or potential litigation. Whether or not there is evidence of association with work or causation by certain work activities is often a key factor should litigation ensue. It behoves the occupational health practitioner to ensure that statements made in clinical records and in reports to management concerning conditions that are work related can be fully substantiated on clinical grounds.

An integrated team approach to managing sickness absence

The occupational health service usually operates as a team with a number of professional disciplines and with some clerical and administration support. The professional team may include physicians, nurses, occupational hygienists, physiotherapists, psychologists, counsellors, exercise physiologists, ergonomists and safety managers.

Cross-communication between all professional members of the team is important and the involvement of the support team is also vital as they provide access to the team by employees and managers. They should be as equally aware of the aims and objectives, or 'mission' in management terms, of the service as are the professional members of the team. The support staff may also have much to contribute in managing and improving operational processes within the team, given their high profile as a contact point with customers at all levels.

Liaison is also vital between the occupational health team and managers in managing absence, so that actions can be agreed and progress in individual cases can be monitored. A useful approach to this is a case conference, where the progress of cases can be discussed on a regular (say monthly) basis, without revealing clinical details but concentrating on functional and temporal interpretation of the clinical assessments. If these meetings include occupational health professionals, human resources managers and appropriate line managers, much can be done to agree individual responsibilities and actions in each individual case of absence. The involvement of managers from different functions within the organization may facilitate cross-functional placement of those with temporary or permanently impaired health and help to maximize appropriate placement of individuals and minimize unnecessary retraining and recruitment costs.

References

1. Prins, R. Sickness absence in Belgium, Germany and The Netherlands; a comparative study. *Ph.D. thesis*, Rijksuniversiteit Limburg te Maastricht (1990)
2. Davies, N.V. and Teasdale, P. *The costs to the British Economy of Work Accidents and Work-Related Ill Health.* HSE Publications, Sudbury (1994)
3. Clinical Standards Advisory Group. *Back Pain.* HMSO, London (1994)
4. Malcolm, R.M. Effects of changing the pattern of sickness absence referrals in a local authority. *Occupational Medicine*, **43**(4), 211–215 (1993)
5. Sharp, C. and Watt, S. A study of absence rates in male and female employees working in occupations of equal status. *Occupational Medicine*, **45**(3), 131–136 (1995)
6. Industrial Society. *Wish You Were Here.* The Industrial Society, London (1992)
7. Cox, R.A.F., Edwards, F.C. and McCallum, R.I. *Fitness for Work; The Medical Aspects.* Oxford University Press, Oxford (1995)

Chapter 9

Biological monitoring: general principles

P Hoet, V Haufroid, A Bernard and R Lauwerys

Introduction: definition and role of biological monitoring

The objective of biological monitoring is to prevent excessive exposure to chemicals that may cause acute or chronic adverse health effects [1]. In a first approach, the health risk may be assessed by comparing the value of the measured parameter with its currently estimated maximum permissible value in the medium analysed (the so-called biological limit value). This approach is called *biological monitoring of exposure*. Biological monitoring of exposure directly assesses the amount of a chemical effectively absorbed by the organism. Depending on the characteristics of the selected biological parameter and the conditions under which it is measured, the biological monitoring of exposure may be subdivided into two groups: the biological monitoring of internal dose and the biological monitoring of the target or biologically effective dose. The former relies on the determination of the chemical or its metabolites in body fluids and assesses the exposure of the whole organism. The latter is based on the determination of the amount of chemical bound to biologically relevant molecules and is therefore an indicator of the extent of exposure of what is believed to be the target tissue/organ in the body. The second approach is called *biological monitoring of early effects*. The marker of effect may be an endogenous component (such as enzyme) or a measure of the functional capacity of the body or organ system. There is a very large number of potential markers for assessing the bio-

logical effects of chemicals. They can be broadly divided into those that indicate toxic effects, such as biomarkers of liver dysfunction (e.g. serum enzymes) or renal dysfunction (e.g. microglobulinuria) and those detecting early biochemical changes or responses which are considered as reversible, non-adverse effects such as the inhibition of the erythrocyte enzyme delta-aminolaevulinic acid deshydratase by lead. These latter tests are often included in the biological monitoring programme of exposure.

The third approach is based on the use of susceptibility markers. The *biological monitoring of susceptibility* is a more recent approach which enables it to be verified whether an individual is particularly sensitive to the effect of a xenobiotic or to the effects of a group of compounds. This characteristic may be inherited or acquired.

A biological monitoring programme is usually reserved for chemicals which penetrate into the organism and exert systemic effects. For systemically active chemicals, biological monitoring represents the most effective approach for assessing the potential health risk, since a biological index of internal dose or effective dose is necessarily more closely related to a systemic effect than any environmental measurement. Very few biological tests have been proposed for the identification or the monitoring of chemicals present at the interface between the environment and the organism (the skin, gastrointestinal mucosa or respiratory tract mucosa), but the analysis of nickel in the nasal mucosa and the counting of asbestos bodies in sputum may be considered as examples of such tests.

Contrary to atmospheric monitoring, biological monitoring integrates the chemical absorption by all routes (pulmonary, oral, cutaneous) and from all possible sources (occupational, environmental, dietary, etc.). This is particularly useful when assessing the overall exposure to widely dispersed pollutants. Even for elements present in the environment under different chemical forms with different toxicities (e.g. inorganic arsenic in water or in the industrial setting and organic arsenic in marine organisms), it may still be possible correctly to estimate the health risk by speciation of the element in the biological medium analysed. Moreover, biological monitoring of exposure takes into account the various individual factors which influence the uptake or the absorption of the chemical, such as sex, age, physical activity, hygiene and nutritional status.

In general, the proper application of a biological test for determining the internal dose of a chemical requires the collection of relevant information on its metabolism (absorption, distribution, excretion), its toxicity and on the relationships between internal dose, external exposure and adverse effects. The knowledge of the latter permits the direct (from the internal dose–adverse effect relationship) or indirect (from the threshold limit value and the internal dose–external exposure relationship) estimation of the maximum permissible internal dose (biological limit value) [1,2]. Unfortunately, for many industrial chemicals, one or all of the preceding conditions are not fulfilled, which limits the possibilities of biological monitoring. As mentioned above, biological monitoring is usually not applicable to substances acting locally, nor is it useful for detecting peak exposures to rapidly acting substances. The detection of excessive exposure to these chemicals should mainly rely on the continuous monitoring of the pollutant concentration in the environment.

Methods in biological monitoring

Biological monitoring of internal dose

The great majority of the tests currently available for biological monitoring of exposure to industrial chemicals (*Table 9.1*) rely on the determination of the chemical or its metabolites in biological media. In practice, the biological samples most commonly used for analysis are urine, blood and to a lesser extent alveolar air. Analysis of other biological materials such as milk, fat, saliva, hair, nails, teeth and placenta is less frequent. As a general rule, urine is used for inorganic chemicals and for organic substances which are rapidly biotransformed to more water-soluble compounds; blood is used for most inorganic chemicals and for organic substances poorly biotransformed; alveolar air analysis is reserved for volatile compounds.

Tests measuring the chemical or its metabolites in biological media can be classified into two broad categories: *selective tests* and *non-selective tests*.

Selective tests

This category includes the majority of tests currently used in occupational medicine. The unchanged chemical is measured in biological media when the substance is not biotransformed (which is the case for nearly all inorganic chemicals), when it is poorly biotransformed (e.g. some solvents such as methylchloroform or tetrachloroethylene), when the exposure is too low for a significant amount of metabolite to be produced (such as very low exposure to benzene), or when a high degree of specificity is required. The determination of the unchanged chemical may indeed have a greater specificity than that of a metabolite that may be common to several substances.

Most organic chemicals are rapidly metabolized in the organism to more water-soluble compounds that are easily excreted via the urine or bile. Exposure to these chemicals is generally monitored by measuring specific urinary metabolites. These tests are more readily accepted by the workers because they do not require blood collection. Furthermore, they offer the advantage that when urine is collected at the appropriate time (at the end of a shift or in the morning of the next day), the concentration of the metabolite in urine is much less influenced by very recent exposure than that of the unchanged chemical in blood or in alveolar air.

Non-selective tests

These tests are used as non-specific indicators of exposure to a group of chemicals. Examples of

Table 9.1   Proposed methods for the biological monitoring of exposure to industrial chemicals

Chemical agent	Biological parameter	Biological material	Reference value	Tentative maximum permissible concentration	Remarks
A. INORGANIC AND ORGANOMETALLIC SUBSTANCES					
Aluminium	Aluminium	Serum	< 1 µg/100 ml	150 µg/g creatinine	
	Aluminium	Urine	< 50 µg/g creatinine		
Antimony	Antimony	Urine	< 1 µg/g creatinine	35 µg/g creatinine	
Arsenic	Total arsenic	Urine	< 40 µg/g creatinine		Influence of arsenic from marine origin
	Total arsenic	Blood	< 1 µg/g		
	Total arsenic	Hair	< 10 µg/g creatinine		
	Sum of inorganic arsenic and methylated metabolites	Urine		50 µg/g creatinine if TWA: 50 µg/m³ 30 µg/g creatinine if TWA: 10 µg/m³	Little interference of arsenic from marine origin
Barium	Barium	Urine	< 15 µg/g creatinine		
	Barium	Blood	< 0.8 µg/100 ml		
Beryllium	Beryllium	Urine	< 2 µg/g creatinine	5 µg/g creatinine	Non-smokers
Cadmium	Cadmium	Urine	< 2 µg/g creatinine	0.5 µg/100 ml	
	Cadmium	Blood	< 0.5 µg/100 ml		
	Metallothionein	Urine			
Carbon disulphide	Iodine-azide test	Urine		> 6.5 (Vasak index)	To detect exposure > 100 mg/m³
	2-Thiothiazolidine-4-carboxylic acid (TTCA)	Urine	< 1 mg/g creatinine	4 mg/g creatinine	
Chromium VI (soluble compounds)	Chromium	Urine	< 1 µg/g creatinine	30 µg/g creatinine	
	Chromium	Red blood cells			
Cobalt	Cobalt	Urine	< 2 µg/g creatinine	20 µg/g creatinine	
	Cobalt	Blood	< 0.2 µg/100 ml		
	Cobalt	Serum	< 0.05 µg/100 ml		
Copper	Copper	Serum	< 50 µg/100 ml		
	Copper	Serum	< 0.14 mg/100 ml		
Fluoride	Fluoride	Serum			
	Fluoride	Urine	< 0.5 mg/g creatinine	3–4 mg/g creatinine	Post-shift minus pre-shift value
Germanium	Germanium	Urine	< 1 µg/g creatinine		
Lead	Lead	Blood	< 25 µg/100 ml	40 µg/100 ml	
	Lead	Urine	< 50 µg/g creatinine	50 µg/g creatinine	
	Lead (after 1 g EDTA iv or 2 g DMSA po)	Urine	< 600 µg/24 h	600 µg/24 h	

Table 9.1 Proposed methods for the biological monitoring of exposure to industrial chemicals (*cont'd*)

Chemical agent	Biological parameter	Biological material	Reference value	Tentative maximum permissible concentration	Remarks
Lead (*cont'd*)	Free porphyrin	Red blood cells	< 75 µg/100 ml RBC	80 µg/100 ml RBC	
	Zinc protoporphyrin	Blood	< 40 µg/100 ml	40 µg/100 ml	
			< 2.5 µg/g Hb	3 µg/g Hb	
	δ-Aminolaevulinic acid (ALA)	Urine	< 4.5 mg/g creatinine	5 mg/g creatinine	
	Coproporphyrins	Urine	<100 µg/g creatinine	100 µg/g creatinine	
	ALA dehydratase	Red blood cells			
	Pyrimidine-5′-nucleotidase	Red blood cells			
Lead tetraethyl	Lead	Urine	< 50 µg/g creatinine	100 µg/g creatinine	
Manganese	Manganese	Urine	< 3 µg/g creatinine		
	Manganese	Blood	< 1 µg/100 ml		
Mercury inorganic	Mercury	Urine	< 5 µg/g creatinine	50 µg/g creatinine	
	Mercury	Blood	< 1 µg/100 ml	2 µg/100 ml	
	Mercury	Saliva			
Methylmercury	Mercury	Blood	< 1 µg/100 ml	10 µg/100 ml	
	Mercury	Hair			
Nickel (soluble compounds)	Nickel	Urine	< 2 µg/g creatinine	30 µg/g creatinine	
	Nickel	Plasma	< 0.05 µg/100 ml		
Nickel carbonyl	Nickel	Urine		60 µg/g creatinine	
Nitrous oxide	N₂O	Urine			
	N₂O	Expired air			
Selenium	Selenium	Serum	< 15 µg/100 ml		
	Selenium	Urine	< 25µg/g creatinine		
Silver	Silver	Urine	< 1 µg/g creatinine		
	Silver	Serum	< 0.5 µg/100 ml		
Tellurium	Tellurium	Urine	< 1 µg/g creatinine		
Thallium	Thallium	Urine	< 1 µg/g creatinine	50 µg/g creatinine	
	Thallium	Blood	< 0.1 µg/100 ml		
Uranium	Uranium	Urine	< 0.1 µg/g creatinine		
	Uranium	Blood	< 0.01 µg/100 ml		
Vanadium	Vanadium	Urine	< 1 µg/g creatinine		
	Vanadium	Blood	< 0.1 µg/100 ml		
Zinc	Zinc	Urine	< 0.9 mg/g creatinine		
	Zinc	Serum	<170 µg/100 ml		

Table 9.1 Proposed methods for the biological monitoring of exposure to industrial chemicals (*cont'd*)

Chemical agent	Biological parameter	Biological material	Reference value	Tentative maximum permissible concentration	Remarks
B. ORGANIC SUBSTANCES					
1. Non-substituted aliphatic and alicyclic hydrocarbons					
n-Hexane	2-Hexanol	Urine		0.2 mg/g creatinine	End first day of work
	2,5-Hexanedione	Urine		2 mg/g creatinine	End of workweek
				4 mg /g creatinine	During exposure
	n-Hexane	Blood		15 µg/100 ml	During exposure
	n-Hexane	Expired air		50 ppm	
2-Methyl-pentane	2-Methyl-2-pentanol	Urine			
	2-Methylpentane-2,4 diol	Urine			
	2-Methyl-pentane	Expired air		1500 µg/l	
	2-Methyl-pentane	Blood		35 µg/100 ml	
3-Methyl-pentane	3-Methyl-2-pentanol	Urine			
	3-Methyl-pentane	Expired air		1500 µg/l	
	3-Methyl-pentane	Blood		35 µg/100 ml	
Cyclohexane	Cyclohexanol	Urine		3.2 mg/g creatinine	
	1,2-Cyclohexane diol	Urine			
	1,4-Cyclohexane diol	Urine			
	Cyclohexane	Blood		45 µg/100 ml	During exposure
	Cyclohexane	Expired air		220 ppm	During exposure
2. Non-substituted aromatic hydrocarbons					
Benzene	Phenol	Urine	< 20 mg/g creatinine	45 mg/g creatinine	If TWA: 10 ppm
	Muconic acid	Urine		<20 mg/g creatinine	If TWA: 1 ppm
	Phenyl mercapturic acid	Urine	< 0.5 mg/g creatinine	1.4 mg/g creatinine	If TWA: 1ppm
	Benzene	Expired air		<0.022 ppm	If TWA: 1ppm (during exposure)
	Benzene	Blood		<2 µg/100 ml	If TWA: 1ppm (during exposure)
Toluene	Hippuric acid	Urine	< 1.5 g/g creatinine	2.5 g/g creatinine	If TWA: 100 ppm
				1.5 g/g creatinine	If TWA: 50 ppm
	O-cresol	Urine	< 0.3 mg/g creatinine	1 mg/g creatinine	If TWA: 100 ppm
				0.6 mg/g creatinine	If TWA: 50 ppm
	Toluene	Expired air		20 ppm	During exposure (if TWA: 100 ppm)
	Toluene	Blood		0.05 mg/100 ml	During exposure (if TWA: 100 ppm)
				0.005 mg/100 ml	18 h after end of exposure

Table 9.1   Proposed methods for the biological monitoring of exposure to industrial chemicals (*cont'd*)

Chemical agent	Biological parameter	Biological material	Reference value	Tentative maximum permissible concentration	Remarks
Ethylbenzene	Mandelic acid	Urine		1 g/g creatinine	
	Phenylglyoxylic acid	Urine			
	Ethylbenzene	Blood		0.15 mg/100 ml	During exposure
	Ethylbenzene	Expired air			
Cumene (isopropylbenzene)	2-Phenylpropanol	Urine		200 mg/g creatinine	
	Cumene	Expired air			
	Cumene	Blood			
Trimethylbenzenes (mesitylene, pseudocumene, white spirit)	Dimethylbenzoic acids	Urine			
Styrene	Mandelic acid	Urine		800 mg/g creatinine	16 h after end of exposure
	Phenylglyoxylic acid	Urine		250 mg/g creatinine	
	Styrene	Blood		0.1 mg/100 ml 0.002 mg/100 ml	
	Styrene	Expired air		9 ppm	
	Styrene	Urine		50 µg/l	
α-Methylstyrene	Atrolactic acid	Urine		1.5 g/g creatinine	
Xylene	Methylhippuric acid	Urine			
	Xylene	Blood		0.3 mg/100 ml	During exposure
	Xylene	Expired air			
Naphthalene	1-Naphthol	Urine			
Biphenyl	2- and 4-Hydroxy-biphenyl	Urine		1.5 mg/g creatinine	
Polycyclic hydrocarbons	1-Hydroxypyrene	Urine	<2 µg/g creatinine (<1 µmol/mol creatinine)	2.7 µg/g creatinine (<1.4 µmol/mol creatinine)	
	Haemoglobin adducts	Red blood cells			
	DNA adducts	Lymphocytes			
3. Halogenated hydrocarbons					
Monochloromethane (methylchloride)	S-methylcysteine	Urine			
Monobromomethane (methylbromide)	S-methylcysteine	Urine			
	Bromide	Blood	< 1 mg/100 ml		
	Bromide	Urine	< 10 mg/l		
Dichloromethane	HbCO	Blood	< 1%	2%	Non-smokers
	Dichloromethane	Blood		0.05 mg/100 ml	
	Dichloromethane	Expired air		15 ppm	
1,2-Dibromoethane	N-acetyl-S-(2-hydroxyethyl) cysteine	Urine			

Table 9.1 Proposed methods for the biological monitoring of exposure to industrial chemicals (cont'd)

Chemical agent	Biological parameter	Biological material	Reference value	Tentative maximum permissible concentration	Remarks
Vinyl chloride	Thiodiglycolic acid	Urine	< 2 mg/g creatinine		
Trichloroethylene	Trichloroethanol	Urine		150 mg/g creatinine	
	Trichloroacetic acid	Urine		75 mg/g creatinine	After 5 d exposure
	Trichloroethanol	Plasma		0.25 mg/100 ml	16 h after the end of exposure
	Trichloroethylene	Expired air		0.5 ppm	During exposure
				10 ppm	After 5 d exposure
	Trichloroacetic acid	Plasma		5 mg/100 ml	During exposure
	Trichloroethylene	Blood		0.06 mg/100 ml	End of workweek
1,1,1-Trichloroethane (methylchloroform)	Trichloroethanol + trichloroacetic acid	Urine		40 mg/g creatinine	
	Trichloroacetic acid	Urine		10 mg/g creatinine	End of workweek
	Trichloroethanol	Urine		30 mg/g creatinine	
	Trichloroethanol	Blood		0.1 mg/100 ml	
	Trichloroethane	Blood		100 µg/100 ml	
	Trichloroethane	Urine		800 µg/g creatinine	
	Trichloroethane	Expired air		30 ppm	16 h after the end of exposure
	Tetrachloroethylene	Expired air		60 ppm	During exposure
Tetrachloroethylene	Tetrachloroethylene	Blood		8 ppm	16 h after the end of exposure
	Tetrachloroethylene	Urine		100 µg/100 ml	16 h after the end of exposure
	Trichloroacetic acid	Urine		70 µg/g creatinine	16 h after the end of exposure
				5 mg/g creatinine	End-of-week
Hexachloroethane	Hexachloroethane	Plasma			
Hexachlorobutadiene	Hexachlorobutadiene	Blood			
Monochlorobenzene	4-Chlorocatechol	Urine			
	4-Chlorophenol	Urine			
p-Dichlorobenzene	p-Dichlorobenzene	Urine			
	2,5-Dichlorophenol	Urine		250 µg/g creatinine	
o-Dichlorobenzene	2,3- and 3,4-Dichlorophenols	Urine			
	3,4- and 4,5-Dichlorocatechols	Urine			
Halothane	Trifluoroacetic acid	Urine		10 mg/g creatinine	After 5 d exposure (if TWA: 5 ppm)
	Trifluoroacetic acid	Blood		0.25 mg/100 ml	After 5 d exposure (if TWA: 5 ppm)
	Halothane	Urine		90 µg/g creatinine	If TWA: 50 ppm
				10 µg/g creatinine	If TWA: 5 ppm
	Halothane	Expired air		0.5 ppm	If TWA: 5 ppm
Enflurane (Ethrane)	Enflurane	Urine			
1,1-Dichloro-2,2,2-trifluoroethane (HCFC-123)	Trifluoroacetic acid	Urine		3.5 µg/l	

Table 9.1 Proposed methods for the biological monitoring of exposure to industrial chemicals (*cont'd*)

Chemical agent	Biological parameter	Biological material	Reference value	Tentative maximum permissible concentration	Remarks
1-Chloro-1,2,2,2-tetrafluoroethane (HCFC-124)	Trifluoroacetic acid Fluoride	Urine Urine			
1,2,2,2-Tetrafluoroethane (HCFC-134a)	Trifluoroacetic acid	Urine			
2,3,7,8-Tetrachloro-dibenzo-p-dioxine (TCDD)	TCDD TCDD	Serum Blood			
Polychlorinated biphenyl	Polychlorinated biphenyl	Serum Adipose tissue Blood			
	Trichlorobiphenyl	Blood			
Other volatile halogenated hydrocarbons (carbon tetrachloride, chloroform, halogenated anaesthesics, etc.)	substances	Expired air Blood			
4. Amino- and nitroderivatives					
Triethylamine (TEA)	TEA + triethylamine-*N*-oxide	Urine		60 mg/g creatinine	If TWA: 2.5 ppm
Dimethylethylamine (DMEA)	DMEA + dimethylethylamine-*N*-oxide	Urine		90 mg/g creatinine	If TWA: 5 ppm
Aniline	Aniline	Urine			
	p-Aminophenol	Urine		30 mg/g creatinine	
	Methaemoglobin	Blood	<2%	5%	
	Aniline released from haemoglobin adducts	Blood		10 µg/100 ml	
Nitroglycerine	Nitroglycerine	Blood			
Ethyleneglycol dinitrate	Ethyleneglycol dinitrate	Urine			
	Ethyleneglycol dinitrate	Blood			
Isopropylnitrate	Isopropylnitrate	Blood			
	Isopropylnitrate	Urine			
	Isopropylnitrate	Expired air			
Several aromatic amino- and nitro-compounds	Methaemoglobin	Blood	<2%		
	Diazo-positive metabolite	Urine			
	Parent compounds, e.g. benzidine, β-naphthylamine	Urine			
	Haemoglobin adducts	Blood			
Nitrobenzene	*p*-Nitrophenol	Urine		5 mg/g creatinine	
	Methaemoglobin	Blood	<2%	5%	

Table 9.1 Proposed methods for the biological monitoring of exposure to industrial chemicals (*cont'd*)

Chemical agent	Biological parameter	Biological material	Reference value	Tentative maximum permissible concentration	Remarks
4,4'-Methylene bis (2-chloroaniline) or MO-CA	MOCA	Urine			
Methylene dianiline or MDA	MDA	Urine			
Benzidine-derived azo compounds	Benzidine	Urine			
Monoacetylbenzidine derived azo compounds	Monoacetylbenzidine	Urine			
2,4-Dinitrotoluene	2,4-Dinitrobenzoic acid	Urine			
Hydrazine	Hydrazine	Urine			
Trinitrotoluene	2,4 and 2,6-Dinitroaminotoluene	Urine			
	Trinitrotoluene	Urine			
5. Alcohols					
Methanol	Methanol	Urine	< 2.5 mg/g creatinine	25 mg/g creatinine	
	Methanol	Blood			
	Formic acid	Urine	< 60 mg/g creatinine		
	Formic acid	Blood			
Isopropanol	Acetone	Urine	< 2 mg/g creatinine	30 mg/g creatinine	
	Isopropanol	Expired air		500 mg/m^3	
Furfuryl alcohol	Furoic acid	Urine	< 65 mg/g creatinine		
6. Glycols and derivatives					
Ethyleneglycol	Oxalic acid	Urine			
	Glycolic acid	Urine	< 50 mg/g creatinine		
	Ethyleneglycol	Serum			
Ethyleneglycol monomethylether (methylcellosolve)	Methoxyacetic acid	Urine			
Ethyleneglycol monoethylether (ethylcellosolve or 2-ethoxyethanol)	Ethoxyacetic acid	Urine		150 mg/g creatinine	If TWA: 5 ppm
Ethyleneglycol monoethylether acetate (2-ethoxyethanol acetate)	Ethoxyacetic acid	Urine		150 mg/g creatinine	If TWA: 5 ppm
Ethyleneglycol monobutylether (butylcellosolve)	Butoxyacetic acid	Urine			
Ethyleneglycol phenylether (phenylcellosolve)	Phenoxyacetic acid	Urine			

Table 9.1 Proposed methods for the biological monitoring of exposure to industrial chemicals (*cont'd*)

Chemical agent	Biological parameter	Biological material	Reference value	Tentative maximum permissible concentration	Remarks
Propyleneglycol monomethylether γ-isomer (1-methoxy-2-propanol)	Propyleneglycol (1,2-propanediol)	Urine			
	Propyleneglycol monomethylether	Blood		4 mg/100 ml	
	Propyleneglycol monomethylether	Urine		10 mg/g creatinine	
Propyleneglycol monomethylether β-isomer (2-methoxy-1-propanol)	Methoxypropionic acid	Urine			
Dioxane	β-Hydroxyethoxyacetic acid	Urine			
7. Ketones					
Acetone	Acetone	Urine	< 2 mg/g creatinine	30 mg/g creatinine	
	Acetone	Blood	< 0.2 mg/100 ml	5 mg/100 ml	
	Acetone	Expired air			
Cyclohexanone	Cyclohexanol	Urine		20 mg/g creatinine	
	1,2-cyclohexane diol	Urine			
	1,4-cyclohexane diol	Urine			
Methylethylketone	Methylethylketone	Urine		2.5 mg/g creatinine	
	Methylethylketone	Blood			
	Methylethylketone	Expired air			
	3-Hydroxy-2-butanone	Urine			
Methyl-*n*-butylketone	2,5-Hexanedione	Urine		4 mg/g creatinine	End of the workweek
Methylisobutylketone	Methylisobutylketone	Urine		0.5 mg/g creatinine	
8. Ethers					
Tetrahydrofurane	Tetrahydrofurane	Urine			
9. Aldehydes					
Furfural	Furoic acid	Urine	<65 mg/g creatinine	80 mg/g creatinine	
10. Amides and Anhydrides					
Dimethylformamide	*N*-methylformamide†	Urine		30 mg/g creatinine	
	Dimethylformamide	Blood		0.15 mg/100 ml	
	N-methylformamide†	Blood		0.1 mg/100 ml	
	Dimethylformamide	Expired air		2.5 ppm	
	N-acetyl-*S*-(*N*-methylcarbamoyl) cysteine	Urine		40 mg/g creatinine	During exposure
Dimethylacetamide	*N*-methylacetamide	Urine		35 mg/g creatinine	
Acrylamide	*S*-(2-carboxyethyl cysteine)	Urine			
	Haemoglobin adducts	Red blood cells			
Maleic anhydride	Maleic acid	Urine	< 1.5 mg/g creatinine		

Table 9.1 Proposed methods for the biological monitoring of exposure to industrial chemicals (*cont'd*)

Chemical agent	Biological parameter	Biological material	Reference value	Tentative maximum permissible concentration	Remarks
Phthalic anhydride	Phthalic acid	Urine		8 mg/g creatinine	If TWA: 1 ppm
Hexahydrophthalic anhydride	Hexahydrophthalic acid	Urine		8 mg/g creatinine	If TWA: 0.1 ppm
11. *Esters*					
Phthalic acid esters	Phthalic acid	Urine			
Methylmethacrylate	Methacrylic acid	Urine			
12. *Phenols*					
Phenol	Phenol	Urine	<20 mg/g creatinine	250 mg/g creatinine	
p-tert-Butylphenol	p-tert-Butylphenol	Urine		2 mg/g creatinine	
13. *Asphyxiants*					
Carbon monoxide	Carboxyhaemoglobin	Blood	< 1%	3.5%	Non-smokers
	Carbon monoxide	Blood	< 0.15 ml/100 ml	7 ml/100 ml	Non-smokers
	Carbon monoxide	Expired air	< 2 ppm	12 ppm	Non-smokers
Cyanides and aliphatic	Thiocyanate	Urine	< 6 mg/g creatinine		Non-smokers
nitriles	Thiocyanate	Plasma	< 0.6 mg/100 ml		Non-smokers
	Cyanide	Blood	<10 µg/100 ml		Non-smokers
		Blood	<50 µg/100 ml		Smokers
	SCN (mg/g creatinine) Urine + blood			3	
Acrylonitrile	HBCO (%) Acrylonitrile	Urine			
	Thiocyanate	Urine	< 6 mg/g creatinine		Non-smokers
Methaemoglobin-forming agents except for specific compounds mentioned elsewhere	Methaemoglobin	Blood	< 2%	5%	
14. *Pesticides*					
Organophosphorus	Cholinesterase	Red blood cells		30% inhibition	
	Cholinesterase	Plasma		50% inhibition	
	Cholinesterase	Whole blood		30% inhibition	
	Dialkylphosphates	Urine			
Parathion	p-Nitrophenol	Urine		0.5 mg/g creatinine	
Carbamates insecticides	Cholinesterase	Red blood cells		30% inhibition	
	Cholinesterase	Plasma		50% inhibition	
	Cholinesterase	Whole blood		30% inhibition	
Carbaryl	1-Naphthol	Urine		10 mg/g creatinine	
Baygon	2-Isopropoxyphenol	Urine			

Table 9.1 Proposed methods for the biological monitoring of exposure to industrial chemicals *(cont'd)*

Chemical agent	Biological parameter	Biological material	Reference value	Tentative maximum permissible concentration	Remarks
DDT	DDT	Serum			
	DDT+DDE+DDD	Blood	<10 µg/100 ml	15µg/100 ml	
	DDA	Urine			
Dieldrin	Dieldrin	Blood	< 1 µg/100 ml	1 µg/100 ml	
	Dieldrin	Urine			
Lindane	Lindane	Blood		2 µg/100 ml	
Endrin	Endrin	Blood		5 µg/100 ml	
	Anti-12-hydroxy-endrin	Urine	< 1 µg/g creatinine	0.13 mg/g creatinine	
Hexachlorobenzene	Hexachlorobenzene	Blood	< 0.3 µg/100 ml	30 µg/100 ml	
	2,4,5-Trichlorophenol	Urine			
	Pentachlorophenol	Urine	<30 µg/g creatinine		
Pentachlorophenol	Pentachlorophenol	Urine	<30 µg/g creatinine	1 mg/g creatinine	
	Pentachlorophenol	Plasma		0.05 mg/100 ml	
Chlorophenoxyacetic acid derivatives (2,4-D; 2,4,5-T; MCPA)	2,4-D	Urine			
	2,4,5-T	Urine			
	MCPA	Urine			
Synthetic pyrethroids	Cyclopropane carboxylic acid	Urine			
Dinitroorthocresol	Dinitroorthocresol	Blood		1 mg/100 ml	
	Amino-4-nitro-orthocresol	Urine			
Chlordimeform	2-Methyl-4-chloroaniline	Urine			
Captan	Tetrahydrophthalimide	Urine			
Ethylene oxide	Ethylene oxide	Expired air		0.5 mg/m³	During exposure
	Ethylene oxide	Blood		0.8 µg/100 ml	During exposure
	N-acetyl-*S*-(2-hydroxyethyl) cysteine	Urine			
15. *Hormones* Diethylstilboestrol	Diethylstilboestrol	Urine		30 mg/g creatinine	24-h urine collection
16. *Mutagenic and carcinogenic substances*	• Mutagenic activity	Urine		Comparison with a control group	
	• Thioethers	Urine			
	• Chromosome analysis	Lymphocytes			
	• Spermatozoa analysis	Sperm			
	• Protein adducts	Blood			
	• DNA adducts	Lymphocytes			
	• Nucleic acid adducts	Urine			
	• Oncogen proteins	Serum			

Table 9.1 Proposed methods for the biological monitoring of exposure to industrial chemicals (*cont'd*)

Chemical agent	Biological parameter	Biological material	Reference value	Tentative maximum permissible concentration	Remarks
17. Other substances					
Cyclophosphamide	Cyclophosphamide	Urine			
Ethylene oxide	Ethylene oxide	Expired air		0.5 mg/m³	
	Ethylene oxide	Blood		0.8 µg/100 ml	
	N-acetyl-S-(2-hydroxyethyl) cysteine	Urine			
Toluene diisocyanate	Toluenediamine	Urine			
Hexamethylene diisocyanate	Hexamethylenediamine	Urine			
4,4'-Methylenedipheny-l diisocyanate	4,4'-Methylenedianiline	Urine			
Tobacco smoke	Cotinine	Urine			

Analyses performed on biological materials collected at the end of the workday unless otherwise indicated.
†The metabolites measured as N-methylformamide by gas chromatography is mainly N-hydroxymethyl-N-methylformamide.

non-selective exposure tests currently available are given below.

Determination of diazopositive metabolites in urine

This test has been proposed to monitor exposure to aromatic amines.

Analysis of thioethers in urine

The urinary excretion of thioethers increases following exposure to electrophilic substances and has been proposed to monitor occupational exposure to carcinogenic or mutagenic substances. The specificity of this test is, however, limited: the urinary excretion of thioethers may be increased by several compounds that are not carcinogenic or mutagenic (e.g. toluene, *o*-xylene or biphenyl), various endogenous substances are also eliminated in urine as thioethers, and finally, smoking is an important confounding factor.

Determination of the mutagenic activity in urine

An enhanced mutagenic activity has been observed in the urine of many groups of workers such as rubber workers, coke plant workers, workers exposed to epichlorhydrin, anaesthetists and nurses handling cytostatic drugs. As with the thioether test, smoking is an important confounding factor. In smokers, the mutagenic activity of the urine is increased proportionally to the daily cigarette consumption.

Because of their lack of specificity and the existence of a large individual variability, non-selective tests cannot be used to monitor exposure on an individual basis. However, when an adequate control group is used as a reference, they may be useful qualitatively to identify groups at risk.

Non-invasive methods have also been developed for measuring the *in vivo* metal content of selected tissues. These methods, which are usually based on neutron activation or on X-ray fluorescence techniques, have been applied for the determination of cadmium in kidney or liver, of lead in bones and of mercury in the central nervous system and bones [3,4]. They enable the monitoring of the long-term retention of heavy metals in the organism and, in some cases, the target organ dose (e.g. cadmium in the kidney).

Biological monitoring of effective dose

The most useful biological monitoring methods are those which directly measure the amount of active chemical bound to the target molecule (the target dose). When feasible, that is, when the target site is readily accessible, these methods may assess the health risk more accurately than any other monitoring test. The most known test of this category is the determination of carboxyhaemoglobin in venous blood induced by exposure to carbon monoxide (or dichloromethane metabolized into carbon monoxide). However, one should remember that exposure to carbon monoxide is certainly not specific to occupational activities and that tobacco smoking is a major source of exposure to carbon monoxide.

Progress in this approach comes from the determination of macromolecule adducts mainly in relation with exposure to potentially genotoxic substances. DNA adducts can be measured in blood as indicators of the target tissue's DNA exposure to reactive substances. In some cases, however, the amount of DNA obtained from white blood cells or lymphocytes may be insufficient and, more importantly, DNA adducts can be removed by DNA repair processes or by cell death. An alternative consists of measuring the adducts formed with non-target macromolecules such as proteins (albumin, haemoglobin). These are present in large quantities in human blood. Since they are not repaired, haemoglobin adducts reflect the cumulative exposure during the lifetime of the protein (4 months). However, as chemicals may vary in their ability to cross the erythrocyte membrane, the degree of alkylation of serum albumin (lifetime 21 days) might constitute a better index of exposure, at least for some electrophilic compounds. Macromolecule adducts have been used recently for the biomonitoring of occupational exposure to aromatic amines, ethylene oxide, styrene, 1,3-butadiene, to complex mixtures of polycyclic aromatic hydrocarbons (PAH) in iron foundries, coke oven, aluminium plants, among roofers and surface-coating workers [5,6].

They seem very promising methods, but much research is still needed before they can be introduced into the routine biological monitoring of industrial workers.

Biological monitoring of early non-adverse effect(s)

Biological effect monitoring is defined as the measurement of a reversible biochemical change caused by the absorption of the substance, the degree of change being below that associated with toxic injury and not associated with a known irreversible pathological effect [7]. Thus, the biological monitoring of effects relies on the identification and the quantification of reversible, non-adverse biological effects related to the internal dose. A biological effect is considered as non-adverse if the functional or physical integrity of the organism is not diminished, if the ability of the organism to face an additional stress (homeostasis) is not decreased or if these impairments are not likely to occur in the near future (delayed toxicity). These tests might predict the occurrence of adverse effects if exposure is not reduced, but are to be distinguished from the tests identifying health effects. However, the distinction between adverse and non-adverse biological effects is not always clear cut and is sometimes arbitrary, since it may be difficult to evaluate the health significance of an effect.

There is a very large number of potential markers for determining the non-adverse biological effects of chemicals and only a few examples are indicated mainly:

1 The inhibition of pseudocholinesterase by organophosphorus pesticides.
2 The inhibition of the erythrocyte enzyme δ-aminolaevulinic acid dehydratase by lead.
3 The determination of the 6β-hydroxycortisol/17-hydroxycorticosteroid ratio as an index of exposure to chemicals inducing microsomal enzymes (e.g. organochlorine compounds and polycyclic hydrocarbons [8]).

The determination of the activity of most enzymes in blood (e.g. transaminases) or proteins and enzymes in urines (e.g. β_2-microglobuline, *N*-acetyl-β-D-glucosaminidase) usually indicates adverse effects rather than reversible biochemical changes. These tests are therefore more adequate for an early detection of a health impairment programme than for biological monitoring of non-adverse reversible effects.

Biological monitoring of susceptibility

Based on presumed aetiology, susceptibility can often be separated into three categories: genetic (inherited factors seem to be involved in determining many toxic effects of xenobiotics), constitutional (sex, age, pregnancy are possible determinants of individual susceptibility) and environmental (an individual's resistance toward chemical toxicity may also be affected by other environmental exposure, e.g. diet and lifestyle) [9].

Increasing interest has focused on determining the role of genetic variations in toxic responses and hence variations in susceptibility. Genetic variations in glutathione S-transferases, N-acetyltransferases, paraoxonase, cytochrome P_{450} exemplify the relationship of metabolic variations to individual susceptibility to cancer and other diseases of environmental origin (for review see [10]). The possibility that subjects with high paraoxonase activity may be protected from the toxic effects of parathion has indeed been suggested. An excess of slow acetylators among workers exposed to aromatic amines with urinary bladder cancer and rapid acetylators with colorectal cancer has also been observed.

Human cytochromes P_{450} constitute a great family of mixed function mono-oxygenases. The major tissue contributing to cytochrome P_{450} activity is the liver, but many other tissues express these enzymes in a tissue-specific manner. A number of cytochromes P_{450} involved in the metabolism of xenobiotics are known to be polymorphically expressed in humans [11,12].

Criteria for selecting biological tests

In practice, only a few biological tests can be used routinely to monitor exposure to industrial chemicals. Before a biological monitoring programme is implemented, the most appropriate parameter (or parameters) must be selected by taking into account:

1 Its specificity.
2 Its sensitivity; there should be a strong relationship between the parameter and external exposure, and this relationship must exist at exposure levels below those associated with adverse effects.

3 The analytical and biological variability of the test.
4 The applicability of the test, including cost and possible discomfort for the subject.
5 The capability of the test to evaluate a risk to health.

In this context, the existence of a biological limit value is an important element which must be taken into account when selecting a biological monitoring test. Tests which can estimate the target dose or the target organ dose should be preferred to assess the risk to health. When a chemical is not toxic by itself and must be metabolically activated before affecting the target site, the determination of the reactive chemical may be more relevant than that of the parent compound or of any other metabolite not directly related to the toxic effects. For example, to assess the risk linked with exposure to *n*-hexane or methyl-*n*-butylketone, it might be more relevant to measure 2,5-hexanedione in blood or in urine than to determine these solvents directly in blood or expired air.

Interpretation of results

Results can be interpreted on an individual basis. However, this is only possible if the intra-individual variability of the parameter is small and its specificity is high. The results may also be interpreted on a group basis by considering their distribution. If all the observed values are below the biological limit value, the working conditions are satisfactory. If all, or the majority, of the results are above the biological limit value, the overall exposure conditions must certainly be corrected. A third condition may also occur: the majority of the workers may have values below the biological limit level, but a few have abnormally high values (the distribution is bimodal or polymodal). Two interpretations can be put forward:

1 Either the subjects with the high values perform activities exposing them to higher levels of the pollutant, in which case the biological monitoring programme has identified job categories for which work conditions need to be improved.
2 These workers do not perform different activities and, in this case, their higher internal dose must result from different hygiene habits, or from non-occupational exposure or polymorphism if a metabolite is measured.

When interpreting the results, it must be kept in mind that the metabolism of xenobiotics may be influenced by various endogenous or exogenous factors. As mentioned above, endogenous factors may be genetic or pathophysiological, such as age, sex and diseases. For instance, hepatic insufficiency may be associated with a decreased biotransformation of xenobiotics, whereas renal diseases may impair their elimination in the urine. Alcohol consumption is a frequent exogenous confounding factor. In the body, ethanol is transformed to acetate by two successive oxidations, one catalysed by alchohol dehydrogenase and the other by aldehyde dehydrogenase. This metabolic pathway is not specific to ethanol, and many other organic compounds including some solvents may be oxidized by the same enzymes. When these substances are absorbed concomitantly with ethanol, metabolic interferences may occur. In man, ethanol has been shown to inhibit the oxidation of methanol, ethyleneglycol derivatives, trichloroethylene, xylene, toluene and styrene.

This inhibition of the biotransformation of a solvent following the ingestion of a large dose of alcohol may also result in a rise of the blood levels of the solvent. But when alcohol is regularly consumed, the opposite may be observed. In workers exposed to toluene, Waldron and colleagues [13] found that blood toluene concentrations were lower in those who drank regularly. Presumably, this results from the induction by alcohol of the microsomal oxidizing system of the liver. The interference of alcoholic beverage consumption with biological monitoring to chemicals has been recently reviewed [14]. The author concludes that 'because of the possible profound change in biological levels of exposure indicators, intake of alcoholic beverages should be avoided on the day when samples for biological monitoring are collected'.

Many other substances, for example barbiturates, polycyclic hydrocarbons and the organochlorine pesticides, are inducers of microsomal enzymes, and may therefore interfere with the biotransformation of xenobiotics.

Smoking may also be a confounding factor. For example, it may increase the urinary excretion of orthocresol or of trans, trans-muconic acid and other benzene-related compounds, probably because cigarette smoke contains orthocresol and benzene [15,16]. Smoking must also be taken into account when monitoring the mutagenic activity of urine or its thioether concentration. Finally, confounding may also arise from the diet, the consumption of drugs, or the exposure to several industrial chemicals, such as mixed exposure to phenol and benzene.

Analytical aspects

In any monitoring programme, the analytical aspect is of paramount importance. The parameter selected must be sufficiently stable to allow the transportation of the sample and possibly its storage for a few days. Therefore, before a new programme of biological monitoring is implemented, preliminary investigations must be conducted to test its stability under the conditions of sampling (including the type of container, stability in the biological fluid and the effect of physical factors). The laboratory responsible for the analysis must adopt good laboratory practices, which involves the use of a well-standardized method and the implementation of regular internal and external quality-control programmes.

Ethical aspects

Finally, it must be kept in mind that in biological monitoring, humans are used as an integrator of exposure. The ethical aspects must receive a great deal of attention [17]. In particular, biological monitoring of susceptibility has raised many problems, such as the risk of its use for worker selection. The monitoring procedure itself must also be without health risks. Sufficient information must be given to the subjects before and after monitoring and the individual results must remain confidential.

References

1. Lauwerys, R. and Hoet, P. *Industrial Chemical Exposure: Guidelines for Biological Monitoring.* Lewis Publishers, Boca Raton, Florida (1993)
2. Bernard, A. and Lauwerys, R. General principles of biological monitoring of exposure to organic chemicals. In *Biological Monitoring of Exposure to Chemicals*, Vol. 1, *Organic Compounds* (eds M.H. Ho and H.K. Dillon). John Wiley, New York (1986)
3. Lauwerys, R. *In vivo* tests to monitor body burdens of toxic metals in man. In *Chemical Toxicology and Clinical Chemistry of Metals* (eds S. Brown and J. Savory). Academic Press, New York (1983)
4. Nilsson, U. and Skerfving, S. *In vivo* X-ray fluorescence measurements of cadmium and lead. *Scandinavian Journal of Work and Environmental Health*, **19** (Suppl. 1), 54–58 (1993)
5. Adamkiewicz, J., Nehls, P. and Rajewsky, M.F. Immunological methods for detection of carcinogen-DNA adducts. In *Monitoring Human Exposure to Carcinogenic and Mutagenic Agents.* IARC, Lyon (1984)
6. Hemminki, K., Dipple, A., Shuker, D. *et al.* (eds). *DNA Adducts: Identification and Biological Significance.* IARC, Lyon (1994)
7. Health and Safety Executive, UK. Biological monitoring for chemical exposures in the workplace. *Guidance Note EH56 from Environmental Hygiene Series.* HMSO, London (1992)
8. Hugget, R., Kimerle, R., Mehrle, P. *et al.* *Biomarkers. Biochemical, Physiological and Histological Markers of Anthropogenic Stress.* Lewis Publishers, Chelsea, MI (1992)
9. Grandjean, Ph. Individual susceptibility in occupational and environmental toxicology. *Toxicology Letters*, **77**, 105–108 (1995)
10. Weber, W. Influence of heredity on human sensitivity to environmental chemicals. *Environmental and Molecular Mutagenesis*, **25** (Suppl. 26), 102–114 (1995)
11. Smith, C., Smith, G. and Wolf, C. Genetic polymorphisms in xenobiotic metabolism. *European Journal of Cancer*, **30A**, 1929–1935 (1994)
12. Wrighton, S. and Stevens, J. The human hepatic cytochromes P_{450} involved in drug metabolism. *Critical Reviews in Toxicology*, **22**, 1–21 (1992)
13. Waldron, H.A., Cherry, N. and Johnston, J.D. Effects of ethanol on blood toluene concentrations. *International Archives of Occupational and Environmental Health*, **51**, 365–369 (1983)
14. Fiserova-Bergerova, V. Biological monitoring: VIII: Interference of alcoholic beverage consumption with biological monitoring of occupational exposure to industrial chemicals. *Applied Occupational Environmental Hygiene*, **8**, 757–760 (1993)
15. Dossing, M., Bachum, J., Hansen, S.H. *et al.* Urinary hippuric acid and ortho-cresol excretion in man during experimental exposure to toluene. *British Journal of Industrial Medicine*, **40**, 470–473 (1983)
16. Ong, C., Lee, B., Shi, C. *et al.* Elevated levels of benzene-related compounds in the urine of cigarette smokers. *International Journal of Cancer*, **59**, 177–180 (1994)
17. Rothstein, M. Legal and ethical aspects of medical screening. *Occupational Medicine: State of the Art Reviews*, **11**, 31–39 (1996)

Chapter 10

Biological monitoring and genotoxicity

B Hellman

Introduction

Chemical interactions with DNA, primary DNA damage, gene mutations, chromosomal aberrations and other types of genetic alterations, including various changes in the expression of phenotypes, are increasingly used as 'molecular biomarkers' for exposure, disease, susceptibility and/or mechanisms of action in experimental and epidemiological studies. DNA adducts, DNA strand breaks, base pair substitutions, gene amplifications, chromosomal translocations, genomic mutations and other genetic end-points have, so far, been used mainly for biomonitoring purposes (to increase the precision of exposure data and/or to associate early biological responses with the probability of a disease outcome), and in cancer risk assessments. However, the same types of genetic end-points are also used in studies of the biological mechanisms of tumour development and in studies on the phenotypic expression of genetic diseases. Some of the end-points have also been used as molecular biomarkers in studies of other types of diseases (e.g. infectious and cardiovascular diseases).

It should be emphasized that most researchers using various types of genetic alterations for biomonitoring purposes are working with an inadequate and unbalanced set of genetic end-points and functional polymorphisms. The plethora of genotoxic effects and other genetic alterations that have been suggested as molecular biomarkers for exposure, disease and/or individual susceptibility are indeed promising research tools, and they may very well improve the potentialities of future aetiological cancer epidemiology, but there is still a long way to go before DNA adducts, DNA strand breaks, gene mutations, chromosomal aberrations and other molecular biomarkers based on genetic alterations can be used with confidence for biomonitoring purposes and in cancer risk assessments. The fact that the area of 'molecular epidemiology' is still in its infancy has also been emphasized in a recent report from the WHO Regional Office for Europe [1], stating that: *'The current level of uncertainty related to the contribution to risk for most markers should be strongly emphasized, because many researchers are using these markers in intervention studies as if the relations were clearly understood.'*

'Molecular epidemiology'

Epidemiological studies using various types of genetic alterations as molecular biomarkers to increase the precision of exposure data, to control for confounders when assessing a potential relationship between exposure and disease, to increase the precision of measurements of effects, for early detection of various adverse health effects and diseases and/or to identify particular risk groups in the population, are all examples of studies in molecular epidemiology. However, the concept of 'molecular epidemiology' is not that easy to define unequivocally, and the term is often used in a rather broad sense to describe that some kind of a molecular, biochemical or cellular measurement has been used in epidemiological research.

The main focus in epidemiological studies using various types of genetic alterations as 'molecular biomarkers' is usually directed either towards malignant diseases following from mutations in somatic cells ('molecular cancer epidemiology') or towards genetic diseases following from mutations in germ cells ('genetic epidemiology'). Similar types of genetic alterations are used in both types of study, and they are used both for health risk assessments and for clinical diagnosis of various diseases. If a particular molecular biomarker is going to be used for the purpose of risk assessment, it is an absolute prerequisite that the characteristic parameters of the adverse health effect of interest have been identified and validated, and that the specificity and sensitivity of the molecular biomarker and its method of measurement have been established [2]. A molecular biomarker that is going to be used for diagnostic purposes can only be used with confidence if there is a well-established relationship between the biological marker and the clinical disease of interest.

Molecular epidemiology is obviously a multi-disciplinary science focusing on the importance of various interactions between genetic and environmental factors, and the subsequent development of different types of complex diseases. It is a typical hybrid science, requiring a combination of both laboratory techniques and traditional epidemiological methods. If this type of study is to be successful, it should involve both laboratory scientists and field researchers. Depending on the techniques used, the laboratory researchers are typically experts in analytical chemistry, genetic toxicology or molecular biology. Depending on the issue at question, the field researchers are typically geneticists (focused on hereditary diseases, pedigrees and genetic counselling), oncologists (trying to understand the genesis of various malignant diseases) or specialists in occupational and environmental medicine (focusing on aetiological factors for tumour development and other common diseases from a preventive public health perspective).

The interaction between the laboratory oriented scientists and the traditionally oriented epidemiologists is not without complications. Differences in traditions and the way of defining basic concepts (such as the meaning of 'validity' and 'control group') will inevitably lead to confusion. The situation becomes even more complex when these scientists communicate their findings to the general public, trying to interpret the meaning of a reported change in a certain type of genetic endpoint in, for example, blood samples from a restricted number of people exposed to a given toxicant.

Genetic alterations as 'molecular biomarkers' in risk assessments

Nowadays, the regulation of new chemicals relies almost completely on toxicological testing using experimental animals. This testing (i.e. hazard identification) is usually performed before any substantial human exposure has occurred. However, animal toxicity data cannot predict with absolute certainty the final outcome for human exposure when it comes to, for example, occupational exposures at various industrial settings. There are also many chemicals for which there is only limited knowledge about their toxicological profiles. This means that the final information about the potential human health hazards of many chemicals have to be obtained from epidemiological studies.

Studies in occupational and environmental epidemiology suffer from many problems. One of the most notorious is that precise assessments of relevant exposures are difficult to undertake, and it is therefore a great hope that the use of various molecular biomarkers will make the exposure assessments more specific in future studies. The general idea is that population groups at risk may be identified by deviations from the normal values for the various biomarkers of exposure.

Molecular biomarkers can be classified in various ways. The most common classification scheme is based on the idea that the development of any given environmentally-related disease constitutes a sequence of events starting with the exposure and ending with the clinically manifest disease, and that various genetic and functional polymorphisms can be used as molecular biomarkers in this disease process. This type of classification scheme becomes rather obvious when it comes to the use of genetic alterations as molecular biomarkers in cancer risk assessments. Substantial experimental evidence has accumulated indicating that the development of an environmentally-induced cancer follows a multistage process. The disease process starts with an exposure, leading to an 'internal dose', and subsequently to a 'biologically effective dose' ('target dose'). The interaction between the ultimate toxicant and DNA can lead to a 'premutagenic' lesion, and subsequently to various types of permanent genetic alterations (i.e. mutations). These mutations may subsequently lead to altered cellular structures and functions, subclinical changes and finally to a clinically manifest malignant disease.

Independent of which type of genetic end-point is used for biological monitoring, any given end-point can always be used as a molecular biomarker of exposure (providing a measure of the biologically effective dose). This is one of the major objectives of biological monitoring. However, this assessment will normally rely on measurements made in various 'surrogate tissues' (typically blood) or 'surrogate media' (typically urine), because tissues from suspected target organs are seldom available. Some of the genetic end-points used as molecular biomarkers for the biologically effective dose are rather specific (i.e. the DNA adducts), others (e.g. DNA strand breaks, gene mutations and sister chromatide exchanges) are clearly non-specific biomarkers of exposure, showing also naturally occurring cellular events and damage induced by genotoxic agents other than the one under study.

There is growing evidence to suggest that the multistage process of tumorigenesis involves changes in at least two different classes of naturally occurring cellular genes, the proto-oncogenes (which may become activated to oncogenes which start to produce proteins that are important for the cellular growth and differentiation) and the tumour suppressor genes (which may become inactivated so that the cells are liberated from their normal growth restraints). Proto-oncogenes can become activated, and tumour suppressor genes can become inactivated by single point mutations, gene amplifications and chromosomal translocations. Screening of mutations in the p53 tumour suppressor gene has been suggested as a possible diagnostic tool for early stage neoplasias (i.e. as a 'surrogate end-point', 'disease' or 'tumour' biomarker), and it seems as if investigations of various genetic and functional polymorphisms related to oncogene activation and tumour suppressor gene inactivation are becoming increasingly used as molecular biomarkers of early changes in tumour development.

Gene mutations and other genetic end-points can also be regarded as molecular biomarkers of 'susceptibility'. Using the classical epidemiological terminology, a susceptibility marker would be equivalent with an 'effect modifier' [4]. For bio-monitoring purposes, an ideal molecular biomarker of susceptibility should be able to identify individuals in a population having an acquired or inherited difference in susceptibility towards the adverse effects of chemical exposures. The molecular biomarkers that have been used as biomarkers of susceptibility are usually genetic in origin, and one should not forget that there are many other factors (e.g. age, ongoing and previous diseases, medication and concomitant exposures to other toxicants) that can affect an individual's susceptibility to a given chemical [2].

The most commonly used molecular biomarkers of individual susceptibility, at least when it comes to human biomonitoring and cancer risk assessments, are based on studies of genetic polymorphisms of various enzyme systems. Genetic polymorphisms for drug metabolism have been studied using assays involving the measurement of drug clearance (making it possible to separate the population into, for example, one group of slow acetylators and one group of rapid acetylators). Genetic polymorphisms of the cytochromes in the cytochrome P_{450} family (involved in the metabolic bioactivation of many genotoxic carcinogens) have also been used as molecular biomarkers of susceptibility. The DNA repair capacity represents an extremely important parameter when it comes to an individual's susceptibility towards genotoxic carcinogens. It is, for example, well known that inherited diseases affecting the efficiency of DNA repair may lead to increased risk for the development of tumours. The DNA repair capacity is not easy to measure directly in biomonitoring studies, but the urinary output of DNA adducts has been used as an indirect measure of DNA repair.

Consequently, each individual genetic end-point that has been used as a molecular biomarker in cancer risk assessments represents an event in a continuum between external exposure and a clinically manifest disease. The relationship between the different end-points (e.g. DNA adducts → DNA strand breaks → gene mutations and chromosomal aberrations → altered phenotype expression), is influenced by various genetic and host related factors that reflect susceptibility to any of the events in this continuum [3,4].

Genetic end-points used for biomonitoring purposes

The genetic alterations that have been used as molecular biomarkers to monitor internal exposures to genotoxic agents (biological effective doses), early biological responses, surrogate end-point markers (also referred to as 'genetic markers', 'tumour markers' or 'disease markers'), to stratify subjects according to their susceptibility towards various diseases ('susceptibility markers') and/or to clarify the mechanisms behind both acquired and inherited diseases, include a wide range of genetic 'end-points' requiring a whole battery of laboratory techniques for their detection. As indicated in *Table 10.1*, the end-points used for biomonitoring purposes are actually the same as those usually screened for when testing for genotoxic effects of chemicals. However, whereas the testing for genotoxicity usually is performed using a battery of well-established *in vitro* and *in vivo* assays strictly following the protocols given in internationally accepted testing guidelines, the biomonitoring of the various genetic end-points is usually performed using one test only, and often there are no specific testing guidelines available for the assays and techniques used.

The genetic end-points used for biological monitoring include chemical interactions with DNA, primary DNA damages, gene mutations, structural chromosomal aberrations, numerical chromosomal mutations, and other genetic events such as recombinations (i.e. gene conversion, reciprocal exchanges between homologous chromosomes, and sister chromatide exchanges), gene amplifications and insertion mutations. A short description of some of the genetic end-points that have been used as molecular biomarkers in biomonitoring studies is given below. Interest has been focused on DNA adducts, primary DNA damage, gene mutations and structural chromosomal aberrations.

DNA adducts are chemical modifications of DNA following from the covalent binding of a reactive electrophilic chemical species with a nucleophilic site in the DNA molecule. Many genotoxic carcinogens induce primary DNA damage through the formation of DNA adducts. If the DNA adducts and the primary DNA lesions are not correctly repaired before DNA replication, some of these adducts will lead to base-pair substitutions, deletions, insertions, recombinations and other replication errors. These errors will become permanent genetic alterations once the cell undergoes mitosis (somatic cells) or meiosis

Table 10.1   A representative sample of genetic end-points and laboratory techniques used for biomonitoring purposes

Genetic end-point	Techniques used for biomonitoring purposes
Covalent DNA binding Alkylated DNA Bulky aromatic DNA adducts	^{32}P-postlabelling assay; immunoassays, synchronous fluorescence spectroscopy
Primary DNA damage DNA cross linking DNA double strand breaks DNA single strand breaks Oxidative DNA damages	Alkaline elution technique, nick translation, alkaline single cell gel electrophoresis (for registration of DNA strand breaks) Determination of 8-oxy-deoxyguanosine and other modified DNA bases in the urine using HPLC-techniques (for registration of oxidative DNA damage)
Gene mutations Point and gene mutations Mutational spectrum Activation of oncogenes Inactivation of tumour suppressor genes	Selection of mutants with an altered phenotype Detection and amplification of specific DNA sequences using specific restriction enzymes, and PCR-technique Studies of genetic and functional polymorphisms
Structural chromosomal aberrations Chromatide aberrations Chromosome aberrations Micronuclei	Classical cytogenetic methods in cells arrested in metaphase Balanced translocations and inversions are usually quantified using chromosome banding analysis The micronucleus assay
Other genetic alterations Gene amplification Sister chromatide exchanges Activation of oncogenes Inactivation of tumour suppressor genes	Genetic and functional polymorphisms (for registration of gene amplification) Sister chromatide exchange assays

(germ cells). The central dogma of molecular biology and genetic toxicology is that information flows from DNA to RNA (transcription), and from RNA to proteins (translation), and that the genetic information flows between different generation cells via mitosis and meiosis. This means that permanent changes in DNA can be studied indirectly as altered phenotype expressions.

DNA adducts

The DNA adducts are mainly used as 'molecular dosimeters' (i.e. as molecular biomarkers of exposure), but they have also been used to assess the genotoxic potential of chemicals (i.e. as molecular biomarkers of effect). The biological significance of the DNA adducts must be assessed both on the basis of adduct heterogeneity, and of the cell and tissue specificity for adduct formation, persistence and repair [2]. In studies on humans, it is important that the duration and timing of the exposure is known for a proper evaluation of the biological significance of a given adduct concentration. Some adducts result in mutations, others do not. Some DNA adducts are repaired quickly, others hardly at all.

Sensitive techniques based on physicochemical or immunological methods have been developed for the detection of various types of DNA adducts in human samples. The most frequently used methods are the ^{32}P-postlabelling method, various immunoassays, GC-MS technique (gas chromatography coupled with mass spectrometry) and synchronous fluorescence spectroscopy. Each of these techniques has advantages and disadvantages. The ^{32}P-postlabelling technique (which is actually not one specific assay, but rather several different assays using quite different protocols), is extremely sensitive, at least when it comes to the detection of non-polar, rather bulky DNA adducts. However, the laboratory procedures are very complicated, and some DNA adducts cannot be detected at all (mainly because of a low 'labelling efficiency' when the radioactive isotope is introduced into the nucleotides after the DNA digestion). Whereas immunoassays can be both specific and sensitive for some type of adducts, these assays are less specific for other DNA adducts because of the fact that many of the antibodies used tend to cross-react with other adducts [2]. The quantitative aspects of these techniques have not been satisfactorily resolved, and there are often substantial inter-laboratory differences in the results obtained. Different assays do not necessarily measure the same type of adducts. The relationships between adduct levels in surrogate tissues and target organs is poorly established, and so is the relationship between the adducts and disease outcome [1].

Protein adducts

Most, if not all, genotoxic carcinogens that form DNA adducts can also form adducts with other cellular macromolecules. Various types of protein adducts have therefore been used as surrogate measures of DNA binding. There are several proteins that have been used as molecular biomarkers of exposure, but the most extensively used are those circulating in the blood, i.e. haemoglobin (with a life span of 120 days), and albumin (with a life span of approximately 20–25 days). Haemoglobin adducts (which are the most commonly used protein adducts for biomonitoring purposes) are usually quantified using chemical methods to release the adducts from the protein. The hydrolysis with acids or bases is followed by derivatization, and the the final analysis is performed using GC-MS or immunological techniques [2].

Primary DNA damages

In comparison to DNA adducts, primary DNA damage may be looked upon as a further refined molecular biomarker of exposure. However, since primary DNA damage is an actual indicator of a biologically active process, it can also be used as a molecular biomarker of a biological response. So far it seems as if most epidemiological studies using DNA strand breaks, oxidative DNA damages and other types of DNA damages have used them as end-point markers (effect markers), rather than exposure markers for the purpose of exposure assessment [6]. The recorded levels of DNA damage have then been related to the specific exposure of interest.

Oxidative DNA modification has been the focus of interest for several reasons, and this type of damage (which can be induced by both endogenous and environmentally-induced reactive oxygen species) has been used in molecular epidemiology for biomonitoring purposes, both as an exposure marker and an effect marker. In comparison to most other laboratory techniques used for the assessment of various types of genetic alterations in human samples, it is relatively easy to determine 8-oxy-deoxyguanosine, one of the most important molecular biomarkers for oxidative DNA damage. This is usually done using HPLC (high performance liquid chromatography) with electrochemical detection. Urinary excretion of 8-oxy-deoxyguanosine has been suggested to be an attractive candidate for a non-invasive biomarker of oxidative modifications to the DNA molecule [1].

DNA single strand breaks and DNA double strand breaks are typical representatives of DNA damages which are both naturally occurring and induced by genotoxic carcinogens, including, for example, ionizing radiation. DNA strand breaks are used both as exposure markers and effect markers in studies of induced damage. They can also be used as biomarkers of DNA repair. Several techniques have been used to monitor DNA strand breaks in human samples (e.g. the alkaline elution technique, the nick translation assay, and neutral or alkaline single cell gel electrophoresis). Alkaline single cell gel electrophoresis (also known as the 'comet assay') is an increasingly popular method for the detection of DNA single strand breaks. In comparison to most other methods used when screening for genotoxicity in human samples, the 'comet assay' is a sensitive, simple and rapid technique. Because of its unique design, it is possible to determine whether all cells show the same degree of damage, or if there is a heterogeneous response to the genotoxic insult of interest.

Gene mutations

Current somatic gene mutation assays used for biomonitoring purposes usually select for a change or a loss of a normal protein produced by specific genes. The most commonly used assays for detection of base-pair substitutions (i.e. transitions and transversions) and frameshift mutations (i.e. deletions or additions of individual bases in DNA), are based on mutations in the X-linked HGPRT-locus (hypoxanthine guanine phosphoribosyl transferase) in cloned T-lymphocytes, and in the autosomal locus for HLA-A (the human leukocyte antigen-A). Both these genes are used to monitor mutation frequencies and mutational spectra [2]. It is the location and type of point mutations in a specific sequence of nucleotides that define a mutational spectrum, and, judging from the literature, it

seems as if the determination of mutational spectra is an increasingly popular method in molecular epidemiology.

By definition, all permanent changes in a DNA sequence will lead to an altered genotype. Some of these changes will also lead to phenotypic alterations that can be selected for. Other changes in the genotype will not lead to any changes in the expression of the phenotype. An alternative approach for the measurement of induced point and gene mutations, which does not require a prior selection of mutant cell populations, is the use of the restriction site mutation technique. This technique, which is commonly used in molecular biology, is based on the detection of DNA sequences that are resistant to the cutting action of specific restriction enzymes. When the resistant sequences have been found, they are amplified using the PCR technique (polymerase chain reaction) and then sequenced so that any potential mutation can be detected.

Structural and numerical chromosomal aberrations

The structural and numerical chromosomal aberrations represent two different types of chromosomal mutation. Whereas structural chromosomal aberrations have been used for biomonitoring purposes for several years, numerical chromosomal mutations are almost never used for this purpose, at least not when it comes to the determination of genetic alterations in somatic cells and cancer risk assessments. Whereas the numerical chromosomal mutations follow from the failure of homologous chromosomes or sister chromatides to separate during the meiosis or mitosis (this phenomenon is called 'non-disjunction' and does not involve any direct damage to the genetic material), structural chromosomal aberrations probably arise as a result of an erroneous repair of DNA damages in a certain stage of the cell cycle (the G0-phase). The structural chromosome aberrations (including acentric fragments, dicentric chromosomes, ring chromosomes, and chromatide breaks, intrachanges and exchanges) are usually monitored using classical cytogenetic methods. However, balanced translocations and inversions can be difficult to monitor without a so-called banding analysis.

Depending on their ability to persist in dividing cell populations, the structural chromosomal aberrations are either balanced (stable) or unbalanced. Most unstable aberrations (acentric fragments, ring chromosomes and other asymmetrical rearrangements) will most certainly lead to cell death. Since many of the stable chromosomal aberrations (e.g. balanced translocations and other symmetrical rearrangements) can be transmitted to the next cell generation at cell division, these will be more biologically significant than the unbalanced ones, and they can very well be involved in the multistage process of tumour development, for example, by activating proto-oncogenes, or by inactivating tumour suppressor genes.

Some frustrations and unresolved issues in 'molecular epidemiology'

Most genetic end-points that have been used for biomonitoring purposes are used as 'exposure markers', providing an estimate of the biologically effective dose. However, in other studies, the same type of genetic end-points may be used as molecular biomarkers of effect or even individual susceptibility. The fact that there seems to be no clear distinction between these three major categories of molecular biomarkers in biomonitoring studies may indeed be rather confusing for an uninitiated reader. Is a given molecular biomarker a biologically significant event in a disease process in itself, or is it a correlate, or a predictor of a significant event? In some instances, molecular biomarkers of effects are not mechanistically related to chemically-induced lesions, but they may represent concomitant independent changes [2]. Therefore, although an effect (e.g. sister chromatide exchanges) is being analysed, the use in human biomonitoring is conceptually more close to the assessment of exposure.

DNA adducts are usually regarded as exposure markers in biomonitoring studies, representing the biologically effective dose of a genotoxic agent interacting directly with the genetic material. The formation of DNA adducts can also represent an early biological effect forming the basis of primary DNA damages, possibly leading to a critical mutation. Moreover, if there is a true correlation between high levels of DNA adducts, and an increased risk for cancer or other diseases, then it should, at least in theory, be possible to use

DNA adducts as a susceptibility marker indirectly showing the DNA repair capacity.

It should be emphasized that, so far, there is a real gap in our knowledge when it comes to the biological relevance of most of the genetic end-points that have been used for biomonitoring purposes. DNA adducts, for example, are formed in many tissues and in response to many exposures (including 'endogenous' ones). How do we know which are relevant to study? Are individuals with increased levels of endogenous DNA adducts actually at an increased risk for cancer? Are all genotoxic agents interacting with the genetic material forming DNA adducts that can be adequately detected with present techniques? Are all DNA adducts equally important for the induction of DNA damage and mutations?

From experimental studies it is well known that DNA binding and other types of interactions with the genetic material are closely associated with an increased rate of mutations, and that some of these mutations may lead to various diseases if they occur at critical sites of the genome. At the same time, it is also known that most mutations are without biological consequences, and that many of the genetic and functional polymorphisms that have been used as molecular biomarkers are unrelated to the disease process of interest.

For most environmentally-related diseases, there is a continuum of events starting with exposure and ending with the clinical manifestation of the disease. For each of the individual steps involved, there are both genetic and functional polymorphisms. Even if we had the resources to use a whole battery of techniques measuring various types of genetic end-points when monitoring for biologically effective doses, 'early biological effects' and/or altered structures and functions in various organs and tissues, it seems rather unlikely that it will be possible to control for all the genetic and functional polymorphisms that can be expected in a normal population with regard to, for example, various pathways of bioactivation and detoxification, DNA-repair capacity, hormonal and immunological status.

It is rather obvious that changes in the structure of DNA can be critical in the long chain of events leading to the development of a clinically manifest malignant disease. Malignant cells contain a genome in which the genes are either altered or wrongly expressed, and there are numerous studies showing that many DNA damaging agents are carcinogenic when tested in chronic cancer bioassays. However, the process of tumorigenesis is a complex multistage process, also involving epigentic (non-genotoxic) events. There are many chemical carcinogens that act by some other mechanisms than by inducing direct DNA damage and mutations. The biologically effective doses of non-genotoxic carcinogens, and the early biological responses following epigenetic events in the multistage process of tumorigenesis, will not necessarily be detected using various types of genetic alterations as molecular biomarkers in cancer risk assessments.

The situation is further complicated by the fact that the occurrence of DNA damage is a quite common phenomenon in our cells. It has, for example, been estimated that endogenous factors alone may induce around 4000 DNA lesions per day per cell [5]. Obviously, only a limited number of these lesions will be of biological importance. Some of them might lead to critical genetic alterations, but most will either be repaired or associated with cell death.

Some of the issues that have to be resolved before 'genotoxicity' can be used with confidence as a biomarker of exposure, effect or susceptibility in field studies on workers with an occupational exposure to low levels of suspected genotoxic chemical carcinogens, are related to the strategies used for the sampling, handling and storage of the biological samples. Logistics and conditions that have been proved to be optimal for one type of genetic end-point, using one specific type of assay, could be devastating when using another type of genetic end-point or another type of assay measuring the same type of end-point. Another problem in molecular epidemiology relates to the difficulty of transforming the rather complicated and often very time-consuming laboratory techniques into routine methods that are capable of handling a large number of specimens in a cost-effective and timely manner [3].

Other critical issues are related to the half-life and specificity of the molecular biomarker. Markers with short half-life reflecting very recent exposures should be used with caution, and it is often a good idea to use repeated sampling in order to establish whether or not a single measurement is representative of long-term prevalent exposures [1]. An appropriate sampling of biological specimens requires that the temporal relationships between the molecular biomarker, and the external exposure (for exposure markers) or the disease (for effect markers) are understood. For the purpose of risk assessment, it is important to know whether a certain molecular biomarker reflects recent short-term or cumulative long-term exposures [1]. Most measures of biologically effective doses based on genetic alterations reflect recent exposures.

Usually there is only a limited number of tissues available for routine analysis, at least in human biomonitoring studies. Easily accessible tissues or body fluids (typically whole blood and/or urine) are therefore often used as surrogates for the known or presumed target organs. The possible limitation of the use of molecular biomarkers in surrogate media should always be considered in biomonitoring studies. Other parameters that should be known before performing a biomonitoring study (but seldom are in reality), are the 'background range' of the molecular biomarker of interest, and its intra- and interindividual variations over time in a supposedly 'non-exposed' reference population. All human biomonitoring studies suffer from variability of the 'baseline frequency' due to the presence of both endogenous factors such as age, gender, medical history, ongoing diseases, etc., and exogenous factors, such as smoking, drinking and eating habits and lifestyle factors, etc. [2].

Little is known about the validity of most, if not all, molecular biomarkers in relation to both the exposure and the disease of interest, and this seems to be true also when it comes to the relevance of both the study design and the laboratory procedures that have been used in too many papers that have been published in the field of molecular epidemiology. Valid molecular biomarkers of exposure, for example, would be those with a biological relevance, defined pharmacokinetics, temporal relevance and defined 'background' variability [1]. Even if most of the genetic alterations that have been used as molecular biomarkers of exposure have biological relevance (i.e. are representing parts of a chain of events that are a subset of exposure opportunities and a pool from which outcome events are likely to occur [1]), it is rather doubtful if all the other criteria are fulfilled. Quite often it seems as if measurements based on molecular biomarkers are difficult to reproduce, and often there are no standard procedures available for most of the assays used for biomonitoring purposes. Inter-laboratory comparisons are often hampered by the fact that many assays are semiquantitative by nature.

Conclusion

Despite the recent developments in 'molecular biology', we have still to acknowledge that there is a substantial gap in our knowledge when it comes to the mechanisms behind the development of most malignant and inherited diseases. The development of these diseases is highly complex, involving both genetic and epigenetic changes. Most diseases follow from interactions between both endogenous factors (largely determined by the genotype) and environmental factors (including both cultural and lifestyle factors). Genes interact with each other, and so do the environmental factors. Many diseases are inevitably linked to natural ageing, and the status of one organ system (e.g. the immune system) can be important for the development of a disease in another organ system.

Consequently, since most malignant and genetic diseases are likely to be the result of multiple mechanisms of actions involving both genetic and environmental factors, following many alternative pathways, one should not be surprised that there are no universal 'molecular biomarkers' available that can be used as an all-embracing 'disease marker'. The fact that the 'hybrid discipline' referred to as 'molecular epidemiology' is in a rapid phase of development should not be concealed, and we have to realize that there are several issues that have to be considered before genetic alterations can be used with confidence as molecular biomarkers of exposure, disease and/or individual susceptibility.

The use of molecular biomarkers involves complex ethical, social and legal issues which must be resolved before they are used for any application. All researchers using molecular biomarkers for biomonitoring purposes should be aware of the fact that the validity of any given biomarker is dependent on its relationship to both the external exposure and the disease of interest, and that this relationship is almost impossible to prove in epidemiological studies. Therefore, with the present level of understanding, any discussion regarding possible adverse health effects following from a slight change in the levels of any molecular biomarker should be restricted to a discussion of group risks only. To use a slightly increased level of DNA adducts, DNA strand breaks, gene mutations, chromosomal aberrations, sister chromatide exchanges or other genetic alterations, in, for example, peripheral lymphocytes, to assess individual cancer risks would be directly unethical given our present level of understanding.

References

1. WHO Regional Office for Europe. Guiding principles for the use of biological markers in the assessment of human exposure to environmental factors: an integrative approach of epidemiology and toxicology. *Toxicology*, **101**, 1–10 (1995)
2. IPCS/WHO. *Biomarkers and Risk assessment: Concepts and Principles*, Environmental Health Criteria 155. World Health Organization, Geneva (1993)
3. Schulte, P.A. A conceptual and historical framework for molecular epidemiology. In *Molecular Epidemiology. Principles and Practices*. (eds P.A. Schulte and F.P. Perera). Academic Press, San Diego (1993)
4. Hulka, B.S. and Wilcosky, T. Biological markers in epidemiologic research. *Archives of Environmental Health*, **43**. 83–89 (1988)
5. Lohman, P.H.M., Morolli, B., Darroudi, F. *et al.* Contributions from molecular/biochemical approaches in epidemiology to cancer risk assessment and prevention. *Environmental Health Perspectives*, **98**, 155–165 (1992)
6. Wahrendorf, J. Design of studies for validation of biomarkers of exposure and their effective use in environmental epidemiology. *Toxicology*, **101**, 89–92 (1995)

Further reading

Schulte, P.A. and Perera, F.P. (eds) *Molecular Epidemiology. Principles and Practices*. Academic Press, San Diego (1993)

Chapter 11

Current occupational health problems

C Edling

Today, there is a change in pattern of work in many industrialized countries, a change that has resulted in a decrease in the 'old' traditional occupational diseases, such as lead poisoning and pneumoconiosis and an increase in what are now called 'work-related' diseases, that is, diseases that can occur regardless of any occupational exposure, e.g. musculoskeletal disorders, asthma and cardiovascular diseases. Moreover, the occupational physician or nurse, nowadays sees an increasing number of patients who present different symptoms without any sign of disease. The complaints are often polysymptomatic and the symptoms tend to be chronic. It is often possible to distinguish different clinical subgroups, such as multiple chemical sensitivity, sick building syndrome and symptoms related to exposure to mercury from dental amalgam or hypersensitivity to electricity. The care of these patients is an increasing challenge to the occupational health service. It is essential not to question the patient's complaints and symptoms but the explanation of the symptoms. This chapter briefly describes the current basis for these 'new diseases', together with some practical advice for their management as well as current knowledge with regard to exposure to electric and magnetic fields and cancer and pregnancy outcome.

Multiple chemical sensitivity syndrome

Multiple chemical sensitivity (MCS) syndrome, known also as environmental illness, ecological illness, environmental hypersensitivity or total allergy syndrome, has been described as 'the most puzzling clinical entity emerging in the 1980s'. Patients with MCS are characterized by the manifestation of an array of symptoms that follow low-level exposure to a variety of common substances. The most common symptoms are headache, tiredness, nausea and dizziness. There has been considerable debate in the medical community as to whether MCS is a distinct diagnostic entity and about whether the sufferers of this condition share a common aetiology. Multiple chemical sensitivity lacks a standard case definition, but that given by Cullen in 1987 is widely used. He outlined seven criteria aimed to distinguish patients with MCS from patients with acute occupational diseases:

1 The disorder is acquired in relation to some documentable environmental exposure(s), insult(s) or illness(es).
2 Symptoms involve more than one organ system.
3 Symptoms recur and abate in response to predictable stimuli.
4 Symptoms are elicited by exposures to chemicals of diverse structural classes and toxicological modes of action.
5 Symptoms are elicited by exposures that are demonstrable (albeit of low level).
6 Exposures that elicit symptoms must be very low, by which is meant standard deviations below 'average' exposures known to cause adverse human responses.
7 No single widely available test of organ function can explain the symptoms.

However, other case definitions for multiple chemical sensitivity have been proposed, for example, by the National Research Council and the Agency for Toxic Substances and Disease Registry Working Groups in USA.

The origins of MCS are unknown but highly controversial in the medical community. Unfortunately, the lack of a uniform case definition for individuals with MCS has hampered investigations of its aetiology. Some researchers claim that MCS is primarily a psychiatric or behavioural problem; an expression of a psychosomatic disorder, an obsessive or paranoid illness, or an anxiety or depressive illness. Others have pointed to possible biological mechanisms for MCS that might involve the nervous system, the immune system, the endocrine system, or some combination of these. It has been proposed that chemicals contacting the olfactory nerves in the nose, may cause a disturbance in the limbic system and may result in several symptoms.

Clinical management and treatment

MCS patients who suspect that their symptoms are initiated and/or exacerbated by workplace exposures are likely to consult an occupational physician. However, patients may seek help from many different specialists, including internists, allergists, psychiatrists and environmental medicine physicians. A careful and emphatic history is critical to the evaluation of the individual with multi-organ symptoms, provoked by low-level chemical exposure. Acknowledgement of symptoms and the establishment of a trusting relationship is important. Approaching the history with the suspicion that the patient with MCS is suffering from a psychiatric disorder or is seeking monetary benefits is not helpful in establishing a therapeutic relationship. The individual with MCS typically reports symptoms after exposure to common environmental irritants, such as gasoline, perfumes or household cleaners. Symptoms of headache, fatigue, lethargy, myalgia and difficulty in concentrating may persist for hours to days or even weeks, with typical 'reactions' reported after these common exposures. The patient might be suffering from disabling symptoms, and varying degrees of restrictions in social and work activities may be reported, including problems driving a car, shopping or entering particular workplaces.

The physical examination is almost always normal and there are no diagnostic tests that will be helpful in diagnosing MCS, but some tests may reveal other treatable diseases. An evaluation of the patient's workplace is important, in order to identify if the patient is exposed to chemicals above permissible exposure levels or not.

Often the individual will already have identified a variety of irritants that result in symptoms, and will have initiated an avoidance regimen or is sometimes desperately seeking advice and support regarding treatment. Equal to the controversy about what causes MCS is the uncertainty about the most effective treatment. Consequently, a variety of methods have been utilized for the treatment. Exposure minimization through environmental modification is a reasonable recommendation, as well as the advice to the patients to avoid exposures to substances that cause them permanent harm. Regardless of the cause of MCS, it appears that psychological symptoms play a prominent role in the syndrome. Until the cause of MCS is definitely identified, behavioural techniques aimed at the reduction of symptoms appear to be the most promising treatment approach.

The sick building syndrome

Indoor air quality is of concern because most people in the western world spend about 90% of their time indoors. From most countries in the industrialized western world there are now reports of sick buildings and of people suffering from the sick building syndrome (SBS). The term 'sick building syndrome' came into use in the 1970s because of complaints from office workers. A group of symptoms was found to be more prevalent than normal among office workers in certain buildings, and the symptoms resolved quickly when the worker left the implicated building. Although the symptoms are common and non-specific, the group comprising the SBS has been defined by a working group of the WHO. The syndrome includes mucous membrane irritation (irritative symptoms from eyes, skin and upper airways), central nervous system symptoms (headache, fatigue, nausea and dizziness), chest tightness (cough and shortness of breath) and skin complaints (dryness, itching, erythema).

The cause of SBS is unknown. Factors contributing to perceived indoor air quality include temperature, humidity, odours, air movements and ventilation, lighting, workplace organization, personal risk factors and bioaerosol and volatile hydrocarbon contamination. Over the years, it has been common to distinguish SBS from building-related illness. This is defined as an illness related to a known specific cause. The SBS relates to the medical manifestations experienced predominantly within the buildings. 'Sick building', however, is the term given to those buildings which appear to be places in which its occupants experience symptoms at a higher prevalence than the general population. Even the increased morbidity and mortality in asthma and allergy found in several countries has been suggested to be due to raised concentrations of indoor pollutants in modern buildings.

Information on SBS has been gathered in anecdotal reports, cross-sectional questionnaire surveys, in quasi-experimental field studies and in population-based questionnaire surveys. Furthermore, experimental chamber studies have provided information on mechanisms of symptom generation, markers of exposure or effects, and on population characteristics.

Not everyone who works in a building that is described as sick will suffer from symptoms that are related to SBS. Many of the buildings where SBS occurs are sealed, energy efficient and designed with outside ventilation by means of a recirculating air-conditioning system. Epidemiological studies have shown that a large proportion of the workforce perceive the indoor air quality at work to be inadequate, particularly females working in offices and hospitals. Complaints about poor indoor air quality should be considered as an early indication of disturbances in the indoor environment. There are also reports that poor indoor air quality may affect productivity. This suggests that investments aimed to improve indoor air quality may be profitable, even if productivity is increased by only a few percent.

Research into the causes of SBS has produced a variety of conflicting findings. There are, however, generally consistent findings indicating an association between the prevalence of symptoms and air-conditioning, carpets, more workers in a space, use of visual display terminals, and ventilation rates at or below 10 litres per second per person. The SBS is multifactorial and, in addition to several external factors, individual factors also determine the expression of the syndrome. It is worth emphasizing that epidemiological studies have not found any excess of allergic individuals in problem buildings.

Clinical management and treatment

Patients frequently confront their primary care physicians with non-specific complaints, temporarily related to indoor environments, both at work and at home. Some symptoms and symptom complexes may represent a disease that is identifiable by the usual history-taking, physical examination and laboratory testing. There is no detailed knowledge about the factors in the indoor environment that may cause the symptoms. However, from epidemiological studies there are some descriptions about relations between symptoms and various building-related factors.

The definition of SBS describes the condition of a building and the term 'sick building syndrome' is applicable only if there are more symptoms than expected among the residents in a specific building. Thus, the syndrome is a 'group-diagnosis'. The individuals are the 'markers' of some defect in the building and, in principle, one cannot speak about the SBS with reference to a single individual. Consequently, the investigation must be carried out differently if it is a building with many people complaining, or if it is just one or a few persons who present with symptoms. In any case, a collaboration between a physician and specialists on buildings and chemical measurements will be necessary for a complete investigation.

The first step should be to ensure cooperation from all who may be involved in either the investigation or the actions necessary to improve the indoor environment. In particular, those who are to pay for the repair or reconstruction that may turn out to be necessary should be involved from the beginning. An adequate investigation and correct information are important to avoid unnecessary and costly repairs of the building. However, sometimes it may be cheaper to proceed with repair work immediately, without any extensive investigation. The second step is then to decide upon strategies for the investigation. As in other areas of occupational and environmental medicine, an approach to disease management must include the formulation of a diagnosis, strategies for causal linkage or exclusion, definition of the risk of disease to co-workers, adequate characterization of patient risk and employee communication needs and intervention strategies. Investigation of a group of individuals with SBS symptoms in a building or workplace must be studied with epidemiological methods, preferably with the help of validated questionnaires. The building must be inspected and environmental measurements may be necessary.

The ventilation and air-conditioning system must be inspected, and perhaps adjusted to ensure proper function. The need for physical, chemical or biological measurements may be determined on the basis of the inquiry and the findings from the building inspection. The measurements may be directed towards factors likely to cause the problems. Environmental factors often measured are air temperature, carbon dioxide, air exchange rate, respirable dust, formaldehyde, volatile organic compounds, mould and bacteria. The measures can be compared with existing limit values or, if these do not exist, with 'normal' values for buildings, as presented in the literature. Specific measurements without reference values are dubious. Since SBS symptoms may have many different causes, and different persons have different sensitivity, one must interpret negative results with care. If deviating environmental measures have been identified, a follow-up with new measurements after correction of the building is appropriate.

Single persons with symptoms should initially be examined by a physician. If no obvious cause for the symptoms is found in the medical examination, SBS may be considered. There are no specific diagnostic tests for the syndrome. The SBS manifests itself through several unspecific symptoms and the history is the most important part of the medical examination. A reasonable lowest level for the medical investigation is to search for an atopic predisposition and, if bronchial hyperreactivity is suspected, a provocation test may be appropriate. The association between the symptoms and the building must be shown. Inspection and measurements may be performed in accordance with the guidelines presented above.

Although there are conflicting views concerning the cause(s) of SBS, there is now enough information to form the basis for a preventive strategy. Reduced room temperature and effective cleaning routines are simple means to reduce the prevalence of SBS symptoms. It is important to clean not only the floors, but also other horizontal surfaces. Moreover, carpeting and other textile materials should be minimized, unless it

can be clearly demonstrated that they are properly cleaned. The outdoor air supply rate in buildings should be kept at about 10 litres per second per person, which is somewhat higher than most current ventilation standards. Return air should be avoided, since it enhances the indoor level of volatile organic compounds and other indoor pollutants. Exposure to microorganisms, which may grow in damp houses, or be spread by air-conditioning systems, should also be minimized. Chemical emissions from building materials should be reduced by the selection of low-emitting materials and products. In particular, the introduction of irritative semi- volatile compounds should be discouraged, since such compounds may be bound to dust and lead to a higher chemical dose on the airway mucosa than more volatile compounds.

Symptoms related to exposure to mercury from dental amalgam

Dental amalgam has been used for more than 100 years and is still the most frequently used material for dental restoration. The alloy consists of mercury, silver and tin (50%, 35% and 15%, respectively). In some modern amalgams silver has been partly replaced by copper. It is well known that chronic mercury poisoning may occur from occupational exposure to small amounts of mercury over a long period of time. Neurological or psychiatric symptoms include depression, irritability, exaggerated response to stimuli, excessive shyness, insomnia, emotional instability, forgetfulness and confusion. Other neurological signs include spasms of the arms, legs or facial muscles, lack of muscle coordination and mental retardation. Additional symptoms found are excessive perspiration, uncontrollable blushing, and a fine tremor of the fingers, eyelids, lips and tongue.

One of the controversies regarding dental amalgam is whether any mercury is released and taken up by inhalation. However, it has been shown that mercury vapour is released during the insertion, polishing and removal of amalgam. Furthermore, mercury vapour is continuously released from dental amalgam during toothbrushing, chewing and intake of hot drinks. This mercury can be measured in expired air and saliva. From different studies it can be estimated that mercury from amalgam accounts for a small percentage of the total intake of mercury, and represents less than 10% of the daily intake of mercury from food and other non-dental sources. It is estimated that the average uptake of mercury from amalgam fillings in Swedish adults is within the range 4–19 µg/day. This rather broad range reflects the uncertainty inherent in the model and the data used. The mercury is distributed and taken up by the central nervous system.

Because of the well-known toxicity of mercury and the demonstrated release of mercury from amalgam filling, a controversy now exists as to whether amalgam fillings are toxic. There are many studies where no significant correlation has been found between amalgam load and subjective symptoms, but there are also studies where such relationships have been reported of major concern for kidney dysfunction, neurotoxicity, classical problems associated in the past with occupational exposure, and speculative involvement in the cause of multiple sclerosis and Alzheimer's disease, reduced immune competence resulting in varied disorders, increase in stillbirth and birth defects, and general health.

Despite several studies there is, as yet, no evidence that amalgam fillings can cause any disease, except for allergic reactions to the filling materials. Nor are there any studies to indicate that removing the amalgam leads to better health. The hope of regaining health by removing amalgam fillings is not a new phenomenon. Even as early as 1850, in the USA, there were dentists who claimed that removal of amalgam fillings could result in miraculous cures among patients with chronic diseases. However, the general conclusion is that dental amalgam does not constitute any hazard to health in individuals who are not allergic to mercury.

Occupational exposure to elemental mercury in dentistry is a well-known phenomenon that has gained considerable recent attention. The primary source of occupational exposure to practising dentists is inhaled elemental mercury vapour. The varied factors that are thought to contribute to mercury exposure in dentists can be categorized into groups of characteristics: personal, professional practice and office. Personal characteristics include items such as diet, age and non-occupational mercury exposure. Professional characteristics include items such as the number of fillings carried out per week, the techniques used during the operation and how scrap amalgam is stored. Office characteristics include such

features as prior accidental mercury spills, flooring material and the number of operations.

Clinical management and treatment

The patients often complain of neuraesthenic symptoms, headache, tiredness, memory disturbances, difficulties in concentration, insomnia, dizziness and myalgia. Patients with symptoms referable to the mouth should also be examined by a dentist. The measurement of mercury in blood or urine is not recommended as a routine procedure. Removal of amalgam fillings is not recommended. There is no specific treatment.

Exposure to electric and magnetic fields

The biological effects and possible health outcomes of low-frequency electromagnetic fields have been under discussion for more than 15 years. Strictly speaking there are no 'electromagnetic fields', but there is an electromagnetic force (EMF) effect which is the sum of the electric field and the magnetic field. Physically, electric and magnetic fields can be defined as part of the low-frequency electromagnetic radiation spectrum. The low-frequency fields have two components, an electric field (proportional to the voltage) and a magnetic field (proportional to the strength of the current). Both fields are capable of generating an induced current in exposed people. The low-frequency fields can also be divided into two subgroups as regards frequency. Extremely low-frequency (ELF) fields are usually defined to include 1–300 kHz and of most interest are the 50–60 Hz fields associated with alternating currents in electric power distribution systems. The high frequencies in the kilohertz domain are called very low frequencies (VLF). The amplitude of the electric field is expressed in terms of volts per metre (V/m), and the magnetic field amplitude or magnetic flux density in tesla (T). Most exposures to man-made sources are in the ranges up to 100 kV/m and 20 mT. Wherever there are electric wires, electric motors and electric equipment, electric and magnetic fields are created. Exposure to electric and magnetic fields occurs throughout society, in homes, at work, in schools, and by electrically powered means of transport.

Some occupational groups are more exposed than others. The following list presents 'electrical' occupations in the order roughly corresponding to the degree, from highest to lowest, of exposure to magnetic fields during a workday: welders, linemen and substation operators (electric power industry), electronic engineers and technicians, locomotive engineers, train conductors and railway station workers, radio and television repair men, foundry- and furnaceworkers, miners, telephonists, telephone repair men and installation engineers. Naturally, people in other occupations can also be exposed, e.g. exposure to both electric and magnetic fields in the proximity to a video display terminal (VDT). From studies in which dosimetry has provided information on exposure, $0.1\,\mu T$ seems to represent an average exposure to magnetic fields during a workday.

Experiments *in vitro* have shown different effects of electric and magnetic fields on the cell membrane. The US Office of Technology Assessment summarizes how the fields may affect cell function in the following ways:

- modulation of ion and protein flow across the cell membrane
- chromosome damage and interference with DNA synthesis and RNA transcription
- interaction with the cell response to different hormones and enzymes
- interaction with the cell response to chemical neurotransmitters
- interaction with the immune response of cells.

There are some human data which indicate that exposure to high levels of electric and magnetic fields can decrease the heart rate, and produce changes in the EEG and impairment in psychometric tests.

The lack of realistic mechanisms to couple exposure to EMF and biological events has resulted in much unfocused research, inconsistent observations and interpretations. Most studies have considered the introduction of cancer, neurobehavioural reactions and pregnancy outcomes, but during the last few years a discussion as to whether exposure to EMF can cause electrical hypersensitivity has emerged.

Health outcomes

Pregnancy outcome

Concern about the potential reproductive effects of occupational exposure to electric and magnetic fields has been related to the use of VDTs, and was first raised in 1980 when adverse pregnancy outcomes among women working with VDTs were reported. Exposure to the low-frequency electromagnetic fields, 15–30 kHz, of VDTs has been suggested as one causal factor, along with psychological stress and ergonomic factors, for the possible effects of VDT work on pregnancy outcome. Over the years a number of epidemiological studies have been conducted on the potential effects of working with VDTs on the risk of an adverse pregnancy outcome. In most of the well-designed studies no statistical association has been found between the use of VDTs and spontaneous abortion or congenital malformations. However, in a few studies, women with long VDT work times, more than 20 hours per day, had an increased risk of spontaneous abortion compared to those with no VDT work. Experiments performed on chicken embryos, pregnant mice and rats have failed to confirm suspicions of any teratogenic properties of electric and magnetic fields. The overall evaluation of existing data is that there is no evidence for an effect of VDT work on pregnancy outcome (see also Chapter 14).

Cancer

In 1979 a study was published, indicating that children with leukaemia tended to live closer to electric transmission lines with a so-called highcurrent configuration. This finding prompted other studies of electric and magnetic fields and cancer. Since the configuration was thought to be a surrogate for exposure to magnetic fields, most attention has been paid to the magnetic fields in epidemiological studies. In 1982, the result of the first occupational epidemiological study was published. Electrical workers were found to have an increased risk of leukaemia, possibly due to their workplace exposure to electric and magnetic fields. Subsequent studies were based on census information or some other routinely collected register information. Both leukaemia (especially acute myeloid leukaemia) and brain cancer in diverse populations and across a range of workplaces have generally, but not always, been associated with a small increase in risk related to job titles, such as, lineman, electrician and electrician engineer. These exploratory studies were gross, the numbers were small, the exposure was ill-defined, both with regard to magnetic fields and other workplace carcinogens, the statistical analyses were often very weak and no confounders were controlled for. However, a number of well-designed case control studies seem to support and even strengthen the possible association between leukaemia and working in 'electrical occupations', but because of the gross estimates of exposure, they say little about its association with electromagnetic fields.

There are also several case control studies and cohort studies of occupational exposure to EMF and cancer. Most have shown elevated risk ratios for brain cancer and leukaemia in electrical-related occupations: telephone operators, electronic industry workers, electrical engineers, telecommunication industry workers, linemen, station operators, electricians, amateur radio operators, telephone company workers, electrical utility workers and radio men. Some studies indicate a dose–response relationship between EMF exposure and brain cancer. Even for these studies, however, exposure has in most cases been estimated based on remote information, usually through occupations reported on register files or secured through postal questionnaires. Although the consistency of finding is notable, the key question is whether the association with job title is due to magnetic fields or some other agent in the work place. Overall, the available epidemiological data on magnetic field and cancer are too inconsistent to establish a cause and effect relationship.

This view is also supported by the Swedish criteria group for physical risk factors at the National Institute for Work Life Research. In a recent criteria document on magnetic fields and cancer, they stated that 'an overall evaluation of both animal and epidemiological studies is that occupational exposure could possibly be a human carcinogen. There is, however, a lack of data to determine whether a dose–response relationship exists. The criteria group summarizes the situation that the scientific data base is insufficient to develop limits of exposures.'

Hypersensitivity to electricity

At the end of the 1960s and beginning of the 1970s reports were received from researchers in the former Soviet Union, who had found that individuals experiencing occupational exposure to EMFs showed an increased frequency of diffuse problems relating to the heart and gastro-intestinal tract. These reports were soon forgotten, but in the 1980s the occurrence of skin symptoms and signs among operators of VDTs was reported by different investigators in Sweden. An increase in some mild non-specific skin symptoms was found, but there was no consistency in the diagnoses. The symptoms are not exclusively related to work at VDTs, and the persons affected have themselves defined the condition as 'hypersensitivity to electricity', since the common denominator appears to be nearness to things that have something to do with electricity. Electrical sensitivity, electrical hypersensitivity and electrical allergy are all terms describing one and the same condition. There are several thousands of persons today in Sweden claiming this hypersensitivity. The Swedish National Board of Health and Welfare has recommended the term 'electrical sensitivity' be used, to emphasize that this condition is not an allergic reaction, which terms like 'hypersensitivity' and 'allergy' might imply.

Individuals sensitive to electricity can experience problems when working at a VDT, spending time in rooms with electrical fittings, preparing food at the stove, watching television, travelling by car, train or plane or being in any way exposed to electromagnetic radiation. Sensitive individuals exhibit a very wide range of symptoms, hardly ever limited to one organ system. The most common symptoms experienced are dizziness, headache, fatigue, memory and difficulty in concentration, skin problems, eye problems, heart palpitations and swelling of the legs. The hypersensitivity is believed to be multifactorial in origin. It is not clear whether electrical or magnetic fields are involved or not. Chemical, ergonomic, stress and work organization factors have been proposed to contribute to the aetiology, and it seems as if a mismatch between company organization and possibilities for an individual career at work definitely plays a role in the development of symptoms. Hypersensitive persons have also been found to produce higher levels of stress hormones at work with VDTs than referents, a finding which together with the clinical picture led the authors to diagnose 'techno-stress' in these persons.

The Swedish National Board of Health and Welfare has concluded, after reviewing available data, that there is no support for a causal relationship between exposure to electric and magnetic fields and perceived symptoms. At the same time the board emphasizes strongly that these patients neither simulate nor imagine their illness.

Clinical management and treatment

There are no specific tests available to diagnose this condition and of major importance is that treatable diseases are ruled out. Patients with skin complaints should see a dermatologist. The workplace should be visited and inspected, with special attention being paid to the indoor climate and organizational structure, factors which are known to give rise to problems similar to those experienced by individuals with electrical sensitivity. Since there is no causal relationship between exposure to electric and magnetic fields and different symptoms, measurement of electric and magnetic fields at the workplace is not recommended. On the contrary, measuring may only lead to increased anxiety. However, a more simple 'clean-up' at the workplace, such as the minimizing of electric cords, should be performed.

The eye problems experienced by many individuals working at visual display units are mostly related to the visual ergonomy and can in most cases be considered as a physiological reaction. It is also important to notice that magnetic fields about 0.5 mT and higher can be responsible for flicker on the VDT screen, thereby affecting the quality of the picture which may add to eye strain.

Those changes which are most likely to be successful according to our judgement are a combination of taking a complete survey of the organizational structure, ergonomic relationships (including sight!) and indoor climate, where necessary correcting any potential existing deficiencies and problems, as well as the application for cognitive therapy. The purpose of such a therapy, of course, is not to question a patient's symptoms nor to convince him or her that he or she is not sensitive to electromagnetic radiation, but to teach the patient to deal with these problems, seeing them in the proper perspective. Measurement of EMF levels and the undertaking of extensive measures to reduce electromagnetic radiation at the workplace are not a part of the treatment programme.

Conclusion

Many patients manifest somatic symptoms that are impossible to diagnose as being caused by somatic disorders. These include headache, dizziness, muscular pain, backache, eye irritation, nasal congestion, memory disturbances, poor concentration and tiredness. The patients often relate the symptoms to some type of occupational exposure, particularly to chemicals or physical components. However, these symptoms are normally present at some level in non-occupationally exposed people and may not be directly or mechanistically related to a specific exposure. Patients' attitudes and beliefs about their illness have a bearing on the symptoms they report and also on their behaviour. The complaints are often polysymptomatic and may even be chronic. The name 'environmental somatization syndrome' (ESS) has been proposed for this illness, indicating that the patients experience and communicate psychogenic distress in the form of physical symptoms. This is not a new phenomenon in occupational and environmental medicine and there are examples, during the last century, of widespread ESS epidemics. In the middle of the nineteenth century there were reports of patients who attributed their diffuse symptoms (fatigue, headache, dizziness, insomnia, eye irritation) to exposure to arsenic in homes and household utensils. During the Second World War the same type of symptoms were attributed to chronic carbon monoxide poisoning, and more recent long-term occupational exposure to organic solvents has been claimed to cause tiredness, concentration difficulties and memory impairment.

In this chapter MCS, SBS, amalgam poisoning and electrical hypersensitivity have been discussed. They all have in common a polysymptomatic picture similar to ESS, and there are no tests that can confirm a diagnosis. Whether these disorders are today's example of the ESS may be too early to decide, but there are close resemblances. However, one has to bear in mind that both physical factors and personality have an input on the response to an exposure. This response can be an interaction between a physiochemical pathway with a direct effect on health and a psychophysiological pathway mediated by stress and anxiety and manifested in non-specific symptoms. We still do not know enough of the mechanisms involved, but future research in the field of biochemistry, genetics and psychology may give us a better understanding of the mechanisms as well as individual susceptibility – an understanding that is important for the management and support of our patients.

Further reading

Cullen, M.R. (ed.) Workers with multiple chemical sensitivities. Occupational medicine. *State of the Art Reviews*, **2**, no 4 (1987)

Fasciana, G.S. *Are Your Dental Fillings Poisoning You?* Keats Publishing, New Canaan, Connecticut (1986)

Göthe, C.-J., Molin, C. and Nilsson, C.G. The environmental somatization syndrome. *Psychosomatics*, **36**, 1–11 (1995)

Knave, B. Electric and magnetic fields and health outcomes – an overview. *Scandinavian Journal of Work and Environmental Health*, **20** (special issue), 78–89 (1994)

Molin, C. Amalgam – fact and fiction. *Scandinavian Journal of Dental Research*, **100**, 66–73 (1992)

Rothman, A.L. and Weintraub, M.I. The sick building syndrome and mass hysteria. *Neurology Clinics*, **13**, 405–412 (1995)

Seltzer, J.M. (ed.) Effects of the indoor environment on health. Occupational medicine. *State of the Art Reviews*, **10**, no 1 (1995)

Spurgeon, A., Gompertz, D. and Harrington, J.M. Modifiers of non-specific symptoms in occupational and environmental syndromes. *Occupational and Environmental Medicine*, **53**, 361–366 (1996)

Verschaeve, L. Can non ionizing radiation induce cancer? (Review). *The Cancer Journal*, **8**, 237–249 (1995)

Chapter 12

Cancer in the workplace

H Vainio

Occupational cancer in the aetiology of human cancer

'Cancer' is a group of diseases that will strike many of us, directly or indirectly, since cancer accounts for more than 20% of all deaths in industrialized societies and is becoming a major cause of death in many developing countries [1]. Exposures in workplaces are a substantial cause of cancer in industrialized societies, although the precise fraction of cancers attributable to occupational exposures is difficult to assess: estimates range from 1% to 40%, depending on the time and place; a figure of 4–5% has been widely presented as a reasonable figure for industrialized countries [2,3]. These estimates are proportions and are therefore dependent on the contribution of causes other than occupational exposures to the overall burden of cancer. The estimates do not apply uniformly to people of each sex or to people of different social classes. If only the segment of the adult population with occupational exposures – manual workers in agriculture, industry and mining – are considered, the proportion increases substantially.

To date, 70 chemicals, complex mixtures and exposure circumstances have been determined to cause cancer in humans (*Tables 12.1* and *12.2*) [4,5]. Historically, many of these were first identified in the workplace under conditions of heavy exposure, chimney sweepers' exposure to soot being the classical example. In 1775, Percival Pott first described scrotal cancer in chimney sweepers, which he associated with heavy exposure to soot at a young age. Pott did not, however, have a clear idea of the underlying process, nor did he probably pay much attention to the specific features or severity of the disease [6]. It took more than a century before reports of skin cancers induced by occupational exposures to coal-tars and mineral oils started to appear in the literature. But the first clue as to the causative agent was provided by the publication of experimental results in which the painting of coal-tar onto rabbits' ears was shown to induce cancer [7]. When Passey, in 1922, induced skin tumours in mice by painting them with coal-tar, final proof was given that Pott's observations of a century-and-a-half previously were correct [8].

In the first half of this century, therefore, it was expected that epidemiological observations would always be corroborated by experimental results in animals. However, after the first epidemiological data were published in 1950 on the association between lung cancer and tobacco smoking [9,10], the relative weights of experimental and epidemiological data in the identification of human carcinogens changed: it was the incapacity to reproduce in experimental animals the striking finding of the carcinogenicity of tobacco smoke in humans that led epidemiologists to lay down criteria for assessing the causation for chronic diseases on the basis of epidemiological evidence alone [11]. The prevailing opinion has since been that only epidemiological studies can provide unequivocal evidence that an exposure is carcinogenic to humans; experimental studies of cancer in rodents can nevertheless *predict* an occupational carcinogen. Such predictions are not perfect; however, long-term carcinogenicity studies in animals are still the best tool we have for predicting carcinogenic effects before they occur at unacceptably high levels in the human population [12].

During the last two decades, progress in the understanding of the process of carcinogenesis has been fast, starting with the early historical observations, through the development and exploitation of animal models, cell and tissue models *in vitro*, and, most recently, to advances in molecular genetics [13,14]. Several of the genes involved in the multistage process of carcinogenesis are components of pathways in the control of normal growth and differentiation [15–18]. It is now known that chemical agents can act at different stages in carcinogenesis, probably by very different mechanisms [19,20]. An agent is considered to be carcinogenic when an alteration in the frequency or intensity of exposure is followed by a change in the frequency of occurrence of cancer at a particular site. Such scientific progress may make it possible to rely on the predictive data from the molecular epidemiological and biological sources in the prevention of occupational cancer.

Identifying occupational carcinogens

In 1969 the International Agency for Research on Cancer (IARC) initiated a programme to identify agents that pose a carcinogenic risk to humans. So far, 66 volumes of monographs have been published, containing the evaluations of over 800 agents. The evaluations are made with the assistance of international groups of experts, who assemble periodically to review current information on the role of an agent in the aetiology of cancer in humans. As a first step, the group assesses information on human exposure and experiments in animals. Each type of information is judged to provide 'sufficient', 'limited' or 'inadequate' evidence of carcinogenicity in animals and in humans, or evidence suggesting lack of carcinogenicity. Other relevant data on mechanisms and other aspects are also reviewed and summarized. The second step is to integrate these three pieces of evidence into a scientific judgement: the agent is judged to be 'carcinogenic' (Group 1), 'probably carcinogenic' (Group 2A), 'possibly carcinogenic' (Group 2B) or 'probably not carcino-

genic to humans' (Group 4); or it may be judged to be 'not classifiable' as to its human carcinogenicity (Group 3). This process underscores the judgemental basis of a risk assessment and provides clear-cut categories at a point in time.

During the past 25 years, some 70 chemicals, mixtures of chemicals, occupational exposure circumstances, and physical and biological factors that cause cancer in humans, have been identified by IARC working groups. The agents include: industrial processes, environmental agents (such as solar radiation), therapeutic agents (such as alkylating cancer chemotherapeutic agents), specific chemicals encountered in the workplace, culturally determined factors (such as alcoholic beverages), parasitic infections (such as infection with *Schistosoma haematobium*) and chronic viral infections (such as hepatitis B and hepatitis C viruses).

Table 12.1 lists the industrial processes and occupations that have been evaluated with regard to their carcinogenic risk to humans in IARC monographs. Categorization of a process or industry into Group 1 indicates that the working circumstances entail exposures that are carcinogenic to humans. Group 2A contains exposure circumstances that are probably carcinogenic and Group 2B those that are possibly carcinogenic to humans. *Table 12.2* provides information on chemicals, groups of chemicals and mixtures encountered predominantly in occupational settings and which have been considered to be causally linked to human cancer. The target sites are also presented. *Table 12.3* presents industries and occupations in which the presence of a carcinogenic risk is considered to be well established, with relevant cancer sites and known or suspected causal agent(s).

Recognition of occupational cancer

Recognition of work-related factors is vital for the effective diagnosis, treatment and prevention of ill-health. The alert clinician is in a key position to identify associations between exposures in the workplace and disease. Sometimes, problems are identified by workers. Cancer, with its long latency (often extending to two or three decades), is unlikely to be recognized as work-related, however, unless previous local events have sensitized the

Table 12.1 Industrial processes and occupations associated with cancer in humans (in IARC monographs, volumes 1–66)

Group	Exposure	Target organ*
1	Aluminium production	Lung, bladder
	Auramine, manufacture of	Bladder
	Boot and shoe manufacture and repair	Nasal cavity, leukaemia
	Coal gasification	Skin, lung, bladder
	Coke production	Skin, lung, kidney
	Furniture and cabinet making	Nasal cavity
	Haematite mining (underground) with exposure to radon	Lung
	Iron and steel founding	Lung
	Isopropanol manufacture (strong-acid process)	Nasal cavity
	Magenta, manufacture of	Bladder
	Painter (occupational exposure as a)	Lung
	Rubber industry (certain occupations)	Bladder, leukaemia
	Strong-inorganic-acid mists containing sulphuric acid (occupational exposure to)	Lung, larynx
2A	Art glass, glass containers and pressed ware, manufacture of	(Lung, stomach)
	Hairdresser or barber (occupational exposure as a)	(Bladder, lung)
	Non-arsenical insecticides (occupational exposures in spraying and application of)	(Lung, myeloma)
	Petroleum refining (occupational exposures in)	(Leukaemia, skin)
2B	Carpentry and joinery	(Nasal cavity)
	Dry cleaning (occupational exposures in)	(Bladder, oesophagus)
	Printing processes (occupational exposures in)	(Lung, oropharynx, bladder, leukaemia)
	Textile manufacture (work in)	(Nasal cavity, bladder)

* Target organs shown in parentheses are not confirmed.

workers and occupational health personnel to look for it. In the case of rare tumours, physicians may be able to identify new associations, such as that between exposure in the manufacture of polyvinyl chloride and hepatic angiosarcoma [21]. Common tumours, such as lung cancer, may go unrecognized even in occupationally exposed workers because of other confounding exposures, such as tobacco smoking: a superficial evaluation would automatically incriminate smoking as the (only) cause, although this may not be true, as well exemplified among asbestos insulators [22]. Owing to the multiplicative interaction of asbestos and smoking in the causation of lung cancer, a reduction in either causative agent can have a large impact on the excess risk for lung cancer [23]. Thus, whenever there is a positive interaction between two (or more) hazardous exposures, there is a greater possibility for effective prevention; the effect of the joint exposure can be attacked two or more ways, each requiring removal or reduction of one of the exposures. Interactions have also been demonstrated between tobacco smoking and several other occupational agents, such as arsenic, nickel and ionizing radiation [23].

Many patients, even in the Nordic countries where there are well-functioning occupational health services and efficient cancer registries, fail to be registered as having had an occupational cancer. For instance, in a Danish study of two cancers well-recognized as being occupationally related – pleural mesotheliomas and sinonasal adenocarcinomas, associated with occupational exposures to asbestos and wood dust, respectively – the estimated under-reporting was around 50% [24]. In Sweden also, reporting of mesothelioma has been found to be low (36%) [25]. In most cases, there was insufficiently detailed information about the occupational exposures. This is a universal problem that should be addressed in medical schools and particularly in the training of occupational physicians.

Regulation of occupational cancer hazards

Efforts to regulate occupational carcinogenic hazards are at their best when they can

Table 12.2   Chemicals, groups of chemicals and mixtures encountered predominantly in occupational settings that have been conclusively associated with cancer in humans (in IARC monographs volumes 1–66)

Group 1 exposure	Target organ*	
	Human	Animal†
4-Aminobiphenyl	Bladder	M, Liver, bladder, mammary glands intestine; D/Rb, Bladder
Arsenic and arsenic compounds	Lung, skin	M/H (Lung, larynx)
Asbestos	Lung, pleura, peritoneum	M, Peritoneum (mesothelioma); R, Lung, pleura, peritoneum
Benzene	Leukaemia	M, Lung, lymphoma, leukaemia, Zymbal gland; R, Oral cavity, Zymbal gland, skin, mammary gland, fore-stomach
Benzidine	Bladder	M, Liver, mammary gland, Zymbal gland; H, Liver
Beryllium and beryllium compounds	Lung	R, Lung; Rb, Bone (osteosarcoma)
Bis(chloromethyl)ether and chloromethyl methyl ether (technical-grade)	Lung	M, Lung, skin; R, Lung, nasal cavity; H, Lung
Cadmium and cadmium compounds	Lung (prostate)	M, Testis (lung); R, Testis, lung, local, prostate
Chromium (VI) compounds	Lung	M/R, Lung, local
Coal-tar pitches	Skin, lung, bladder	M, Skin
Coal-tars	Skin, lung	M/Rb, Skin; R, Lung
Mineral oils, untreated and mildly treated	Skin	M/Rb/Mk, Skin
Mustard gas (sulphur mustard)	Pharynx, lung	M (Lung, local)
2-Naphthylamine	Bladder	M, Lung, liver; R/H/Mk, Bladder
Nickel compounds	Nasal cavity, lung	R, Lung, local
Shale-oils	Skin (colon)	M/Rb, Skin
Soots	Skin, lung	M, Skin; R, Lung
Talc containing asbestiform fibres	Lung	–
Vinyl chloride	Liver, lung, blood vessels	M, Liver, lung, mammary gland, blood vessels; R, Liver, Zymbal gland, blood vessels; H, Liver, blood vessels, skin
Wood dust	Nasal cavity	–

* Target organs shown in parentheses are not confirmed.
† M, mouse; R, rat; H, hamster; Mk, monkey; D, dog; Rb, rabbit.

be based on adequate epidemiological data. Epidemiological studies are clearly a valuable source of information for regulations and offer the best basis for validating risk assessment models that rely on extrapolation of data from experimental systems.

Although epidemiology has provided important information about occupational cancer risks, it is not an ideal approach to public health, since cancer will already have occurred at least in some segments of the population. These segments are often people who are occupationally exposed, as such exposure is far more intensive than that of other segments of society [26]. The general population may also be exposed to carcinogens that occur in the workplace, as potentially carcinogenic materials and processes introduced into the workplace may be released into the general environ-

ment. The effects of exposure to new chemicals and other agents and exposure restricted to small populations or low levels are very difficult to detect, since epidemiology is a fairly blunt tool, and cancer excesses below 20–30% are practically impossible to detect. Cancer risk estimates based on epidemiology are available for fewer than 30 agents, and the estimates are highly uncertain [12].

In view of the limitations of epidemiology, much effort has recently been put into developing predictive approaches in the laboratory. Long-term carcinogenicity studies in animals are commonly used to predict human cancer hazards. Although the accuracy of the risk estimates derived from such studies is open to question, this protocol provides good indications of occupational cancer risk, as measures of carcinogenic activity (potency) derived from occupational

Table 12.3 Occupations and industries recognized as presenting a carcinogenic risk

Industry	Occupation/process	Cancer site/type	Known (or suspected) causative agent
Agriculture, forestry and fishing	Vineyard workers using arsenical insecticides	Lung, skin	Arsenic compounds
	Fishermen	Skin, lip	Ultraviolet radiation
Mining and quarrying	Arsenic mining	Lung, skin	Arsenic compounds
	Iron-ore (haematite) mining	Lung	Radon decay products
	Asbestos mining	Lung, pleural and peritoneal mesothelioma	Asbestos
	Uranium mining	Lung	Radon decay products
	Talc mining and milling	Lung	Talc containing asbestiform fibres
Chemical	Bis(chloromethyl)ether and chloromethyl methyl ether production and use	Lung (oat-cell carcinoma)	*Bis*(chloromethyl)ether and chloromethyl methyl ether
	Vinyl chloride production	Liver angiosarcoma	Vinyl chloride monomer
	Isopropyl alcohol manufacture (strong-acid process)	Sinonasal	Not identified
	Pigment chromate production	Lung, sinonasal	Chromium (VI) compounds
	Dye manufacture and use	Bladder	Benzidine, 2-naphthylamine, 4-aminobiphenyl
	Auramine manufacture	Bladder	Auramine and other aromatic amines used in the process
	para-Chloro-*ortho*-toluidine production	Bladder	*para*-Chloro-*ortho*-toluidine and its strong-acid salts
Leather	Boot and shoe manufacture	Sinonasal, leukaemia	Leather dust, benzene
Wood and wood products	Furniture and cabinet making	Sinonasal	Wood dust
Pesticide and herbicide production	Arsenical insecticide production and packaging	Lung	Arsenic compounds
Rubber	Rubber manufacture	Leukaemia	Benzene
		Bladder	Aromatic amines
	Calendering, tyre curing, tyre building	Leukaemia	Benzene
	Milling, mixing	Bladder	Aromatic amines
	Synthetic latex production, tyre curing, calendering, reclaim, cable making	Bladder	Aromatic amines
	Rubber film production	Leukaemia	Benzene
Asbestos production	Insulated material production (pipes, sheeting, textile clothes, masks, asbestos-cement products)	Lung, pleural and peritoneal mesothelioma	Asbestos
Metals	Aluminium production	Lung, bladder	Polycyclic aromatic hydrocarbons, tar volatiles
	Copper smelting	Lung	Arsenic compounds
	Chromate production	Lung, sinonasal	Chromium (VI) compounds
	Chromium plating	Lung, sinonasal	Chromium (VI) compounds
	Iron and steel founding	Lung	Polycyclic aromatic hydrocarbons, silica
	Nickel refining	Sinonasal, lung	Nickel compounds
	Pickling operations	Larynx, lung	Inorganic acid mists containing sulphuric acid
	Cadmium production and refining, nickel–cadmium battery manufacture, cadmium pigment manufacture, cadmium alloy production, electroplating, zinc smelting, brazing and polyvinyl chloride compounding	Lung	Cadmium and cadmium compounds
	Beryllium refining and machining, production of beryllium-containing products	Lung	Beryllium and beryllium compounds

Table 12.3 Occupations and industries recognized as presenting a carcinogenic risk (*cont'd*)

Industry	Occupation/process	Cancer site/type	Known (or suspected) causative agent
Shipbuilding, motor vehicle and railroad equipment manufacture	Shipyards and dockyards, motor vehicle and railroad manufacture	Lung, pleural and peritoneal mesothelioma	Asbestos
Gas	Coke plant works	Lung	Benzo[a]pyrene
	Gas works	Lung, bladder, scrotum	Coal carbonization products, β-naphthylamine
	Gas-retort house works	Bladder	β-Naphthylamine
Construction	Insulating and pipe covering	Lung, pleural and peritoneal mesothelioma	Asbestos
	Roofing, asphalt work	Lung	Polycyclic aromatic hydrocarbons
Other	Medical	Skin, leukaemia	Ionizing radiation
	Painting (construction, automotive industry and other use)	Lung	Not identified

studies are generally similar to those derived from long-term rodent studies [27,28]. For a number of reasons, however, sole reliance on such data may not protect workers' health sufficiently. For example, numerous agents found in the workplace have not been tested in long-term carcinogenicity studies, and many others have been inadequately tested. Furthermore, some quantitative estimates of risk derived from experimental studies understate the risks for susceptible individuals. In addition, significant differences in sensitivity between species have been observed for some compounds. As homogeneous strains are usually used in experimental studies, they may provide little information on the range of responses that occur in the more heterogeneous human species.

While few compounds have been shown to cause cancer in humans in occupational settings, several hundred chemicals are known to be carcinogenic in rodents. For most of them, no data are available on exposed humans, and the exposure levels at which these carcinogens will have carcinogenic effects in humans are unknown. Occupational exposures can be high – sometimes equal to the levels used in animal cancer studies; therefore, the argument that animal data obtained at maximally tolerated doses cannot be used to predict human cancer hazard is not valid for occupational settings.

One proposed strategy for using data from experimental studies is to calculate a rough index for comparing and ranking the possible hazards of chemicals that have been demonstrated to cause cancer in rodents on the basis of their potency in animals and the anticipated or permitted exposure in humans. Such indexes are known as human exposure/rodent potency (HERP) or permitted exposure/rodent potency (PERP) indexes [29]. The PERP index expresses the permitted lifetime exposure of a worker (in mg/kg body weight per day) to a chemical that is carcinogenic in animals as a percentage of the lifetime dose that induces tumours in 50% of animals (TD_{50} in mg/kg body weight per day). Gold and co-workers [30] showed that, in the USA, the PERP indexes for 75 rodent carcinogens differed by more than 100 000-fold from one another. For nine of these 75 carcinogens, the permitted exposure of workers is greater than 10% of the dose that induces tumours in one-half of animals that would otherwise have been tumour-free (*Table 12.4*). Although permissible exposure levels differ somewhat from country to country, some of the permitted exposures in workplaces are close to the levels that have been shown to cause cancer in rodents [31].

The wide variation in PERP values reflects the fact that carcinogenic effects are rarely the basis for establishing permissible exposure levels. For instance, the US Occupational Safety and Health Administration reported that, of the hundreds of permissible exposure levels that had been set, only 15 were set on the basis of cancer; seven of these are among the 75 chemicals studied by Gold and colleagues [30]. Many of the permissible exposure levels were set, at least in part, on the basis of the threshold limit values recommended

Table 12.4 Ranking of some 'rodent carcinogens' as the ratio of permitted exposure/rodent potency (PERP) on the basis of the permissible exposure levels (PEL) allowed by the US Occupational Safety and Health Administration (OSHA) and the TD_{50}, the chronic dose rate in mg/kg body weight per day that halves the proportion of tumourless test animals by the end of a standard lifetime (after Gold *et al.* [30])

Chemical	OSHA (ppm)	PEL (mg/m³)	TD_{50} (species) (mg/kg bw per day)	PERP (%)
Ethylene dibromide	20	153	1.52 (rats)	540
1,3-Butadiene	1000	2200	26.2 (mice)	456
Tetranitromethane	1	8	0.45 (rats)	94
Glycidol	25	75	4.28 (rats)	96
Styrene	50	215	23.3 (rats)	50
Bromoethane	200	890	149 (rats)	32
Epichlorohydrin	2	8	2.96 (rats)	15
Bis-2-chloroethyl ether	5	30	11.7 (mice)	14
Methylene chloride	500	1737	724 (rats)	13

by the American Conference of Governmental Industrial Hygienists. As has been stated before [32], these values are generally set at levels that are prevalent in industry, rather than at levels that are below those reported to have adverse health effects in the workplace. The PERP index could be used to select chemicals for which the permissible exposure levels should be reduced. For those of highest priority, exposure assessments, epidemiological studies and perhaps mechanistic studies should be carried out to strengthen extrapolation of data from rodents to humans. In the occupational health context, data from experiments in animals can be used to set priorities for medical surveillance, exposure assessment and epidemiological research.

Human heterogeneity in response to carcinogens

Traditional epidemiology based on 'risk factors' has been successful in identifying a wide variety of chemical and physical carcinogens in the workplace. However, it is one thing to show that benzene is a major cause of leukaemia in exposed populations, but it is altogether a different problem to show which individuals are the unlucky ones or to conclude retrospectively that cases of leukaemia were caused by exposure to benzene. As early as 1823, Henry Earle, one of Percival Pott's grandsons, noted that only a small proportion of exposed chimney sweepers developed scrotal cancer, and conjectured that a 'constitutional predis-

position . . . renders the individual susceptible to the action of soot' [33]. The relationship with genetic factors, however, was not elucidated rapidly; only recently have advances in human genetics and molecular biology allowed such hypotheses to be tested. Recent findings have shown that differences in human response to carcinogens and toxicants are linked to heritable differences in drug-metabolizing enzymes [34,35]. Epidemiological studies have revealed an association between specific alleles of drug- and carcinogen-metabolizing genes and increased cancer risk [36].

Individuals have been shown to respond differently to the same concentration of a given toxicant. Nevertheless, the usual assumption in deriving dose–response relationships in human carcinogenesis is that each person has exactly the same risk for cancer and that those individuals who develop cancer are determined by chance. This assumption may be more appropriate for laboratory animals in a long-term study, as animals are more homogeneous in genetic make-up, diet and other environmental factors. In humans, who have heterogeneous genomes, individual risks may differ substantially. While such heterogeneity in risk is difficult to quantify, measurements of phenotypic and genotypic differences in metabolism can provide information, and investigations of differences in people's ability to activate and detoxify chemicals indicate wide variation [13,37].

The current permissible exposure limits for carcinogenic chemicals do not account for such heterogeneity in responses, and the risk for sensitive members of the population may be substantially understated. This presents a special challenge for occupational health specialists, who have the mandate to protect all workers, including susceptible individuals.

Two well-known examples of polymorphic metabolism (*N*-acetylation and glutathione conjugation) are discussed below, which may influence individual susceptibility to carcinogens.

N-Acetylation and risk for bladder cancer

The molecular basis for inter-individual variations in carcinogen response and metabolism has been well studied with regard to *N*-acetyltransferases [38,39]. Some of the variability is due to inherited polymorphisms, as some people can efficiently carry out *N*-acetylation of 2-naphthylamine and a number of aromatic amines, while others cannot. As some aromatic amines are associated with a high risk for bladder cancer, it has been possible to study the interrelationship of this polymorphism with the risk for bladder cancer in industrial populations. Slow *N*-acetylation activity, as measured by phenotyping, was strongly associated with bladder cancer risk in dye workers, although the specific aromatic amines were not characterized [40,41]. The *NAT2* gene responsible for polymorphic expression of *N*-acetylation has been identified, the activity-associated specific mutations in *NAT2* are largely known, and the structure–function relationship for this gene has been established by studies of the correlation of genotypic and phenotypic activities [42]. Recently, it has been found that the *NAT1* gene, previously thought to be monomorphic, also exhibits polymorphism. *NAT1* is present in most tissues, in contrast to *NAT2*, and is present, for example, in bladder mucosa. Bell and co-workers [43] hypothesized that specific genetic variants in the polyadenylation signal of the *NAT1* gene would alter tissue levels of NAT1 enzyme activity; they were able to show that NAT1 enzyme activity is about twofold higher in bladder mucosa from individuals who inherit a variant polyadenylation signal (NAT1*10 allele).

Glutathione conjugation

Glutathione *S*-transferases are classified into at least four genetically distinct classes of enzyme (alpha, theta, mu and pi), which conjugate xenobiotics and carcinogens with glutathione [44,45]. Several polycyclic hydrocarbon epoxides are known substrates for the mu enzymes (GSTM), including benzo[a]pyrene-diol epoxide. Three allelic variants of *GSTM1* have been found; two of them, *GSTM1*A* and *GSTM1*B*, encode enzymes with activity similar to that of the wild-type allele. In contrast, a null allele, *GSTM1*0*, produces no enzyme and contains a nearly complete deletion of the gene. In most racial groups examined, 20–50% of all individuals are homozygous for the null allele, resulting in no GSTM1 enzyme [46–48]. Phenotypic studies among lung cancer patients have indicated that lack of *GSTM1* is associated with a 2.3-fold increased risk of adenocarcinoma among heavy cigarette smokers but not among light or non-smokers [47,49]. Similar findings have been reported for colorectal cancer but not for breast or bladder cancers [50].

Prevention and future directions

The history of occupational health has been highlighted by the development of methods of prevention of cancer, often long before any specific biological agent has been identified or its exact relationship to human cancer elucidated. A fundamental principle of occupational health is prevention of exposure to known or potential occupational carcinogens.

With the decreasing intensity of occupational exposures, due to improved industrial hygiene, recognition of occupational cancer risks will require new tools. The use of newly developed biomarkers of exposure, effect and individual susceptibility is the greatest promise for isolating and measuring individual exposures in the complex workplace environment and relating them quantitatively to early lesions that herald cancer (without waiting for the actual occurrence of the disease). This will improve our ability to reduce workplace hazards and at the same time provide direct insight into carcinogenic processes in humans. We may even hope that, in the long run, use of biomarkers in studies of humans will allow a link with information from parallel studies in animals, and enable much-needed quantitative risk estimates in models based on biologically interpretable parameters. More and more biomarkers are becoming available, and observational studies based on their use are multiplying; however, unless such studies are clearly targeted to their objectives, thoroughly prepared from a biological viewpoint, and rigorously designed and conducted, they may remain poor surrogates for mechanistic studies, whose experimental approach remains intrinsically superior. Such a slip into irrelevance can be averted by keeping the focus firmly on the principal aim of occupational cancer research: use results arising from both biology and an analysis of behavioural and social determinants of cancer in determining aetiology and preventive strategies.

References

1. Pisani, P. Burden of cancer in developing countries. In *Occupational Cancer in Developing Countries* (eds N. Pearce, E. Matos, H. Vainio *et al.*). International Agency for Research on Cancer, Lyon (1994)

2. Higginson, J. Proportion of cancers due to occupation. *Preventive Medicine*, **9**, 180–188 (1980)

3. Doll, R. and Peto, R. The causes of cancer: quantitative estimates of avoidable risks of cancer in the United States today. *Journal of the National Cancer Institute*, **66**, 1191–1308 (1981)

4. Vainio, H., Wilbourn, J. and Tomatis, L. Identification of environmental carcinogens: the first step in risk assessment. In *The Identification and Control of Environmental and Occupational Diseases* (eds M.A. Mehlman and A. Upton). Princeton University Press, Princeton, N.J. (1994)

5. Boffetta, P., Kogevinas, M., Simonato, L. *et al.* Current perspectives on occupational cancer risks. *International Journal of Occupational and Environmental Health*, **1**, 315–325 (1995)

6. Pott, P. *Chirurgical observations relative to cataract, the polypus of the nose, and cancer of the scrotum, the different kinds of ruptures, and the mortification of the toes and feet* (1775)

7. Yamagiwa, K. and Ichikawa, K. Uber die kunstliche Erzeugung von Papillom. *Verhandlungen Japanischen Pathologischen Gesellschaft*, **5**, 142–148 (1915)

8. Passey, R.D. Experimental soot cancer. *British Medical Journal*, ii, 1112–1113 (1922)

9. Doll, R. and Hill, A.B. Smoking and carcinoma of the lung. *British Medical Journal*, ii, 739–748 (1950)

10. Wynder, E.L. and Graham, E.A. Tobacco smoking as a possible etiologic factor in bronchogenic carcinoma. *Journal of the American Medical Association*, **143**, 329–336 (1950)

11. Hill, A.B. The environment and disease: association or causation? *Proceedings of the Royal Society of Medicine*, **58**, 295–300 (1965)

12. Tomatis, L., Aitio, A., Wilbourn, J. *et al.* Human carcinogens so far identified. *Japanese Journal of Cancer Research*, **80**, 795–807 (1989)

13. Harris, C.C. Chemical and physical carcinogenesis: advances and perspectives for the 1990s. *Cancer Research*, **51**, 5023s–5044s (1991)

14. Weinstein, I.B., Santella, R.M. and Perera, F. Molecular biology and epidemiology of cancer. In *Cancer Prevention and Control* (eds P. Greenwald, B.S. Kramer and D.L. Weed). Marcel Dekker, New York (1995)

15. Bishop, J.M. Molecular themes in oncogenesis. *Cell*, **64**, 235–248 (1991)

16. Bishop, J.M., Capobianco, A.J., Doyle, H.J. *et al.* Proto-oncogenes and plasticity in cell signaling. In *The Molecular Genetics of Cancer.* Cold Spring Harbor Laboratory Press, Cold Spring Harbor, NY (1994)

17. Schlessinger, J. and Bar Sagi, D. Activation of Ras and other signaling pathways by receptor tyrosine kinases. *Cold Spring Harbor Symposia on Quantitative Biology*, **59**, 173–179 (1994)

18. Kinzler, K.W. and Vogelstein, B. Life (and death) in a malignant tumour [news; comment]. *Nature*, **379**, 19–20 (1996)

19. Weinstein, I.B. Mitogenesis is only one factor in carcinogenesis [see comments]. *Science*, **251**, 387–388 (1991)

20. Vainio, H., Magee, P.N., McGregor, D.B. *et al. Mechanisms of Carcinogenesis in Risk Identification.* International Agency for Research on Cancer, Lyon (1992)

21. Creech, J.L., Jr and Johnson, M.N. Angiosarcoma of liver in the manufacture of polyvinyl chloride. *Journal of Occupational Medicine*, **16**, 150–151 (1974)

22. Hammond, E.C., Selikoff, I.J. and Seidman, H. Asbestos exposure, cigarette smoking and death rates. *Annals of the New York Academy of Sciences*, **330**, 473–490 (1979)

23. Saracci, R. The interactions of tobacco smoking and other agents in cancer etiology. *Epidemiology Review*, **9**, 175–193 (1987)

24. Skov, T., Mikkelsen, S., Svane, O. *et al.* Reporting of occupational cancer in Denmark. *Scandinavian Journal of Work and Environmental Health*, **16**, 401–405 (1990)

25. Andersson, E. and Toren, K. Pleural mesotheliomas are underreported as occupational cancer in Sweden. *American Journal of Industrial Medicine*, **27**, 577–580 (1995)

26. Hemminki, K. and Vainio, H. Human exposure to potentially carcinogenic compounds. In *Monitoring Human Exposure to Carcinogenic and Mutagenic Agents* (eds A. Berlin, M. Draper, K. Hemminki and H. Vainio). International Agency for Research on Cancer, Lyon (1984)

27. Crouch, E. and Wilson, R. Interspecies comparison of carcinogenic potency. *Journal of Toxicology and Environmental Health*, **5**, 1095–1118 (1979)

28. Allen, B.C., Crump, K.S. and Shipp, A.M. Correlation between carcinogenic potency of chemicals in animals and humans. *Risk Analysis*, **8**, 531–544 (1988)

29. Gold, L.S., Backman, G.M., Hooper, N.K. *et al.* Ranking the potential carcinogenic hazards to workers from exposures to chemicals that are tumorigenic in rodents. *Environmental Health Perspectives*, **76**, 211–219 (1987)

30. Gold, L.S., Backman, G.M. and Slone, T.H. Setting priorities among carcinogenic hazards in the workplace. In *Chemical Risk Assessment and Occupational Health. Current Applications, Limitations and Future Prospects* (eds C.M. Smith, D.C. Christiani and K.T. Kelsey). Auburn House, Westport, CT (1994)

31. Vainio, H. Syöpävaaraa aiheuttavien aineiden priori-sointi työhygienisten rajaarvojen ja eläintulosten perusteella. *Työ ja Ihminen*, **2**, 41–45 (1988)

32. Roach, S.A. and Rappaport, S.M. But they are not thresholds: a critical analysis of the documentation of Threshold Limit Values [see comments]. *American Journal of Industrial Medicine*, **17**, 727–753 (1990)

33. Schottenfeld, D. and Haas, J.F. Carcinogens in the workplace. *Journal of Clinical Cancer*, **29**, 144–168 (1979)

34. Nebert, D.W. Role of genetics and drug metabolism in human cancer risk. *Mutation Research*, **247**, 267–281 (1991)

35. Nebert, D. W., McKinnon, R.A. and Puga, A. Human drug-metabolizing enzyme polymorphisms: effects on risk of toxicity and cancer. *DNA Cell Biology*, **15**, 273–280 (1966)

36. Idle, J.R. Is environmental carcinogenesis modulated by host polymorphism? *Mutation Research*, **247**, 259–266 (1991)

37. Bolt, H.M. Genetic and individual differences in the process of biotransformation and their relevance for occupational medicine. *Medicina del Lavaro*, **85**, 37–48 (1994)

38. Grant, D.M. Molecular genetics of the N-acetyltransferases. *Pharmacogenetics*, **3**, 45–50 (1993)

39. Badawi, A.F., Hirvonen, A., Bell, D.A. *et al.* Role of aromatic amine acetyltransferases, NAT1 and NAT2, in carcinogen-DNA adduct formation in the human urinary bladder. *Cancer Research*, **55**, 5230–5237 (1995)

40. Cartwright, R.A. Glashan, R.W., Rogers, H.J. *et al.* Role of N-acetyltransferase phenotypes in bladder carcinogenesis: a pharmacogenetic epidemiological approach to bladder cancer. *Lancet*, **2**, 842–845 (1982)

41. Vineis, P. and Ronco, G. Interindividual variation in carcinogen metabolism and bladder cancer risk. *Environmental Health Perspectives*, **98**, 95–99 (1992)

42. Rothman, N., Stewart, W.F., Caporaso, N.E. *et al.* Misclassification of genetic susceptibility biomarkers: implications for case-control studies and cross-population comparisons. *Cancer Epidemiology Biomarkers Prevention*, **2**, 299–303 (1993)

43. Bell, D.A., Badawi, A.F., Lang, N.P. *et al.* Polymorphism in the N-acetyltransferase 1 (NAT1) polyadenylation signal: association of NAT1*10 allele with higher N-acetylation activity in bladder and colon tissue. *Cancer Research*, **55**, 5226–5229 (1995)

44. Ketterer, B., Harris, J.M., Talaska, G. *et al.* The human glutathione S-transferase supergene family, its poly-morphism, and its effects on susceptibility to lung cancer. *Environmental Health Perspectives*, **98**, 87–94 (1992)

45. Mannervik, B. and Danielson, U.H. Glutathione trans-ferases – structure and catalytic activity. *CRC Critical Reviews in Biochemistry*, **23**, 283–337 (1988)

46. Hirvonen, A., Husgafvel Pursiainen, K., Anttila, S. *et al.* The GSTM1 null genotype as a potential risk modifier for squamous cell carcinoma of the lung. *Carcinogenesis*, **14**, 1479–1481 (1993)

47. Daly, A.K. Cholerton, S., Armstrong, M. *et al.* Genotyping for polymorphisms in xenobiotic me-tabolism as a predictor of disease susceptibility. *Environmental Health Perspectives*, **102** (Suppl. 9), 55–61 (1994)

48. Nakajima, T., Elovaara, E., Anttila, S. *et al.* Expression and polymorphism of glutathione S-transferase in human lungs: risk factors in smoking-related lung cancer. *Carcinogenesis*, **16**, 707–711 (1995)

49. Anttila, S., Hirvonen, A., Husgafvel Pursiainen, K. *et al.* Combined effect of CYP1A1 inducibility and GSTM1 polymorphism on histological type of lung cancer. *Carcinogenesis*, **15**, 1133–1135 (1994)

50. Zhong, S., Wyllie, A.H., Barnes, D. *et al.* Relationship between the GSTM1 genetic polymorphism and susceptibility to bladder, breast and colon cancer. *Carcinogenesis*, **14**, 1821–1824 (1993)

Chapter 13

Male reproductive effects

M-L Lindbohm, M Sallmén and A Anttila

Introduction

Data on the adverse effects of occupational exposure on male reproductive health are gradually increasing. The discovery of infertility and sterility among the workers of a pesticide formulating plant exposed to dibromochloropropane (DBCP), in 1977, focused scientific and public attention on this field of research. Thereafter, about 50 occupational sperm surveys on the effects of workplace exposure on male fecundity have been published [1]. Recently, the research has been stimulated by reports on declining sperm count in the past few decades. It has been proposed that this may be due to prenatal exposure of fetal testes to oestrogens or chemicals with oestrogenic activity. The present evidence of the secular changes in semen quality is, however, controversial, as the results from different areas have been inconsistent [2,3].

Infertility caused by male factors is a frequent disorder, the aetiology of which is usually unknown. The male reproductive system has been shown to be highly sensitive to some physical and chemical exposures [4]. The reproductive toxicity of an agent may cause genetic damage to the spermatozoa, reduce sperm quality and quantity, disrupt the neuroendocrine system and inhibit sexual function. The manifestations also include infertility and adverse pregnancy outcome. There is now conclusive evidence that paternal exposure to ionizing radiation and some chemical agents can diminish sperm production and reduce fertility. It is also well recognized that the importance of the father in reproduction goes beyond fertiliza-

tion, although to date there is no well-established male exposure proven to influence pregnancy outcome in humans [5].

Several detailed reviews have been published on the influence of occupational exposure on male reproductive function [6–8] and on male-mediated developmental toxicity [5,9–11]. Information on the methods for assessing male reproductive health is available in other publications [12–14].

Potential mechanisms

There are four major categories of mechanisms of male reproductive toxicity during adulthood: non-genetic, direct or indirect effects on chromosomes or genes, and epigenetic effects on gene expression. In addition, indirect effects are possible by transmission of the agents to the mother via the seminal fluid and maternal exposure to toxicants brought home by the father [5,11,14].

Little is known about how the possible mechanisms contribute to the wide spectrum of reproductive outcomes in humans. Therefore, in this context the possible mechanisms of male reproductive toxicity are presented with minimal reference to specific agent–effect relationships. Some of the most potential agent-specific mechanisms are presented in the reviews of different reproductive hazards (described below).

Non-genetic mechanisms of toxicity include all alterations in the normal physiology and morphology of the male reproductive system, such as abnormalities in spermatogenesis, endocrine function, production of semen and delivery of functional sperm into the female reproductive tract. Several cellular targets of toxicity, depending on the exposure, have been identified: Leydig cells, Sertoli cells, epididymal cells and various cell types in spermatogenesis. Agents acting by non-genetic mechanisms would be expected to diminish the male's fertility potential [14].

Direct genetic mechanisms of male reproductive toxicity involve changes in the germ line DNA that may lead to abnormal sperm, and chromosomal abnormalities or gene mutations in the offspring. This mechanism of effects may result in any of a variety of abnormal reproductive outcomes that manifest themselves during development or after birth (spontaneous abortion, malformations, behavioural or functional abnormalities and cancer).

Indirect genetic mechanisms include alteration of chromatin stability or DNA repair capacity. Alterations of sperm chromatin stability caused by exposure to heavy metals (e.g. lead, copper, cadmium) probably affect the decondensation of the sperm chromatin, thereby interfering with zygote production and the normal fertilization process [15]. This can contribute to reproductive failure or have consequences for fetal development. Exposure to some substances, such as lead, caffeine and alcohol, have been found to act as inhibitors of DNA repair enzymes, and may exert a dominant lethal effect via this mechanism.

Epigenetic mechanisms of male reproductive toxicity refer to non-mutational changes in the germ line DNA that alter the gene activity pattern during development [5]. For example, changes in methylation patterns and genomic imprinting may alter the proper expression of maternal and paternal alleles after fertilization, and thereby lead to abnormal pregnancy outcomes or childhood cancer. There is evidence that genomic imprinting is involved in some human diseases, for example Prader–Willi syndrome and Wilms' tumour [16]. Much more work is needed to define the role that epigenetic mechanisms play in defining developmental outcome after male exposure. The potential for such an effect is greater through these pathways compared to direct genetic mechanisms. For example, the chemical 5-azacytidine is only a weak mutagen in mammalian cells, but has been shown to modify the methylation pattern of genes and thus alter the gene activity pattern by epigenetic mechanisms. Exposure to this agent *in vitro* has caused 10–30% of pre-

viously inactive genes to become reactivated. This effect corresponds to about a millionfold increase over spontaneous reversion mutation rates [17].

The impact of the male in abnormal reproductive outcomes should be viewed in a multigenerational context. The relevant exposure may occur at any point from when the boy was *in utero* until he produced the fertilizing sperm [14]. There is epidemiological evidence suggesting that the prenatal or childhood exposure of male offspring to some agents, including diethylstilboestrol and ethanol, is associated with the reduced ability to produce fertile gametes. In animal experiments, a phenoxy herbicide 2,3,7,8-tetrachloro-dibenzo-*p*-dioxin (TCDD) has shown similar effects [18].

Inorganic lead

Inorganic lead is toxic to the testis in animal experiments [8,19,20]. A wide spectrum of adverse effects has been reported on the reproductive function in male experimental animals, including suppression of spermatogenesis, changes in hormone levels and changes in testicular morphology. Most of these studies have been performed following chronic lead exposure, at levels comparable to those in the occupational environment. In studies where lead is given in doses close to the tolerable maximum, some of the results may be explained by non-specific toxic effects due to the general stress response.

Based mainly on animal models, the biologic rationale for the adverse effects is that lead (and some other toxic metals, such as cadmium or mercury) may partially replace zinc, which is an important component of semen and is needed for sperm head stabilization. Lead has induced changes in the stability of mouse sperm chromatin. Because of the genotoxic potential of lead, the possibility that reproductive capacity may be influenced also by direct changes in the genetic material, e.g. by induction of chromosomal aberrations – particularly in heavy paternal exposure – cannot be ruled out. Some of the alterations in the reproductive function at low lead levels are presumed to result from the lowering of the serum and intratesticular testosterone levels.

The adverse effects of occupational lead exposure on human sperm have been documented in several studies [1,8,19,20] (*Table 13.1*). Semen ana-

Table 13.1 Summary of the effects of inorganic lead on male reproductive function (after [1], [8], [9], [19], [20], [24])

Adverse effect	No. of reports supporting the association	Reported range of blood lead (µmol/l)
Decrease in sperm counts	7	2.0–4.2
Abnormal sperm morphology	6	2.0–3.6
Lowered sperm motility	4	2.0–3.6
Decreased spermatogenesis	2	1.9–NA
Decreased libido	1	1.9
Infertility	1	4.2
Reduced testosterone	3	1.9–3.5
Defects in thyroid function	1	3.5
Increase in prolactin	1	1.9
Testicular dysfunction	1	3.2
Abnormal prostatic function	1	3.5
Increased miscarriage rates in pregnancies fathered by lead workers	3	1.0–3.1
Increased risk of perinatal death or stillbirth in the offspring	2	NA
Increased risk of congenital malformations in the offspring	3	1.0–NA
Increased childhood cancer risk in the offspring	2	NA

NA = data not available.

lysis of workers whose exposure level has been monitored with blood lead concentrations (B-Pb) has shown dose-dependent reductions in the motility, morphology, viability and sperm count. Some functional hormonal and other biochemical effects influencing the production of sperm and semen – such as decreased libido, reduced testosterone, defects in thyroid function and testicular dysfunction – have also been reported. The adverse effects are well manifest in exposure, corresponding roughly to B-Pb levels from 2.0 to 2.4 µmol/l upwards. There is no systematic information available as to the critical exposure level. A study of storage battery workers in Romania reported significantly increased frequencies of asthenospermia, hypospermia and teratospermia when B-Pb levels ranged from 2.0 µmol/l to 3.6 µmol/l [21]. Non-significantly increased frequencies of asthenospermia and hypospermia were seen in a group of workers whose lead exposure stemmed from the polluted environment (current mean B-Pb 1.0 µmol/l). Further studies are warranted for the low exposure level. On the other hand, it has been documented that at very low exposure levels (say, B-Pb < 0.5 µmol/l) seminal plasma lead does not correlate with the concentration of lead in the blood,

and that the concentrations of lead in the seminal plasma are much lower than in the blood [22]. This suggests that there probably are no major direct genetic effects through semen at very low concentrations of lead. The lead concentrations in the seminal plasma are higher than those in the blood at higher exposure levels, as seen in heavy occupational exposure [23].

Only a limited number of epidemiological studies have been performed on the associations between paternal exposure to lead and adverse reproductive outcome. Three studies have reported an increase in the risk of spontaneous abortion following paternal exposure to lead [24] (see *Table 13.1*). Although there is suggestive evidence for a positive association, at least at high exposure levels (B-Pb 2.0–2.4 µmol/l or more), firm conclusions cannot be drawn, due to the small number of exposed cases and difficulties in controlling the potential confounders or effect modifiers. Two of the studies have suggested effects for B-Pb 1.0 or 1.2 µmol/l. Two epidemiological studies have reported that paternal exposure to lead increases the risk of deaths in the perinatal period – late abortion, stillbirth and early neonatal death [25,26]. There is also some weak evidence that paternal lead may increase the risk of congenital malformations in the offspring (reviewed in [20]). Studies on cancer in the offspring have also implicated effects for exposure to heavy metals including lead [9]. Due to the poor information on specific exposures, the available data do not, however, allow reliable identification of the specific aetiological agents.

Most of the studies on lead have been performed among lead smelters or battery manufacturers. Elevated concentrations of lead (whether metallic lead or lead compounds) which could be potentially harmful for the male reproductive function have been documented in several other industries or jobs as well, such as in founding, casting, scrapping, welding, and torch-cutting of leaded metals; car repair and service; glass and pottery manufacture; indoor shooting ranges and stevedoring work; spray painting; and in the use and disposal of various other chemicals.

Mercury

Occupational alkyl mercury has caused reduced sperm counts and terato- and asthenospermia (reviewed in [8]). These effects were seen before other signs of poisoning. A dose-dependent impairment of the fertility index, calculated from semen analytical values, has been documented among men exposed to mercury when working with explosives. The seminal mercury concentrations were 10 times higher than the serum concentrations. Two epidemiological studies relate excess spontaneous abortions with heavy paternal exposure to mercury (reviewed in [10]). In one of the studies performed among heavily exposed power plant workers, there was, as estimated in an exponential model, an increase of about 10% in the risk of abortions per 100 µg/l increase in the paternal urinary Hg concentration (100 µg/l U-Hg corresponds to 500 nmol/l). The other study in a chloralkali plant showed an increase of about 30% in the risk per 20 µg/l (100 nmol/l) of paternal U-Hg.

Other metals

In animals, high doses of hexavalent chromium have caused testicular atrophy and reduced sperm count [8]. Welders constitute a large occupational group with exposure to chromium. Reduced semen quality has been reported in welders in some studies, even though there is no evidence of the potential role of chromium compounds (see the separate section on welding, below). There is no firm evidence in the literature that chromium compounds have caused other effects in male reproductive function.

Other metals potentially harmful for the male reproductive system are manganese, cadmium and possibly arsenic but there are few studies on these metals (reviewed in [1]). Cadmium has not been shown to affect fertility in occupational populations – thus far only one study has focused on this issue. A significant inverse correlation has been documented between blood cadmium levels and sperm density, and a positive correlation between cadmium in the seminal plasma and low semen volume [22] resulting from exposure to cadmium originating mainly from smoking and diet. There is no evidence of the potential effects of these metals on pregnancy outcome. The effects of paternal smoking have not been demonstrated in the epidemiological literature on pregnancy outcome.

It is typical for occupational environments that where exposure to metals occurs there is a complex of metals and other elements in the workplace air.

The potential synergistic effects of such exposures have not been studied adequately. It may also be of importance that the existence of some metals in semen, such as zinc and selenium, may be protective against some adverse effects.

Welding

Exposure to several metals, such as chromates, nickel, manganese, cadmium or lead, occurs during welding, and welding fumes are typically complex mixtures of several metals and gases. Depending on the method used, for example on the apparatus, bar material, feeding rate, and intensity of the electric current, or on the materials processed, there is wide variation in the formation of the aerosols. Exposure to electromagnetic fields or non-ionizing or ionizing irradiation is also possible. In addition, some welders are exposed to a wide range of other chemicals, for example to solvents in cleaning of the metal surfaces, and heat. Thus, there are several potential hazards present in the working environment of welders, and careful assessment of the potential hazards among welding populations is needed. However, one cannot draw any definite conclusions on the role of the specific agents when assessing the risks related to welding work as such.

Decreased fertility, decreased sperm counts and abnormal forms in sperm have been reported among mild steel welders using the manual metal arc (MMA) or metal active gas (MAG) methods [1]. No effects were found among stainless steel welders who used the tungsten inert gas (TIG) method. Decreased fertility has also been reported among metal workers, based on questionnaire information. Several studies have shown associations with childhood cancer in the offspring of male metal workers, including welders. There is no direct information on the specific causative agents, however. No clear increase in the risk of spontaneous abortions or other adverse pregnancy outcomes has been reported for welding occupations and, in general, the evidence concerning potential adverse effects of welding on the paternal reproductive health is not clear cut.

Organic solvents

Data on the adverse effects of organic solvents on male reproductive health are scarce although exposure to organic solvents is common. Hazardous solvent exposure may take place in spray painting, degreasing, furniture manufacture, shoemaking, printing, dry cleaning, metal industries, reinforced plastics industries, and in the production of paints, glues and other chemicals; exposure to a single solvent is uncommon.

Exposure to organic solvents may have adverse effects on semen quantity and quality, sexual function and the reproductive neuroendocrine system. There is human evidence of the reproductive toxicity of some specific solvents, such as carbon disulphide and ethylene glycol ethers. Less convincing evidence exists on the harmful effects of chloroprene, perchloroethylene, styrene, toluene and thinners. In experimental animal studies, *n*-hexane and thinners, particularly the components ethyl acetate and xylene, have caused testicular damage [27,28]. The main metabolite of *n*-hexane, 2,5-hexanedione, has been shown to damage the functioning of Sertoli cells, which are essential for the proliferation and differentiation of all spermatogenic cells. Simultaneous exposure to toluene and xylene, however, seemed to prevent the toxic effects of *n*-hexane exposure. This finding indicates that the outcome of exposure to a solvent mixture cannot necessarily be predicted by summating the individual effects.

Disturbances in sexual function, such as decreased libido and potency, have been reported in male workers exposed to carbon disulphide, used primarily in the production of viscose rayon. Teratospermia, and gonadal and adrenal insufficiency, has also been found in men chronically poisoned with carbon disulphide [7]. At lower levels of exposure, no significant alterations in semen quality or decreases in fertility were indicated [29].

Reproductive toxicity of ethylene glycol ethers (2-ethoxyethanol, 2-methoxyethanol) and their acetates has been documented in several animal studies. The adverse effects include testicular lesions, testicular atrophy, reduced numbers of maturation-stage cells and infertility [30]. In humans, exposure to ethylene glycol ethers has been related to decreased sperm count, increased prevalence of oligospermia or reduced fertility in shipyard painters, metal casters and semiconductor manufacturers (reviewed in [8] and [31]). Ethylene glycol ethers are used in paints, varnishes, thinners, and solvents in resins, in textile printing and in various coating operations.

Only a few studies have been conducted on the effects of other solvents on male fecundity. Subtle changes in semen quality have been reported from exposure to perchloroethylene in dry cleaners and to styrene in workers producing reinforced plastic (reviewed in [4]). There is also some evidence that it may take the wives of dry cleaners slightly longer to conceive, and that more of them seek treatment for infertility than the wives of unexposed workers. No effects on sperm were seen from formaldehyde exposure in autopsy service workers [32].

Paternal exposure to organic solvents has also been related to adverse pregnancy outcome. The present evidence on the developmental effects of paternal solvent exposure is, however, limited and inconsistent. Exposure to solvents in general has been related to early preterm birth in the printing industry, and an increased risk of spontaneous abortions among the wives of exposed workers, in particular among painters and wood workers. The individual solvents associated with spontaneous abortion included toluene, xylene and miscellaneous solvents such as thinners. Exposure to perchloroethylene in dry cleaning or to benzene in chemical plants has not, however, been found to increase the risk of spontaneous abortion among the wives of exposed men (reviewed in [33]).

The findings of the studies on paternal solvent exposure and congenital malformations or birth weight have been contradictory (reviewed in [33]). Male painters have been reported to have an increased risk of fathering offspring with neural tube defects in several investigations. Work as a painter has also been associated with other types of malformations as well as decreased mean weight and length in children at birth. In other fields of industry, paternal solvent exposure has not been related to malformations. Some studies have suggested an increased risk of leukaemia or brain cancer in the offspring of fathers occupationally exposed to solvents or paints [9].

There are several methodological shortcomings, such as inaccurate assessment of exposure, poor response rate and small sample size, in studies on the effects of paternal solvent exposure on pregnancy outcome. Therefore, the present evidence on the developmental effects of male solvent exposure is inconclusive, whereas some individual solvents seem to cause adverse effects on the male reproductive system.

Pesticides

Pesticides are designed to be toxic to a variety of forms of life, including insects, fungi, microbes and plants. Because of the fundamental similarities of organisms at the subcellular level, pesticides often have the potential to cause adverse effects also in humans [34], and the effects of pesticide exposure on male reproduction have been studied extensively (reviewed in [1,8–10 and 35–37]).

The nematocide DBCP (dibromochloropropane) is by far the most impressive occupational testicular toxin in men [8,35]. Research results have shown that DBCP and/or its metabolites are toxic to spermatogonia, thus causing azoospermia or oligospermia, but the precise mechanism of action is not completely understood. Spermatogonia undergo several mitotic divisions to provide the cell numbers essential for a high sperm count [1]. For this reason, even a small amount of DBCP can severely impair spermatogenesis. The hazardous effect has been observed even after a few months of exposure. In testicular biopsies, a complete atrophy of the seminiferous epithelium has been observed among men exposed to DBCP for 2–10 years. Follow-up studies have shown that only some of the affected workers had recovered from azoospermia to a normal sperm count 7–11 years after exposure – the likelihood of recovery being related to the length and level of exposure.

In 1979, the US Environmental Protection Agency (EPA) banned the sale, distribution and commercial use of DBCP, but its use continued in some developing countries, for example Costa Rica and Honduras. During the late 1970s and 1980s, at least 1500 male workers on Costa Rican banana plantations became sterile from the use of DBCP (reviewed in [8]).

Adverse effects of occupational exposure to some other pesticides, e.g. 2,4-dichlorophenoxyacetic acid (2,4-D; asthenospermia, necrospermia and teratospermia), ethylene dibromide (EDP; sperm count, viability and motility), chlordecone (Kepone; oestrogenic effect) and carbaryl (sperm morphology) on semen quality have also been reported (reviewed in [8]).

The herbicide Agent Orange has been widely studied as regards its potential associations between paternal occupational exposure and spontaneous abortion or congenital malformation. Agent Orange is a mixture of 2,4-D and (2,4,5-trichlorophenoxy)acetic acid (2,4,5-T) containing 2,3,7,8-tetrachloro-dibenzo-*p*-dioxin (TCDD) as a contaminant. Studies among the Vietnamese are consistent in reporting an association between paternal exposure to sprayed herbicides and congenital defects, particularly anencephaly and orofacial defects. The findings on miscarriage among the wives of potentially exposed men are conflicting. The sperm quality of American Vietnam veterans was lower compared to non-Vietnam veterans 10–20 years after military service; the aetiology of this observation remained open, however. In occupational settings, paternal exposure to these herbicides has not been found to be related to pregnancy outcome (reviewed in [38]).

There are methodological shortcomings in many of these studies. Reproductive outcomes have been ascertained through maternal or paternal reports, not through medical records. Inaccurate assessment of exposure has been another serious weakness of these studies. A recent study in which past TCDD exposure was estimated on the basis of current blood samples provided little or no support for the hypothesis that exposure to Agent Orange and its dioxin contaminant is associated with adverse pregnancy outcome [39]. In general, the evidence of the adverse effect of dioxin-containing herbicides on male reproduction remains limited in humans.

The findings concerning paternal exposure to pesticides in general and adverse pregnancy outcome are controversial [10]. The highest spontaneous abortion risks have been observed in studies conducted in developing countries where the possibility of conducting high-quality studies is limited. On the other hand, the exposure levels are higher due to poorer working conditions than in developed countries. An association between exposure to pesticides and decreased fecundability (prolonged time to pregnancy) has been observed among Dutch fruit growers [40].

Several studies have focused on paternal work in agriculture and in related occupations or on exposure to pesticides and childhood cancer [36]. There seems to be an association between father's work in agriculture preconceptionally and an increased risk of brain tumours in their children. Besides paternal exposure to pesticides, the risk may be partially attributed to prenatal or postnatal exposure or animal contacts (*Toxoplasma gondii* infection). The results of a recent Norwegian study suggest that pesticide exposure is an independent risk factor for paternally mediated childhood brain cancer [41]. There are also findings on associations between paternal work in agriculture and acute non-lymphocytic leukaemia, Wilms' tumour and retinoblastoma.

Anaesthetic gases

Although several studies on the reproductive effects of exposure to trace concentrations of anaesthetic gases among dentists and physicians have been performed, it is uncertain whether these agents induce reproductive disorders in men. A study of semen quality in anaesthesiologists showed no differences in the number and morphology of the sperm between the exposed group and the controls [42]. The results of epidemiological studies have been contradictory. Some studies have shown a positive association between paternal exposure to anaesthetics and spontaneous abortion or congenital malformations in the offspring, whereas in others there has been no association [10,43]. These studies have been criticized for methodological weaknesses. The concentrations of anaesthetic gases may vary widely with time and place, and relatively high levels of nitrous oxide have been reported in dental clinics. None of the studies, however, has investigated the relationship between reproductive health and the actual concentration of anaesthetic gases in the ambient air of the workplace.

Oestrogens and oestrogenic compounds

Oestrogens or compounds with oestrogen-like activity taken by pregnant women have been suggested as a potential cause of the fall in sperm counts during the past 30–50 years [44]. In animal experiments, oestrogen exposure during an early stage of fetal life has been observed to cause malformation of the male genitalia and reduced fertility after puberty. In humans, the exposure of pregnant women to diethylstilboestrol has induced decreased sperm quantity and quality and increased the incidence of testicular cancer in their sons [8]. Adult men working in the formulation of oral contraceptives using synthetic oestrogens and progestins have been reported to experience symptoms associated with hyperoestrogenism. The exposure has also been related to

decreased libido and impotence [6]. Sexual dysfunction and alterations in male reproductive hormone levels have been observed in men occupationally exposed to a stilbene derivative (4,4′-diaminostilbene-2,2′-disulphonic acid) in the manufacture of fluorescent whitening agents [45]. The present data indicate that occupational exposure to oestrogenic substances may induce adverse male reproductive effects.

Other chemical agents

Other agents reported to affect male reproductive health harmfully include boron, chloroprene, dinitrotoluene and toluene diamine, hydrocarbons, methylene chloride, trinitrotoluene (TNT), and vinyl chloride [6]. Except for TNT, the data on the adverse effects of these agents are scattered and few in number. TNT has induced testicular toxic effects in animals, and TNT exposure at work has been associated with sexual disorders and reduced sperm quality [8]. The literature also points to several potential associations between paternal employment in various occupations or industries and adverse pregnancy outcome [5] and childhood cancer [9]. These suggestive findings warrant further investigation.

Ionizing irradiation

The testis is one of the most radiosensitive tissues of the body; a direct radiation dose as low as 0.15 Gy may cause a significant depression in the sperm count, and temporary azoospermia occur after doses of 0.3 Gy; 2 Gy has caused irreversible azoospermia [46]. The most precise and complete data on radiation effects are from studies on healthy volunteers who received 250 kVp X-rays to the testes in a single dose. Adverse effects have also been documented in cancer patients receiving fractionated irradiation during radiotherapy treatment, and for accidental exposure to beta and gamma irradiation during and after a nuclear reactor accident [46–48].

The effects of protracted exposure to radiation have not been studied adequately. A study among subjects with long-term low-level occupational exposure has reported adverse alterations in spermatogenesis [49]. The periods of exposure among the irradiation-exposed workers varied from 2 to

22 years. The doses received could not be accurately determined, because the film badge records were available for most of the subjects for the last 5–10 years only. For those periods with film badge records, the yearly external doses varied typically between 480 and 3500 mrad (corresponding to 4.8–35 mGy).

Medical radiology personnel, miners (exposed to radon), uranium miners, welders and technicians doing pipe welding, radiographers, and nuclear power plant personnel, are among those with potential occupational exposure. Careful assessments have been made to extrapolate the standards for safe exposure levels, in order to minimize the occupational exposures. If the permissible occupational standard (usually 15 mSv per year in chronic exposure) is not exceeded, major testicular effects are unlikely. The hygienic standard of 15 mSv is roughly equivalent to a threefold yearly increase, compared to the average whole-body dose in the general population. The range of the individual doses in the environmental exposure may vary from < 1 mSv very rarely up to 1000 mSv per year.

Ionizing radiation has been recognized as a highly mutagenic and cytotoxic agent in somatic cells. It is also thought that comparably low doses of irradiation may damage DNA in the germ cells, causing mutations and hereditary defects in the offspring. Indirect or epigenetic pathways in the germ cell alterations cannot be ruled out [50,51]. Early primordial germ cells (prenatal days 13 and 35) are known to be particularly sensitive to the effects of irradiation [1].

It has been much debated whether low-level paternal preconceptional exposure to irradiation causes leukaemias or possibly lymphomas in the offspring. Some positive evidence has been obtained, based on an animal experiment using X-rays, and studies of childhood cancers in the offspring of men receiving irradiation at a nuclear plant, in radiography, and from diagnostic X-rays [52–54]. The suggested evidence should be interpreted with caution, because the numbers on which the risks are based are small, and the possibility of correlations with some unexplored risk factors or population characteristics cannot be ruled out. In the study on nuclear power plant workers [52], the leukaemia risk was associated with paternal preconceptional external doses ranging between 100 and 380 mSv. In particular, the external doses during the 6-month period before the conception were above 10 mSv. No increase in leukaemia rates – also based on a small number of expected cases – has appeared in the offspring of Japanese male survivors from the atomic bombing in Hiroshima and Nagasaki. The atomic bombing survivors had been irradiated instantaneously to an average dose of about 490 mSv.

It is noteworthy that a nation-wide case-control study of childhood cancer revealed an excess of all childhood cancers and leukaemia in the offspring of male nuclear industry workers in the UK [55]. However, there was no estimation of the doses at an individual level, and paternal preconceptional employment appeared to be no more important than postconceptional employment. There was no clear support for potential association with cancer in the offspring of workers exposed to other types of ionizing irradiation (e.g. clinical radiologists or industrial radiographers). Altogether about 30 epidemiological studies have been performed on the potential association between low-dose paternal exposure to radiation and leukaemia. Even though there have been clusters of childhood leukaemias near some nuclear power plants, a causal relationship with radiation cannot be sustained according to these studies [55–57]. Concerning the role of radiation, many of the studies on the paternal component have used flawed methodologies in measuring exposures, and therefore no final conclusions can be drawn.

There also exists growing interest to explore whether paternal exposure to ionizing radiation has any effects on the pregnancy outcome. Several studies published between the 1920s and early 1970s have documented increased miscarriage and stillbirth rates among women married to radiologists (reviewed in [49]). The exposure levels in the past, e.g. if shielding was not used, may have been considerably higher than nowadays. Two studies published after 1970 have shown a slightly increased risk of spontaneous abortion for paternal exposure to ionizing radiation. The evidence from the latter two studies is weak due to the possibility of response bias, and poor documentation of the exposure [10]. In a recent study among medical radiographers, the miscarriage rates did not appear to be in excess [54].

Non-ionizing radiation

There are only a few studies on reproductive hazards related to male exposure to non-ionizing radiation, including optical radiation, radiofrequency radiation, microwaves and low-frequency electromagnetic fields. Reduced sperm quality has been reported for technicians exposed to microwaves. Decreased frequency of 'normal' pregnancy outcome, mainly due to increased frequency of congenital malformations, and fertility difficulties has been observed among high-voltage switchyard workers [6,7]. No association of semen abnormalities was observed with job titles suggesting magnetic field exposure [58]. Paternal employment in electrical occupations involving potential exposure to electromagnetic fields has also been related to childhood cancer [36]. The present data on the reproductive effects of non-ionizing radiation are inconclusive, however.

Heat

The human testes are located outside the body cavity in the scrotum to reduce the intratesticular temperature, since active sperm production is dependent on an environment that is 3–4°C lower than the normal body temperature [8]. A recent history of high fever (more than 38°C) in man may result in temporary impairment of semen quality and reduction of fertility. Also in experimental situations (scrotal heating, sauna bathing), a decrease in sperm quality has been observed. In a small experimental study, mild testicular heating was shown to have contraceptive effects due to decreased motility of sperm [59].

There are only a few studies on the possible effects of occupational heat exposure on sperm production or fertility (reviewed in [4] and [8]). Among couples who were examined or treated for infertility, male exposure to heat was related to sperm abnormalities. The studies conducted among professional drivers, outdoor workers (summer versus winter), welders and oven operators in the ceramic industry suggest that exposure to radiant heat (globe temperature range 31–45°C) or working in a hot environment is associated with a reversible decrease of semen quality. An inconclusive association between high temperature and delayed conception has also been observed.

Summary of the evidence

All in all, the data on the adverse effects of occupational factors on male fecundity and pregnancy outcome are scarce and the present knowledge allows the prevention of only a few male reproductive failures. Further research is needed on the effects of occupational exposure on male reproductive health to prevent potential adverse reproductive and developmental outcomes and to provide a scientific basis for policy-making.

The occupational exposures indicated as harmful for the reproductive health of men in human studies are summarized in *Table 13.2*. There are only a few agents with sufficient evidence of their toxicity to male reproductive function, and for all agents the evidence of their harmful effects on pregnancy outcome is, so far, insufficient. Evidence has been judged here as sufficient if it is based on more than one study of good quality. Lead, mercury, some organic solvents, oestrogens, some pesticides, and trinitrotoluene, as well as heat and ionizing radiation, have been shown to affect the male reproductive function adversely at high exposure levels. The setting of exact exposure limits based on the present data, is, however, difficult.

For most agents, the evidence for their adverse reproductive effects is insufficient. It is based on only one study or on studies with methodological limitations, such as inaccurate data on exposure or outcome, poor participation rate, small sample size and borderline significance. Particularly in studies on paternal effects, pregnancy outcome has often been related to some occupation, industry or a group of chemicals, and less seldom to specifically defined exposures. These findings await the identification of individual hazardous agents.

Prevention

For most of the chemicals potentially harmful to male reproductive health, a systematic and comprehensive risk assessment has not been performed (see Chapter 14). The risk assessment process is essential for prevention, not only on a national but also on the factory level, by evaluating the toxicological data and handling the uncertainties in the human data and in the mechanisms.

Considering the agents and exposures for which there is reasonably consistent evidence that they may impair male reproductive functions (*Table 13.2*, under agents with sufficient evidence), the primary goal of risk prevention is to minimize the prevailing exposure levels towards lower or

Table 13.2 Occupational male reproductive hazards

Exposure	Adverse effects on male fecundity	Adverse effects on pregnancy outcome
Sufficient evidence		
Metals		
lead	+	(+)
mercury	+	(+)
Organic solvents		
carbon disulphide	+	
ethylene glycol ethers and their acetates	+	
Pesticides		
chlordecone (Kepone)	+	
dibromochloropropane (DBCP)	+	(+)
2,4-dichlorophenoxyacetic acid	+	
ethylene dibromide	+	
Synthetic oestrogens and progestins	+	
Trinitrotoluene	+	
Ionizing radiation	+	(+)
Heat	+	
Insufficient evidence		
Metals		
arsenic	(+)	
cadmium	(+)	
manganese	(+)	
Welding	(+)	(+)
Organic solvents	(+)	
benzene	(−)	
methylene chloride	(+)	
perchloroethylene	(+)	(−)
styrene	(+)	
thinners	(+)	
toluene	(+)	
mixtures of solvents	(+)	
Pesticides	(+)	(+)
carbaryl	(+)	
dioxin	(+)	
2,3,7,8-tetrachlorodibenzo-*p*-dioxin (TCDD)	(+)	
Anaesthetic gases	(−)	(+)
Boron	(+)	
Chloroprene	(+)	(+)
Dinitrotoluene and toluene diamine	(+)	(+)
Hydrocarbons	(+)	
Vinyl chloride	(+)	
Non-ionizing radiation	(+)	(+)

+, Positive association; −, No association; Inconclusive data in parentheses.

safe ones. In principle, the knowledge on the critical exposures – even though not complete for many of the adverse effects on male reproductive health – ought to be taken into account in the safety standards. In most countries the paternal component in the adverse effects has not been considered systematically in the standards; for example, the present safety standards for lead are not based on the available data on the male reproductive functions. Instead, the standards in most countries still aim at the prevention of clinical lead poisoning. In some countries separate standards exist for pregnant women, due to the possibility that a very low concentration of prenatal lead may impair neurological development in the fetus. On the other hand, if the safety standard for lead considered such health issues as mild neurotoxic effects in susceptible adult or ageing populations, or possible carcinogenic risks, the new and substantially lower permissible standards might also prevent most of the risks related to male reproductive function.

A variety of industrial hygienic measures are available to minimize effectively harmful exposures at work. These include, for instance, the closing of emission sources (e.g. by providing fume cupboards and chambers, with effective outlets and collectors of the harmful material), improvement of ventilation, proper working methods (e.g. use of water-based methods in cleaning or in working with dusty surfaces; leaving the work rooms empty when the products handled with solvents are drying; picking off metal-painted materials before welding or smelting them); and the use of effective personal protectors. Continuous hygienic and biological measurements of exposure are an important part of the control policy. Sometimes the problems may be solved only by industrial–technological developments, such as the introduction of new automatic production lines and new technology, or substituting harmful materials by safer ones.

For agents on which there is only limited evidence – based on animal data or a single human study, for example – firm regulative guidelines cannot be given. In these situations risk management should include efforts to lower the exposure levels at the workplace, and to keep the employees, supervisors and management informed. Measurements of potential effects on sperm or surrogate somatic cells may sometimes provide detailed additional information for the workplace. Because there is often a lack of confirmed scientific evidence concerning adverse effects on male reproductive health, it is important that occupational health and safety personnel are involved in the development of good workplace practice.

References

1. Bonde, J.P. and Giwercman, A. Occupational hazards to male fecundity. *Reproductive Medicine Review*, **4**, 59–73 (1995)
2. Irvine, S., Cawood, E., Richardson, D. *et al.* Evidence of deteriorating semen quality in the United Kingdom: birth cohort study in 577 men in Scotland over 11 years. *British Medical Journal*, **312**, 467–471 (1996)
3. Fisch, H. and Goluboff, E.T. Geographic variations in sperm counts: a potential cause of bias in studies on semen quality. *Fertility and Sterility*, **65**, 1044–1046 (1996)
4. Bonde, J.P. and Ernst, E. Is male fecundity at risk from occupational and environmental exposures? In *New Epidemics in Occupational Health*. People and Work, Research Reports 1. Finnish Institute of Occupational Health, Helsinki (1994)
5. Olshan, A.F. and Faustman, E.M. Male-mediated developmental toxicity. *Annual Review of Public Health*, **14**, 159–181 (1993)
6. Schrag, S.D. and Dixon, R.L. Occupational exposures associated with male reproductive dysfunction. *Annual Review of Pharmacology and Toxicology*, **25**, 567–592 (1985)
7. Henderson, J., Baker, H.W.G. and Hanna, P.J. Occupation-related male infertility: a review. *Clinical Reproduction and Fertility*, **4**, 87–106 (1986)
8. Lähdetie, J. Occupation- and exposure-related studies on human sperm. *Journal of Occupational and Environmental Medicine*, **37**, 922–930 (1995)
9. O'Leary, L.M., Hicks, A.M., Peters, J.M. *et al.* Parental occupational exposures and risk of childhood cancer: a review. *American Journal of Industrial Medicine*, **20**, 17–35 (1991)
10. Savitz, D.A., Sonnenfeld, N.L. and Olshan, A.F. Review of epidemiologic studies of paternal occupational exposure and spontaneous abortion. *American Journal of Industrial Medicine*, **25**, 361–383 (1994)
11. Ratcliffe, J.M. Paternal exposures and embryonic or fetal loss: the toxicologic and epidemiologic evidence. In *Male-Mediated Developmental Toxicity* (eds A.F. Olshan and D.R. Mattison). Plenum Press, NY (1994)
12. Schrader, S.M., Chapin, R.E., Clegg, E.D. *et al.* Laboratory methods for assessing human semen in epidemiologic studies: a consensus report. *Reproductive Toxicology*, **6**, 275–279 (1992)
13. Comhaire, F.H. Methods to evaluate reproductive health of the human male. *Reproductive Toxicology*, **7**, 39–46 (1993)
14. Wyrobek, A.J. Methods and concepts in detecting abnormal reproductive outcomes of paternal origin. *Reproductive Toxicology*, **7**, 3–16 (1993)
15. Johansson, L. and Pelliciari, C.E. Lead-induced changes in the stabilization of the mouse sperm chromatin. *Toxicology*, **51**, 11–24 (1988)
16. Rainier, S. and Feinberg, A.P. Genomic imprinting, DNA methylation and cancer. *Journal of the National Cancer Institute*, **86**, 753–759 (1994)
17. Holliday, R. The inheritance of epigenetic defects. *Science*, **238**, 163–170 (1987)
18. Peterson, R.E., Theobald, H.M. and Kimmel, G.L. Developmental and reproductive toxicity of dioxins and related compounds: cross-species comparisons. *CRC Critical Reviews in Toxicology*, **23**, 283–335 (1993)
19. Winder, C. Lead, reproduction and development. *Neurotoxicology*, **14**, 303–318 (1993)
20. Bellinger, D. Teratogen update: lead. *Teratology*, **50**, 367–373 (1994)
21. Lancranjan, I., Popescu, H.I., Gavanescu, O. *et al.* Reproductive ability of workmen occupationally exposed to lead. *Archives of Environmental Health*, **30**, 396–401 (1975)
22. Xu, B., Chia, S.-E., Tsakok, M. *et al.* Trace elements in blood and seminal plasma and their relationship to sperm quality. *Reproductive Toxicology*, **7**, 613–618 (1993)
23. von Matthies, J., Schwartz, I. and Donat, H. Einfluss von schwermetallionen auf die männliche fertilität. *Zentralblatt für Gynäkologie*, **111**, 155–166 (1989)
24. Anttila, A. and Sallmén, M. Effects of parental occupational exposure to lead and other metals on spontaneous abortion. *Journal of Occupational and Environmental Medicine*, **37**, 915–921 (1995)
25. Selevan, S.G., Hornung, R., Kissling, G.E. *et al.* *Reproductive Outcomes in Wives of Lead Exposed Workers*. US National Institute for Occupational Safety and Health, Department of Health and Human Services (PB85-220879), Cincinnati, OH (1984)
26. Kristensen, P., Irgens, L.M., Daltveit, A.K. *et al.* Perinatal outcome among children of men exposed to lead and organic solvents in the printing industry. *American Journal of Epidemiology*, **137**, 134–144 (1993)
27. Nylén, P., Ebendal, T., Eriksdotter-Nilsson, M. *et al.* Testicular atrophy and loss of nerve growth factor – immunoreactive germ cell line in rats exposed to n-hexane and a protective effect of simultaneous exposure to toluene or xylene. *Archives of Toxicology*, **63**, 296–307 (1989)
28. Yamada, K. Influence of lacquer thinner and some organic solvents on reproductive and accessory reproductive organs in the male rat. *Biological and Pharmacological Bulletin*, **16**, 425–427 (1993)
29. Vanhoorne, M., Comhaire, F. and de Bacquer, D. Epidemiologic study of the effects of carbon disulfide on male sexuality and reproduction. *Archives of Environmental Health*, **49**, 273–278 (1994)
30. Wess, J.A. Reproductive toxicity of ethylene glycol monomethyl ether, ethylene glycol monoethyl ether and their acetates. *Scandinavian Journal of Work and Environmental Health*, **18**, 43–45 (1992)
31. Correa, A., Gray, R.H., Cohen, R. *et al.* Ethylene glycol ethers and risks of spontaneous abortion and subfertility. *American Journal of Epidemiology*, **143**, 707–717 (1996)

32. Ward, J.B., Jr., Hokanson, J.A., Smith, E.R. *et al.* Sperm count, morphology and fluoroscent body frequency in autopsy service workers exposed to formaldehyde. *Mutation Research*, **130**, 417–424 (1984)

33. Lindbohm, M-L. Effects of parental exposure to solvents on pregnancy outcome. *Journal of Occupational and Environmental Medicine*, **37**, 908–914 (1995)

34. Wilkinson, C.F. Introduction and overview. In *The Effects of Pesticides on Human Health* (eds S.R. Baker and C.F. Wilkinson). Princeton Scientific Publishing Co, Princeton, NJ (1990)

35. Mattison, D.R., Bogumil, R.J., Chapin, R. *et al.* Reproductive effects of pesticides. In *The Effects of Pesticides on Human Health* (eds S.R. Baker and C.F. Wilkinson). Princeton Scientific Publishing Co., Princeton, NJ (1990)

36. Gold, E.B. and Sever, L.E. Childhood cancer associated with parental occupational exposures. *Occupational Medicine: State of the Art Reviews*, **9**, 495–539 (1994)

37. Sever, L.E. Congenital malformations related to occupational reproductive hazards. *Occupational Medicine: State of the Art Reviews*, **9**, 471–494 (1994)

38. Lindbohm, M-L. Paternal TCDD exposure and pregnancy outcome. *Epidemiology*, **6**, 4–6 (1995)

39. Wolfe, W.H., Michalek, J.E., Miner, J.C. *et al.* Paternal serum dioxin and reproductive outcomes among veterans of operation Ranch Hand. *Epidemiology*, **6**, 17–22 (1995)

40. de Cock, J., Westveer, K., Heederik, D. *et al.* Time to pregnancy and occupational exposure to pesticides in fruit growers in The Netherlands. *Occupational and Environmental Medicine* **51**, 693–699 (1994)

41. Kristensen, P., Andersen, A., Irgens, L.M. *et al.* Cancer in offspring of parents engaged in agricultural activities in Norway: incidence and risk factors in the farm environment. *International Journal of Cancer*, **65**, 39–50 (1996)

42. Wyrobek, A.J., Brodsky, J., Gordon, L. *et al.* Sperm studies in anesthesiologists. *Anesthesiology*, **55**, 527–532 (1981)

43. Tannenbaum, T.N. and Goldberg, R.J. Exposure to anesthetic gases and reproductive outcome. *Journal of Occupational Medicine*, **27**, 659–668 (1985)

44. Sharpe, R.M. and Skakkebaek, N.E. Are oestrogens involved in falling sperm counts and disorders of the male reproductive tract? *Lancet*, **341**, 1392–1395 (1993)

45. Grajewski, B., Whelan, E.A., Schnorr, T.M. *et al.* Evaluation of reproductive function among men occupationally exposed to a stilbene derivative: I. Hormonal and physical status. *American Journal of Industrial Medicine*, **29**, 49–57 (1996)

46. Ogilvy-Stuart, A.L. and Shalet, S.M. Effect of radiation on the human reproductive system. *Environmental Health Perspectives, Supplement*, **101** (Suppl. 2), 109–116 (1993)

47. Ash, P. The influence of radiation on fertility in man. *British Journal of Radiology*, **53**, 271–278 (1980)

48. Birioukov, A., Meurer, M., Peter, R.U. *et al.* Male reproductive system in patients exposed to ionizing irradiation in the Chernobyl accident. *Archives of Andrology*, **30**, 99–104 (1993)

49. Popescu, H.I. and Lancranjan, I. Spermatogenesis alteration during protracted irradiation in man. *Health Physics*, **28**, 567–573 (1975)

50. Wiley, L.M. Male mice receiving very low doses of ionizing radiation transmit an embryonic cell proliferation disadvantage to their progeny embryos. In *Male-Mediated Developmental Toxicity* (eds A.F. Olshan and D.R. Mattison). Plenum Press, NY (1994)

51. Nomura, T. Male-mediated teratogenesis: ionizing radiation/ethylnitrosourea studies. In *Male-Mediated Developmental Toxicity* (eds A.F. Olshan and D.R. Mattison). Plenum Press, NY (1994)

52. Gardner, M.J., Snee, M.P., Hall, A.J. *et al.* Results of case-control study of leukemia and lymphoma among young people near Sellafield nuclear plant in West Cumbria. *British Medical Journal*, **300**, 423–429 (1990)

53. Shu, X.O., Reaman, G.H., Lampkin, B. *et al.* Association of paternal diagnostic X-ray exposure with risk of infant leukemia. *Cancer Epidemiology Biomarkers and Prevention*, **3**, 645–653 (1994)

54. Roman, E., Doyle, P. Ansell, P. *et al.* Health of children born to medical radiographers. *Occupational and Environmental Medicine*, **53**, 73–79 (1996)

55. Sorahan, T., Lancashire, R.J., Temperton, D.H. *et al.* Childhood cancer and paternal exposure to ionizing radiation: a second report from the Oxford survey of childhood cancers. *American Journal of Industrial Medicine*, **28**, 71–78 (1995)

56. Rose, K.S.B. A review of epidemiological studies concerning leukaemia and lymphoma among young people and the genetic effects of ionising radiation. *Nuclear Energy*, **33**, 331–336 (1994)

57. Doll, R. Effect of small doses. *Nuclear Energy*, **34**, 15–19 (1995)

58. Lundsberg, L.S., Bracken, M.B. and Belanger, K. Occupationally related magnetic field exposure and male subfertility. *Fertility and Sterility*, **63**, 384–391 (1995)

59. Mieusset, R. and Bujan, L. The potential of mild testicular heating as a safe, effective and reversible contraceptive method for men. *International Journal of Andrology*, **17**, 186–191 (1994)

Chapter 14

Pregnancy and work

H Taskinen and M-L Lindbohm

Introduction

Human reproduction is a complex process which can be disturbed in many phases by host and environmental factors. Therefore, it has been difficult to distinguish the occupational causes of spontaneous abortions and congenital malformations from other factors related to the parents and their living environment. The extrapolation of results of animal studies on humans is often complicated because of the structural and functional differences between the species and because the mechanisms of harmful effects are seldom known. In this chapter, information on the effects of occupational exposure on female reproductive health, pregnancy and the health of offspring are highlighted.

Effects of occupational exposure on menstrual cycle function

Alterations in the menstrual cycle are of many types and quite common for a variety of reasons. Possible effects of occupational exposure to the menstrual function have recently been reviewed [1–3]. Hormone production (synthetic oestrogens and progestagens, diethylstiloestrol; [2]) has been reported to be associated with hormonal imbalance in workers, and exposure to organic chemicals including toluene [3], styrene [1], perchlorethylene, organic solvents in photolithography (such as xylene, n-butyl acetate and glycol ethers), and work as a hairdresser [3] have been reported in association with various types of menstrual disorders. Women exposed to 130 ppm of styrene had high serum levels of prolactin. High prolactin may cause oligo- or amenorrhoea [1].

Mercury, metal dopants such as arsenic in the semiconductor industry, mercury together with noise and shift work, cannery work (cold temperatures and shift work), and psychological stress (reviewed in [3]), lead and manganese (reviewed in [2]) have also been reported to have an association with menstrual disorders.

The effects of ionizing radiation on the menstrual cycle vary with age and dose. An ovarian dose of 4 Gy (in radiotherapy) may cause a 30% incidence of sterility in young women, but 100% sterility in women over 40 years of age [4]. Hyperprolactinaemia and deficiency of other anterior pituitary hormones have been reported after radiotherapy to the hypothalamic–pituitary region. Anticancer chemotherapy, especially with alkylating agents, may cause premature ovarian failure [5]. The alkylating agents damage primary follicles and oocytes, and cause amenorrhoea. Polycyclic aromatic hydrocarbons, including, benzo(a)pyrene, which are present in foundry air and in cigarette smoke, are toxic to ovaries in animal tests and adverse effects on the ovaries in smokers have been suggested [6].

Effects of occupational exposure during pregnancy

Organic solvents

Organic solvents are used widely in various fields of industry, the most important of which are shoe-making, spray painting, furniture manufacturing, the plastics, graphics and metal degreasing industries, the production of paints, lacquers and adhesives, and dry cleaning. Organic solvents are volatile liquids and the main routes of exposure are inhalation and absorption through the skin. Solvents or their metabolites are rapidly distributed by the blood stream to different tissues. In view of their lipid solubility, it is likely that most traverse the placenta into the fetus. The passage of methylene chloride, trichloroethylene and xylene through the placenta has been shown in humans, and placental transfer of several other solvents has been demonstrated in rats and mice [7].

The developmental toxicity of solvents has been examined in animal tests on mammals. Teratogenic effects have been shown, for example, for chloroform and 2-ethoxyethanol. Some solvents have induced retarded growth (e.g. tetrachloroethylene, toluene, trichloroethylene, xylene and methyl ethyl ketone) or caused embryotoxicity (styrene, ethylene glycol ethers) [7]. In humans, maternal occupational exposure to organic solvents has been related to menstrual disorders, reduced fertility, spontaneous abortion, stillbirth, perinatal death and congenital malformation as well as leukaemia and brain tumours in the children of exposed workers [8,9].

The reproductive effects of solvent exposure have been examined in various occupational groups exposed to different levels and types of solvents. Usually, the workers have been exposed to mixtures of solvents and the studies have given varied results. Increased risks of spontaneous abortion or reduced fertility have been observed in industrial populations which are usually exposed to high levels of solvents (*Table 14.1*). These occupational groups include manufacturing work, dry cleaning work, painting, shoe work, pharmaceutical factory work, audio speaker factory work and semiconductor work [10,11a].

No relationship between solvent exposure and spontaneous abortion has been observed among workers whose level of exposure is usually likely to be low, such as laboratory workers, dental assistants, pharmacy assistants, workers in man-

agerial, health care and service sectors, or the general working population. Among laboratory workers, high exposure to solvents, as assessed by industrial hygienists, was, however, associated with spontaneous abortion [12]. In pharmacy assistants, solvent exposure was associated with an increased risk of stillbirth and perinatal death [13].

Occupational solvent exposure has also been related to an excess of congenital malformations among the children of exposed women. The excesses of specific malformations have not been systematic, since in different studies exposure has been related to different types of malformation. Exposure to various solvents has been linked with central nervous system defects, oral clefts, sacral agenesis, omphalocele and gastroschisis, renal–urinary and gastrointestinal defects, and ventricular septal defects (reviewed in [10]). Two recent studies confirm the association between exposure to solvents and oral clefts [14,15].

Maternal exposure to some specific types of solvent, e.g. toluene, styrene, ethylene glycol ethers, tetrachloroethylene and aliphatic hydrocarbons, has been associated with an adverse pregnancy outcome. The results on individual solvents must, however, be interpreted with caution, because simultaneous exposure to several different solvents is common among workers.

Toluene is used in the production of a number of industrial chemicals and as a solvent for paints, lacquers, printing inks, adhesives and rubber. Experimental studies in animals provide evidence that exposure to toluene during gestation can cause decreased late fetal weight and retarded skeletal development. Case reports describe adverse reproductive outcomes that have been attributed to toluene abuse during pregnancy [16]. Occupational exposure to toluene has been related to spontaneous abortion among shoe workers, audio speaker factory workers, and laboratory workers with high exposure to toluene. In addition, an excess of urinary tract defects was reported to follow toluene exposure (reviewed in [10]).

Exposure to *styrene* is common in the reinforced plastics industry. Studies in animals suggest that styrene and styrene oxide have embryotoxic or fetotoxic effects [17]. Some early epidemiological reports suggested that exposure to styrene induces menstrual disturbances, spontaneous abortions and congenital malformations in humans. In more recent studies, however, no risk was observed among workers exposed to styrene in

Table 14.1 Solvent exposure in various occupations and reproductive outcome (after Lindbohm [10])

Occupation	Exposure	Effect
Manufacturing work	Solvents	Spontaneous abortion
Workers monitored for exposure	Solvents, aliphatic hydrocarbons	Reduced fertility, spontaneous abortion
Painters	Solvents	Spontaneous abortion
Dry cleaning work	Tetrachloroethylene	Spontaneous abortion, reduced fertility
Shoe work	Solvents	Reduced fertility
Shoe work	Toluene	Spontaneous abortion
Audiospeaker factory work	Toluene	Spontaneous abortion
Pharmaceutical factory work	Solvents (> 3 solvents), methylene chloride	Spontaneous abortion
Semiconductor work	Ethylene glycol ethers	Spontaneous abortion, subfertility
Laboratory work, high exposure	Solvents	Spontaneous abortion
Laboratory work, high exposure	Toluene	Spontaneous abortion
Pathology and histology laboratories	Formalin and xylene	Spontaneous abortion

the reinforced plastics industry [1]. A suggestive association of high styrene exposure was, however, reported with low birth weight [18].

Ethylene glycol ethers and their acetates are used in a variety of industries (e.g. photography and dyeing, silk screen printing, manufacturing of electronic components) and products (e.g. varnishes, paints, resins, thinners and cleaners). Ethylene glycol ethers have caused adverse reproductive and developmental effects in various animal species exposed by different routes of administration. In studies among semiconductor manufacturing workers, exposure to ethylene glycol ethers has been associated with increased risks of spontaneous abortion and subfertility [19,20].

Tetrachloroethylene is mainly used as a dry-cleaning agent and a degreaser. Animal studies indicate that tetrachloroethylene is not teratogenic, but may cause retarded development with high levels of exposure [7]. In humans, an increased risk of spontaneous abortion has been linked with high levels of exposure to tetrachloroethylene in dry cleaning work. The findings on the adverse reproductive effects of *aliphatic hydrocarbons* have been inconsistent. High exposure has been related to spontaneous abortion among graphics workers and pharmaceutical factory workers, but not among women working in laboratories. An increased risk of spontaneous abortion has also been linked to exposure to petroleum ether in laboratory work, methylene chloride in pharmaceutical factory work, xylene and formalin in pathology and histology laboratories, and paint thinners (reviewed in [10]).

Epidemiological reproductive studies have several methodological weaknesses, which may decrease their validity. The most serious weakness in studies on the effects of organic solvents has been inaccurate data on exposure which has been usually based on the workers' own reports. A few investigations have used more objective data sources or methods to assess the level of exposure. In some of these studies, exposure was assessed by occupational health care personnel [21] or industrial hygienists [12,22]. In one study, biological monitoring data were used to support the exposure information obtained from the workers themselves [23]. Three of these studies showed an association between solvent exposure and spontaneous abortion.

Overall, the available evidence suggests that maternal exposure to high levels of solvents increases the risk of spontaneous abortion. The findings on congenital malformations and fertility, although less conclusive, also suggest that solvent exposure may represent a hazard to the developing fetus, and impair fertility. The results on individual solvents must be interpreted with caution. Simultaneous exposure to multiple solvents and other agents is common among solvent-exposed workers, and it is difficult to ascribe an adverse effect to an individual agent. Associations of spontaneous abortions observed with some particular solvents or subgroups of solvents are suggestive only. Nevertheless, it would be prudent to minimize exposure to organic solvents, and in some countries the guidelines for occupational health personnel recommend that solvent exposure should not exceed 10% of the threshold limit value during pregnancy [24].

Pesticides

The global use of pesticides in agriculture, greenhouses and forestry is about 2 million tonnes a year. The Environmental Protection agency (EPA) in the USA estimated that there are about 600 active ingredients, and the number of various formulations is about 50 000 [25]. The great number of chemicals, multi-exposure and the possibility of considerable background exposure have made it difficult to investigate the effects of various active ingredients in pesticides, or of occupational exposure to pesticides in general. Pesticide formulations may contain organic solvents, which must also be taken into account when reproductive toxicity is assessed.

Exposure to pesticides from environmental sources or at work has been reported in association with several adverse effects related to pregnancy and offspring. Effect on fertility can be measured by time to pregnancy, that is the number of menstrual cycles or months it takes a couple to conceive, and this can be used to study the effects of exposure on fecundability or fertility. Time to pregnancy was measured among fruit growers in the Netherlands. The couples who tried to conceive during the spraying season took twice as long to conceive as others, and the fecundability ratio (the probability to conceive for each menstrual cycle) was significantly decreased (0.42, 95% CI 0.20–0.92) [26]. It was probably the male partner of the couple who most often sprayed pesticides, but the wives participated in the fruit growing; therefore, the maternal exposure may also have been important. The sex ratio was changed in favour of girls in the children born in the most recent period (1987–90) [27]. In another study, where only female workers were included,

exposure to pesticides seemed to increase the chance to get a boy [28]. According to one hypothesis, the sexes of children are associated with the hormone concentration of the male partner at the time of conception – high testosterone producing boys, high gonadotropin, girls [29]. If this is true, female exposure would show no effect on sex distribution.

An increased risk of spontaneous abortion has been found among women in agricultural occupations (including also horticulture or fur farming) and among gardeners (in indoor gardens, vineyards or in floriculture) who sprayed pesticides during pregnancy (reviewed in [30]). In one study, the increased risk of spontaneous abortion was seen only among those who used pesticides on 3–5 days a week during the first trimester of pregnancy. The risk was not increased, however, when a proper respirator or respirator and protective clothing were used [28]. No specific pesticide or pesticide group was identified as being more harmful than others. In another study no increase in spontaneous abortion was seen, but stillbirths without birth defects were increased among women who worked in agriculture or horticulture for more than 30 h/week [31]. Environmental exposure to malathion, and to insecticides and herbicides was also associated with stillbirths (reviewed in [30]).

Congenital malformations have been studied more than other outcomes in relation to pesticide exposure (reviewed in [30]). An increase in birth defects has been associated with some individual pesticides or with work where pesticides or pesticide mixtures are used (*Table 14.2*). Limb anomalies and orofacial clefts have been reported in several studies, but not in all. The varying results may be due to methodological problems, e.g.

Table 14.2 Congenital malformations and exposure to pesticides (after Nurminen [30])

Type of malformation	Exposure type
Central nervous system defects	Pesticides
Anencephaly, meningomyelocele	2,4,5-Trichlorophenoxyacetic acid (2,4,5-T)
Spina bifida	Agricultural chemicals
Neural tube defects, orofacial clefts, renal agenesis	Insecticides and herbicides
Orofacial clefts	Agricultural work
Cardiac, urogenital and limb-reduction defects	Atrazine
Limb and orofacial anomalies (1st trimester exposure)	Malathion
Gastrointestinal anomalies (2nd trimester exposure)	Malathion
Musculoskeletal defects	Gardeners
Haemangiomas	Pesticides in floriculture

difficulties in assessing exposure, or a lack of information on confounding factors.

The association between parental exposure to pesticides and childhood cancer has been investigated in several studies (reviewed in [32]). In some, an increased risk for all cancers, and for leukaemia, lymphomas, brain and nervous system tumours, has been found, but not in others. In Norway, a significant association between the purchase of pesticides for farm use and testicular cancer and brain tumours in the offspring was found [33]. Although it is not possible to draw firm conclusions from the results, some caution should be exercised until more reliable data are to hand.

Despite the many uncertainties in interpreting these results, they do suggest that exposure to pesticides, at least during pregnancy, may be harmful (reviewed in [30]). In animal experiments some pesticides have been shown to have harmful effects (e.g. carbaryl, benomyl, ethylenthiourea, maneb, zineb, thiram) and these reinforce the view that exposure to pesticides at work during pregnancy should be minimized or avoided.

Metals

In metal industries there is multiple exposure to several metals, and reproductive hazards may exist, although the data do not allow firm conclusions to be drawn. Risks may also exist in the electronics industry and in semiconductor manufacturing (reviewed in [34]). An increased risk of spontaneous abortions and perinatal death, low birth weight, and congenital malformations, has also been found in women working in a copper smelter or living near to it (reviewed in [35]). Emissions in the 1970s contained lead, copper, zinc, gold, silver, cadmium, mercury, arsenic and sulphur dioxide, but the exposure has been reduced considerably over the past 15 years. For the past 20 years no effect on birth weight and perinatal mortality has been seen [36].

Lead

Historical descriptions of the reproductive outcome of women exposed to high levels of lead include high rates of miscarriage, neonatal mortality, premature babies and low birth weight. Recent studies among women occupationally exposed to lead have indicated no decrease in fecundability in terms of time to pregnancy [116], nor an increased risk of spontaneous abortions (reviewed in [35]). The level of the exposure, as measured by blood lead concentrations, is low at present; therefore, the results do not disagree with the reported harmful effects at earlier high exposure levels – lead compounds were formerly used as an abordifacient.

Lead is transferred across the placenta during the 12th to 14th weeks of pregnancy. At birth the blood lead concentration (B-Pb) in the umbilical cord of the child is close to that of the mother. The fact that placental transfer of lead takes place after organogenesis gives biological plausibility to the findings: lead does not cause major birth defects, but an increased risk of minor anomalies has been reported. There is also evidence of outcomes such as low birth weight, prematurity and impaired cognitive development in children exposed to lead during gestation (reviewed in [34]). The risk of worsened postnatal mental development and intrauterine growth retardation may increase when the B-Pb prenatally is $15 \mu g/dl$ or more ($0.7 \mu mol/l$); the risk of lowered birth weight may occur at prenatal B-Pb level of $25 \mu g/dl$ ($1.2 \mu mol/l$) [37,38]. These levels are rather low and do not exceed the work environment limit values. Lead may be mobilized from bones to blood during pregnancy and lactation, and female workers should also avoid heavy exposure before pregnancy. In Finland, it is recommended that the blood lead level of pregnant women should not exceed $0.3 \mu mol/l$ ($6.2 \mu g/dl$), which is the reference value of the non-occupationally exposed female population [39].

Inorganic mercury

The data are scanty on the reproductive effects of inorganic mercury in humans (reviewed in [35]), but it crosses into the fetus and is teratogenic in some animals. A study of 81 women working in dentistry classified the exposure according to the mercury content in their hair. Menstrual disorders were reported by 31% of the exposed women ($n = 45$), spontaneous abortions by 16% (11% in the non-exposed), stillbirth by 2.6% and congenital malformations by 5%, including 5 cases of spina bifida and 1 case of interatrial defect [40]. The relative risk for any adverse effect in all 117 pregnancies among the exposed women was increased. Maternal exposure to inorganic mercury has also been associated with anomalies [41]. In other studies on dental workers and lamp workers no significant increases were found for spontaneous abortion [42,43]. Although the results in humans are inconsistent, mercury is, however, a known potent toxicant, and suspected to be teratogenic and fetotoxic in animal tests. Therefore, occupational exposure should be restricted. Various levels have been suggested; for example, a mercury vapour concentration less than $0.01 \, mg/m^3$ (REPROTOX database 1996) or $0.2 \, \mu g/m^3$ [44]. The occupational limit values in many countries is $0.05 \, mg/m^3$. In Finland, it is recommended that the biological reference values for non-occupationally exposed people (mercury in the urine, U-Hg, $50 \, nmol/l$, and inorganic mercury in the blood, B-Hg, $25 \, nmol/l$) should not be exceeded during pregnancy [45]. Urinary Hg levels of $50 \, nmol/l$ correspond to long-term exposure to mercury vapour at levels of $8 \, \mu g/m^3$.

Nickel

Recently, adverse outcomes of pregnancy have been reported in a preliminary report concerning women working at a nickel hydrometallurgy refining plant in the Kola peninsula in Russia [46]. The rate of spontaneous and threatened abortions and of congenital malformations, especially cardiovascular and musculoskeletal defects, was increased. Only 29% of the pregnancies were reported as normal among the nickel workers, compared with 39% in construction workers in the same region. Nickel concentrations (nickel sulphate) measured in the air were $0.1-0.31 \, mg/m^3$ (in Finland, the occupational limit value for nickel is $1 \, mg/m^3$ and for nickel compounds $0.1 \, mg/m^3$). The nickel content in the urine (U-Ni) of the factory workers ranged from 3.2 to $22.6 \, \mu g/l$ ($= 0.09-0.38 \, \mu mol/l$); not very high compared with the Finnish upper limit for occupationally exposed workers ($1.30 \, \mu mol/l$). The concentrations are, however, above the reference value for the general population in Finland (U-Ni $< 0.06 \, \mu mol/l$). Sulphur dioxide and other metals were also present in the atmosphere and these results need to be confirmed or refuted in further studies. In several animal studies, but not in all, various adverse effects on reproduction have been found. For nickel carbonyl, an exposure limit of $0.035 \, mg/m^3$ is recommended for pregnant workers [44]. Because of the carcinogenicity of nickel and its compounds, restrictions are given for pregnancy in some countries [39].

Cadmium

Some of the effects on the reproductive organs have been studied among smokers, since cigarette smoking significantly elevates the amount of cadmium in the body; for example, from one packet of cigarettes $2-4 \, \mu g$ cadmium is inhaled. Smokers have higher amounts of cadmium in the ovaries than non-smokers, and the placenta of smokers contains more cadmium than that of non-smokers (reviewed in [47]). The lower birth weight of children of smokers has been connected with the possible toxic effects of cadmium to the placenta. Fewer full-term deliveries, more pregnancy complications among women exposed to cadmium, and poorer motor and intellectual development among their children, have been suggested. In animal tests, cadmium has been embryotoxic, fetotoxic and teratogenic, and affects postnatal development (reviewed in [47]). Cadmium is also classified as a carcinogen. There are grounds to restrict the exposure of pregnant women, although there is no firm evidence of reproductive toxicity in humans.

Chromium

There are no reproductive data for chromium in humans, but it crosses the placenta in some animals and is teratogenic to hamsters and mice. Exposure to the carcinogenic forms (hexavalent chromium) and compounds exposure during pregnancy is restricted in some countries [39].

Anaesthetic gases

Occupational exposure to trace concentrations of anaesthetic gases may occur among hospital personnel in operating rooms and delivery wards, and among dental and veterinary personnel. Numerous studies have examined the reproductive effects of these agents, including halothane, nitrous oxide, enflurane and isoflurane. Both animal and human studies have yielded conflicting results.

Animal experiments suggest that exposure to nitrous oxide may increase the risk of growth retardation and fetal loss in subanaesthetic doses similar to those that occur in occupational exposure. Halothane, isoflurane and enflurane have usually not produced an adverse pregnancy outcome at low doses, but embryotoxic and teratogenic effects have been observed at high anaesthetic doses.

Several epidemiological studies have shown an increased rate of spontaneous abortion and congenital malformation among women occupationally exposed to anaesthetic gases [48,49]. It has been suggested, however, that methodological shortcomings have contributed to the reported effects. The main weakness of these studies, and particularly the early studies, has been the lack of reliable exposure and outcome data. A few studies, published in the 1980s, using a more valid study design and more reliable data sources, showed relative risks close to, or slightly above, unity.

One explanation for the contradictory findings of the various studies may be that the type and level of exposure varied, due to differences in the substances being used in operating rooms, methods of administration and in the scavenging equipment employed. Measurements of anaesthetic gases have shown that the concentrations may vary widely with time and place [50], and the levels are high if no scavenging system is used or the ventilation is inadequate.

With the exception of nitrous oxide, the effects of individual anaesthetic gases have generally not been examined in epidemiological studies. Nitrous oxide has been related to an increased risk of spontaneous abortion in dental personnel, although the findings are not entirely consistent. In two recent studies, nitrous oxide exposure was associated with reduced fertility [49,51]. Dental assistants exposed to high levels of unscavenged nitrous oxide and midwives assisting at a high number of nitrous oxide deliveries per month had a lower probability of conception for each menstrual month compared with unexposed women. No data on actual levels were available in these studies. Other measurements showed, however, that peak exposures exceeded 500 ppm in delivery wards and 1000 ppm in dental offices when special scavenging equipment was not in use.

Although the epidemiological evidence on reproductive effects of anaesthetic gases is equivocal, measures to reduce exposure to these gases in operating rooms, delivery wards, dental offices and veterinary surgeries should be pursued. Efficient scavenging equipment, good ventilation and equipment for the administration of anaesthetics are needed to keep the levels of exposure low. When administering an anaesthetic gas by open mask, the risk of peak exposure will remain and it would be prudent to adopt a policy of allowing pregnant women to work in other areas where exposure will not occur.

Antineoplastic agents

Many antineoplastic agents have been shown to be teratogenic or embryotoxic in experimental systems. Workers potentially exposed to these agents include hospital personnel involved in the preparation and administration of antineoplastic drugs and pharmaceutical factory workers in processing and manufacturing these drugs. Laboratory assistants and animal caretakers in animal laboratories may also be exposed to antineoplastic agents.

An increased risk of spontaneous abortion has been observed in epidemiological studies of nurses who prepare antineoplastic drugs for patients. In studies conducted in more heterogeneous populations and using a cruder definition of exposure, the rate of spontaneous abortions has not been increased among exposed hospital personnel. The handling of antineoplastic agents in hospitals has also been associated with congenital malformations in the offspring, slightly lowered birth weight and ectopic pregnancy. An elevated risk of spontaneous abortion has been reported among pharmaceutical factory workers, pharmacy assistants and laboratory workers exposed to these agents (reviewed in [49]).

A Danish study [52] estimated the risk of adverse pregnancy outcome in a well-protected setting, when protective safety measures had been implemented and the level of exposure was probably low. The study found no increased risk of spontaneous abortion, malformation, low birth weight or preterm birth among the nurses handling antineoplastic drugs during pregnancy.

The findings of the epidemiological studies provide some support to the view that occupational exposure to antineoplastic drugs may be associated with an adverse pregnancy outcome. Many of these agents are also carcinogens. Therefore, exposure to antineoplastic drugs for hospital personnel, pharmaceutical factory workers and laboratory workers should be minimized by the use of protective garments and equipment, and good work practices. Centralization of preparation and mixing of antineoplastic agents in well-equipped pharmacies and the use of flow hoods and protective equipment have decreased exposure in hospitals. Current prevention measures do not, however, completely eliminate opportunities for exposure. A study in a hospital following antineoplastic drug-handling guidelines showed few air samples, but multiple surface wipe samples with measurable cyclophosphamide concentrations in oncology, pharmacy and outpatient oncology departments [53]. Surveys on the use of protective equipment have also indicated that the use of protective garments does not always meet the guidelines [54]. A policy of transferring a pregnant worker preparing antineoplastic drug solutions to another job has been adopted in some countries [45].

Ethylene oxide

Ethylene oxide is widely used as a sterilizing agent and in the manufacture of chemicals. In animal experiments it appears to have reproductive toxic effects at very high concentrations [55]. Epidemiological observations among hospital staff engaged in sterilizing instruments with this agent suggest an association between exposure to ethylene oxide and an increased risk of spontaneous abortion [56]. Ethylene oxide is also classified as carcinogenic to humans by the International Agency for Research on Cancer. Thus, exposure should be kept to a minimum.

Ionizing radiation

Exposure to high doses of ionizing radiation is known to be harmful to reproduction. Ionizing radiation, X-rays and gamma rays penetrate tissues and reach the sexual organs and fetus easily. Particulate radiation, such as from alpha (helium nuclei) and beta (electrons) particles, do not penetrate tissues deeply, but generate ions on their short path in the tissue. Radionuclides also emit ionizing radiation, but the type of radiation varies with the chemical species. The distribution of the radionuclide to the organs determines the sites at which radiation energy is active.

Various units are used for measuring the exposure to radiation, in radiation protection and in research reports. The units in common use are as follows. The gray (Gy) is the unit for the dose of energy from ionizing radiation, which is absorbed per mass unit of material (*Table 14.3*). The absorbed dose is not used in radiation protection; instead, the *equivalent dose* and the *effective dose*, in which the potential of various types of radiation to cause adverse health effects (especially cancer

and genetic effects) are taken into account by weighted coefficients, is used. The units of effective dose are the sievert (Sv) and millisievert (mSv). Because the weighted coefficients for the different types of radiation and different organs are based on expert agreement, the sievert unit has no exact counterpart in physics [57].

High exposure, such as radiation therapy to the abdomen, during childhood may cause somatic damage to abdominopelvic structures, leading to difficulties in pregnancy later. High radiation exposures during radiotherapy have caused amenorrhoea and early menopause [58]. High doses, from 0.5 to 2.5 Sv (50–250 rem), may double the natural human mutation rate.

During the pre-implantation period of pregnancy, radiation has an 'all or none' effect, i.e. the embryo either dies or develops normally. In humans, growth retardation, spontaneous abortions and malformation have been observed at radiation doses of 50 mSv [59]. In animal tests, irradiation during organogenesis has caused major congenital malformations and growth retardation; later exposure has caused cataracts, microcephaly, hydrocephalus and skin defects. Microcephaly and central nervous system disturbances were reported in children who were exposed to very large doses of radiation (<250 rad) in the 1960s, and an increased risk of mental retardation and forebrain damage has been reported in children who were exposed *in utero* during the atomic bombing of Hiroshima and Nagasaki to about 1000 mSv. Mental retardation was not seen below an exposure level of 50 rad. In animal tests, microcephaly has not been found with less than 10–20 rad exposure. The high-risk period is suspected to be between 8 and 15 weeks of gestational age, which is the period of neuronal proliferation and migration in the brain [58]. The exposure level in diagnostic procedures during pregnancy has been well below 5 rad, so low exposure is not expected to cause congenital malformations. An increased risk of childhood cancer and leukaemia has been found in association with lower prenatal exposure (<100 mSv radiation dose) [59]. Ionizing radiation has been suggested as one aetiological factor in Down's syndrome [60].

In the occupational setting, an increased risk of spontaneous abortion has been reported among veterinarians and veterinary assistants using diagnostic X-rays and radiology technicians (reviewed in [34]). In two studies on the effects of diagnostic X-rays among nurses, the results were inconclu-

Table 14.3   Units of radioactivity and ionizing radiation

Gray (Gy) = *The dose* of energy from ionizing radiation which is *absorbed to material*, per mass unit.	1 Gy = 1 J/kg
Rad = an old unit which does not belong to SI system	1 rad = 0.01 Gy
Sievert (Sv) = *Equivalent dose*, which is the *product of absorbed dose and weighted coefficient* (agreed for each type of radiation separately)	1 Sv
Rem = an old unit for equivalent dose which does not belong to SI system	1 rem = 0.01 Sv = 10 mSv 1 msv = 0.1 rem
Sievert (Sv) = also unit for *effective dose*, which is the *sum of equivalent doses of exposed organs* (the weighted coefficients for calculation of the equivalent doses for various organs are agreed)	1 msv = 0.1 rem
Becquerel (Bq) = unit of activity of radioactivity, which cannot be translated to units of radiation (Gy or Sv) without exact knowledge of the metabolics of a radioactive substance in the organism	
Curie (Ci) = an old unit of radioactivity which does not belong to SI system	(1 Ci = 3.7×10^{10} Bq)

sive; in one, no excess in spontaneous abortions was found, and in the other, a non-statistically significant increase was found [61]. More malformed children than expected were born to women working in X-ray departments, but this result was not statistically significant.

The evidence of the hazardous effects of radioactive radiation as a whole shows that the fetus is most sensitive to its effects. Recently, the exposure limits have been lowered in some countries following the recommendations of the International Commission of Radiation Protection [62]. In Finland, the mean yearly exposure during 5 years for any worker may not exceed 20 mSv per year (and not > 50 mSv in any year). During pregnancy, the equivalent dose of radiation to the abdominal region may not exceed 2 mSv (corresponding 1 mSv intrauterine dose). The effective dose from radionuclides may not exceed 1 mSv during pregnancy [24].

Non-ionizing radiation

Non-ionizing radiation includes optical radiation, radiofrequency radiation, microwaves and low-frequency electromagnetic fields. Reproductive hazards related to non-ionizing radiation have been investigated among physiotherapists and operators of magnetic resonance imaging (MRI) devices. Several studies have also been made of video display terminal (VDT) workers, and exposure to low-frequency electromagnetic fields of VDTs has been suggested as one causal factor,

along with stress and ergonomic factors, for the potentially harmful effects of VDT work on pregnancy outcome. The magnetic fields produced by modern VDTs, however, are low and often lower than the fields from other sources in the office environment.

Physiotherapists may be occupationally exposed to short-wave radiation, microwaves and ultrasound, but the findings among this group have been inconsistent. In one study, spontaneous abortion was related to the use of short-wave and ultrasound equipment [63] and another to microwave use [64]. A third study showed a low ratio of boys to girls for physiotherapists exposed to high-frequency electromagnetic radiation [65]. Exposure was also associated with a low birth weight for male babies but not with other outcomes. Overall, the evidence on the adverse effects of non-ionizing radiation among physiotherapists is inconclusive.

The increasing use of MRI in diagnostic medicine has raised concerns about workers exposed to electromagnetic radiation. MRI workers may be exposed to strong static magnetic fields ranging from 5 to 100 mT. A survey of MRI technologists did not indicate any major reproductive hazards associated, although a slight but non-significant excess of spontaneous abortions was found [66]. Reports on MRI examinations during pregnancy have also shown no excess of adverse pregnancy outcome. An experimental study in rats exposed to a 30 mT static magnetic field (i.e. within the range of exposure of MRI workers) however, found a slight increase in fetal loss, but no teratogenic effects [67].

Most epidemiological studies of VDT workers have examined the effects according to the amount of time spent working at the terminal. The majority of these studies suggest that VDT work is not associated with spontaneous abortion, congenital malformation, fetal growth retardation or other pregnancy complications (reviewed in [68]). Only a few studies showed an excess of some reproductive outcomes, but the effects of recall bias could not be excluded in these investigations.

The effects of the electromagnetic fields of the terminals were examined in only two studies of VDT work and pregnancy outcome. One found no association between the fields and spontaneous abortion [69], whereas in the other, an increased risk was found for a small group of workers who had used a VDT with a high level ($> 0.3 \mu$T) of extremely low frequency magnetic fields [8]. The findings of the two studies do not necessarily contradict each other, since in the former study there were no VDT models with extremely low frequency magnetic fields reaching the lower bound for the highest exposure category of the latter study. In a recent study among semiconductor workers, no association was seen between extremely low-frequency magnetic fields of 0.2–0.5 or $> 5 \mu$T and spontaneous abortion [19].

Taken as a whole, the epidemiological evidence does not suggest a strong association between exposure to low-frequency magnetic fields and adverse reproductive outcome, although an effect at high levels of exposure cannot totally be excluded. Evidence on the adverse reproductive effects of non-ionizing radiation among physiotherapists and MRI technologists is inconclusive.

Shift work

Shift work has been considered as a potential reproductive hazard, because it may interfere with circadian systems and the temporal pattern of endocrine function. In a study of the internal desynchronization of circadian rhythms, shift work was found to modify the secretory patterns of melatonin, prolactin, cortisol and testosterone [70].

Shift work has been associated with preterm birth and low birth weight in several studies (reviewed in [71]) and an elevated risk of spontaneous abortion has also been indicated, although not consistently in all investigations. Menstrual disorders have been reported in some studies,

and a recent European multicentre study showed an increased risk of subfecundity in women shift workers [72]. It has, however, remained unclear which forms of shift work – rotating or changing schedules, night work, irregular working hours or shift work in general – may be harmful for reproduction. Usually, shift workers are also exposed to other potential reproductive hazards, and in many studies it has been difficult to separate the effects of these other occupational exposures. Nevertheless, shift work should be considered as a risk to reproduction.

Noise

Noise has been suggested to have both direct and indirect effects on pregnancy. Noise is likely to pass through the maternal abdomen and affect the fetus, although the noise energy may be attenuated by the abdomen. Occupational noise exposure during pregnancy has been reported to increase the risk of high-frequency hearing loss in children [73]. Indirectly, noise (like other stressors) has been suggested to increase maternal catecholamine secretion which may further stimulate or retard uterine contractions and affect uteroplacental blood flow.

Most epidemiological studies on the effects of noise exposure concern preterm birth and low birth weight. Elevated risks of these outcomes have been observed among noise-exposed workers, but results showing no adverse relation have also been presented (reviewed in [71]). In two studies, exposure assessment was based on noise measurements at the mothers' workplace or comparable workplaces. The results indicated that noise exposure of around $85 \, dBL_{Aeq(8h)}$ or higher is associated with fetal growth retardation [74,75]. An excess of hormonal disturbances, delayed conception, infertility and spontaneous abortion has also been reported for occupational noise exposure. The current evidence suggests that high noise exposure should be taken into account in the assessment of occupational reproductive hazards.

Physical strain

Pregnancy is a natural and normal physiological state for a woman, and moderate physical activity is beneficial. Physical effort may increase intrauterine pressure and thus decrease the nutritional blood flow to the fetus. In later pregnancy it may also promote contractions, and thus increase the risk of early delivery. If specific risk factors, e.g. illnesses, are threatening the course of pregnancy, or if the work requires considerable physical effort, it may become necessary to restrict the workload and the physical activity. An informative review of relevant studies has been written [76].

Prolonged standing or walking has been found to increase the risk for preterm delivery in several studies. The risk increased if the women also smoked. The evidence is weaker for the effects of prolonged standing and walking on birth weight, but in one study these did lead to smaller birth weight for gestational age. The evidence of the effects of heavy lifting on spontaneous abortions, or gestational length and birth weight, is weaker (reviewed in [76]). Heavy physical work was reported to be significantly associated with malformations, and with malformations of the central nervous system [74], but negative studies also exist. It is recommended that in early pregnancy extremely heavy work (close to the woman's maximal capacity) should be avoided, and during the second and third trimesters the physical workload may need to be decreased, opportunities for rest organized and continuous standing and walking avoided (reviewed in [76]).

Biological agents

Maternal exposure to some microbial agents during pregnancy may result in infection in the fetus. Exposure to the agents causing toxoplasmosis, listeriosis, rubella, herpes, varicella, hepatitis B and C, cytomegalovirus infection, parvovirus infection and HIV infection may occur in health care and child care workers. Many workers have immunity to the common viral illnesses, or have been vaccinated against rubella and hepatitis B. Vaccination is recommended when a vaccine is available (but not during pregnancy or just before it, if the vaccine contains living viruses (e.g rubella, see Table 14.4)). Some conditions can be cured by antibiotics or other procedures if the disease is diagnosed early enough (e.g. toxoplasmosis, complications of parvovirus infection in the fetus). For some conditions there is no other solution than prevention, by ensuring good working practices, but in some cases a job transfer or special maternity leave may be needed.

In an EU directive and some national legislation on the protection of pregnant workers, exposure to toxoplasma and rubella virus are taken into account. In Finland, some other biological agents are also considered potentially riskful for pregnant workers (hepatitis B, herpes, cytomegalovirus, varicella, rubella and HIV, and agents causing listeria and toxoplasma infections), and therefore they are included in the legislation on special maternity leave [45]. A useful review with recommendations has recently been published [77]; in *Table 14.4*, practical advice from the review is summarized.

Much of the prevention of infections in health care workers and those working in child care and schools depends on how well informed the employees and employers are. The occupational health services have an important role in distributing information and planning the measures needed for individual workplaces.

Lifestyle factors

Heavy *alcohol consumption* during pregnancy is known to be teratogenic, causing the fetal alcohol syndrome in humans. The children with the syndrome are characterized by small birth weight, microcephaly, reduction of the width of the palpebral fissures and maxillary hypoplasia. They often have also other malformations. *Smoking* during pregnancy is known to lower the birth weight of the child (reviewed in [34]).

Exposure to chemicals in breast milk

Almost all chemicals which are present in the blood of the mother appear in the breast milk. Substances with short half-lives are important, if the intake occurs during the breast-feeding period. Examples of toxicity to the infant due to maternal exposure (e.g. to tetrachloroethylene at her husband's workplace) have been reported [47]. Acute exposure of breast-feeding mothers to toxic chemicals must, of course, be prohibited. With the increasing length of maternity leave and the number of better informed employers and employees this should not now be expected to occur. Substances with long half-lives, from the occupational or general environment, may be more difficult to detect and may cause exposure to the infant [78]. Some fat-soluble and water-soluble industrial compounds pass into breast milk in sig-

Table 14.4 Infectious agents during pregnancy, and prevention of infection (after Ekblad [77])

Biological agent, effects	Preventive measures at workplace
Hepatitis B Prenatal and perinatal transmission of virus to the infant 50–60% risk of clinical hepatitis of the offspring 25% lifetime risk of dying from liver cirrhosis or hepatocellular carcinoma of the offspring	HBV vaccination of workers at risk HBV vaccination and hepatitis B immunoglobulin to infants of HBV-positive mothers after birth
Hepatitis C Maternal infection in the 3rd trimester may result in neonatal infection in 45–88% Liver disease possible later in life, and clinical course still unknown	No vaccine available Hygienic work habits important for prevention
German Measles (rubella) Twofold risk of spontaneous abortion Congenital heart defects in offspring	In many countries school children, teenage girls and seronegative women after delivery are vaccinated Vaccination (not during pregnancy or 2–3 months before pregnancy)
Zoster virus (varicella or chickenpox) Maternal pneumonia during pregnancy may be life-threatening Congenital malformations possible (infrequent)	Majority of adult women have immunity from childhood In risk occupations (health branch, school teachers, day-care personnel) immunity/seropositivity checking. Job transfer or temporary leave during epidemics, if seronegative Avoid contact with sick children during epidemics Zoster immunoglobulin may be administered after contact with contagious person (Vaccination probably becoming routine procedure in near future, then recommended)
Cytomegalovirus Perinatal infection rate from infectious (often symptomless) mother 50% Neurological symptoms and psychomotor retardation of the child may develop	No vaccination or treatment available Despite earlier immunity reinfections possible Hygienic work habits recommended
Human parvovirus May cause adverse pregnancy outcome Fetal infection may cause hydrops fetalis due to anaemia	No vaccination available Previous immunity protects (screening the female workers at risk occupations during epidemics recommended) Hydrops and anaemia can be treated with fetal blood transfusion Job transfer or temporary leave during epidemics, e.g. at school, if seronegative
Toxoplasma gondii Adverse pregnancy outcome After fetal infection brain, liver, spleen damage, and later eye, ear damage and mental retardation possible	Antibiotic therapy possible Screening for immunity during pregnancy recommended in some countries
Listeria monocytogenes Abortion, stillbirth, premature delivery Pneumonia and septicaemia after birth	Antibiotic (ampicillin) treatment of the maternal infection
Human immunodeficiency virus (HIV) Perinatal transmission rate 10–65%, through breast-feeding 14–29% Low birth weight and increased neonatal and infant mortality HIV infection in the offspring	No vaccine or effective treatment available Occupational risk of infection minimal with a normal handwashing policy

nificant quantities and some chemicals (e.g. pesticides, DDT and eldrin, PCB, tetrachloroethylene) are concentrated in breast milk.

It seems reasonable for occupational health departments to collect information on the potential of chemicals present in the work environment to pass into breast milk and to assess the possibility of health risks to breast-fed children. The comprehensive review [79] may be helpful in this context.

Prevention of reproductive hazards at the workplace

The occupational physician often struggles with the problem of how to translate scientific findings, sometimes sparse, unclear or contradictory, to practical advice to minimize the risk for workers [80]. The current occupational exposure limits, which in many European countries have been adopted from the USA TLV list of 1978, are of limited value, since they are set mostly with regard to health effects other than reproductive health.

In Finland, legislation (the Law on Occupational Safety, 1987) aims to protect the reproductive health of both men and women, as well as the health of the unborn child from harmful effects of occupational exposure. Since 1991, statutes define the practical measures to ensure this is the case, and list chemical, physical and biological agents for which there is evidence of harmful effects on reproduction. The regulations also include mutagenic and carcinogenic agents (warning code R45 and R46) [24] and guidelines recommend exposure levels which should not be exceeded during pregnancy (*Table 14.5*). For non-pregnant workers, no separate exposure levels are defined. At international level, in the amendment of the Council Directive on the classification of hazardous substances, new categories of reproductive hazards were introduced in 1992 [82]. The earlier warning code R47 (teratogenic) was substituted by a group of codes: R60 (may harm fertility), R61 (may harm the unborn child), R62 (potential risk of less fertility), R63 (potential risk to the unborn child) and R64 (may harm lactation) [83].

Risk assessment criteria or guidelines for critical appraisal are needed, especially if the agent is not classified by, for example, the EU or a scientific agency, or is not listed in national regulations. Criteria for assessment have been presented by international agencies such as the OECD and the EU [83], by a Nordic expert group [39] and by individual researchers (e.g. [81]) (*Table 14.5*). Even with good criteria the assessment is complicated, and is often a task for experts, and in the evaluation of reproductive risks occupational health services need help from an expert in a research unit or information service [80]. Here,

Table 14.5   Examples of exposure levels of reproductive risks (see text)

Source	Recommended upper level
Denmark, law on special maternity leave (pregnant women) Finland, guidelines for the law on special maternity leave (pregnant women)	Organic solvents 0.1 TLV Carbon monoxide $14\,cm^3/m^3$ in air corresponding to blood carboxyhaemoglobin concentration of 0.025 Lead, B-Pb, for general population (0.3 µmol/l) Mercury, U-Hg, for general population (50 nmol/l) Organic solvents 0.1 TLV
OECD programme: uncertainty factors (UF) estimated from the no effect level (NOEL) in animal tests	UF = from 100 to 300 of the NOEL if the NOEL for developmental effects is *higher than, or equal to*, the NOEL maternal toxicity UF = from 1000 to 3000 if the NOEL for developmental effects is *lower* than the NOEL for maternal toxicity An additional UF of 5 when a LOEL (lowest observed adverse effect level) is used

Stijkel and van Dijk [81]:
   If calculated result <1/10 of MAC
   If calculated result >1/10 of MAC
   If no inhalationary data
   If no MAC
	Calculated result as such
	 0.1 MAC
	 0.1 MAC
	 $0.1\,mg/m^3$

examples of criteria for extrapolation from research to practice, and recommendations are presented.

The OECD programme on the cooperative investigation of high production volume chemicals suggests following principles for the extrapolation of animal data on reproductive toxicity to humans: in the extrapolation to humans, uncertainty factors (UF) are calculated from the no effect level (NOEL). The uncertainty factors range from 100 to 300 if the NOEL for developmental effects is higher than, or equal to, the NOEL for maternal toxicity. A UF of 1000–3000 is suggested if the NOEL for developmental effects is lower than the NOEL for maternal toxicity. An additional uncertainty factor of 5 is suggested when a NOEL cannot be obtained in the study and a LOEL (lowest observed adverse effect level) has to be used (*Table 14.5*).

Criteria have been developed for the quantitative assessment of reproductive risks of female and male workers, and for various adverse effects corresponding to the EU warning sign categories (from R60 to R64) [81]. The assessment is based on good-quality human and animal studies, where inhalation exposure has been used, and from which the NOEL of exposure can be determined. If NOEL cannot be determined from the data it is extrapolated from lowest effect level (LEL). Other extrapolations, e.g. for exposure time and exposure route, are also carried out based on these criteria. Precautionary occupational exposure limits (OEL) were calculated for 156 substances as follows [44]:

- if the calculated value is lower than 1/10 of the maximum accepted concentration (MAC), that value is suggested as the precautionary OEL
- if the calculated value exceeds 1/10 of MAC, 0.1 MAC should be used as to OEL
- if no inhalatory animal data are available, 0.1 MAC is recommended as to precautionary OEL to prevent reproductive toxicity
- if no MAC is available, $0.1 \, mg/m^3$ should be used as the limit.

The calculation in [44] yielded OEL 0.1 MAC (10% of MAC) for 73 (47%) of the 156 chemicals assessed. The calculations performed OELs *lower than 0.1 MAC* for 28 (18%) chemicals, among those many common organic solvents (ethoxyethanol, ethoxyethyl acetate, ethyl benzene, isopropyl alcohol, methanol, methoxyethanol, methylethyl ketone, perchlorethylene, styrene, toluene, trichlorethane, trichlorethylene,

xylene), carbon monoxide, formaldehyde, halothane and nitrous oxide, and metallic mercury. For metals, for which there are MAC values, including cadmium, copper, lead, molybdenum, nickel carbonyl, selenium, tellurium, thallium, 0.1 MAC is recommended. For most pesticides, 0.1 MAC is accepted, e.g. for aldrin, captan, chlordane, 2,4-D, DDT, demeton, dieldrin, diquat, endrin, heptachlor, malathion, methoxychlor, para- quat, parathion, pentachlorphenol, toxaphene. For many common pesticides there are no MAC values, in which case $0.1 \, mg/m^3$ is recommended as to OEL. The model in [44] allows experimental data to be taken into account better than before, and seems to be worth testing. It remains to be seen which limits will be adopted in use, for example, in the European Union countries.

Occupational exposure to ionizing radiation is also regulated with regard to pregnancy. The International Commission on Radiological Protection recommends that the effective dose to the abdominal region of a pregnant woman should not exceed 2 mSv or 1 mSv to the fetus [62]; this is the legal exposure limit in Finland. According to the EU directive (92/85/EEC) concerning pregnant workers or those who have given birth recently, or are breast-feeding, the employer is also obligated to assess the risk from, for example, non-ionizing radiation, vibrations, noise, and physical and mental strain.

To be able to decide whether a work environment is safe for reproductive health or during pregnancy, quantitative information of exposure, preferably hygienic measurements or biological monitoring results, should be available although if these are lacking, indirect estimations can be used: the amount of the chemical(s), the availability of exhaust hoods or other local ventilation, the number of other workers, and the chemicals in use from the basis of exposure assessment. Comparison with the measurements in similar workplaces elsewhere may also be helpful.

In addition to hazard identification and risk assessment, occupational health services should inform employers and employees about the recognized risks, suggest measures for minimizing the exposure (see Chapter 13), and make recommendations for the enterprise. Occupational health personnel may also help the employee in the negotiations at the workplace, and provide the worker with written documents when they are needed, for example, for special benefits.

Conclusion

So far, reproductive hazards have mainly been understood as problems of pregnant women; accordingly, protective measures have been directed towards them. Recent research points out that occupational exposure may damage the reproductive capacity of women and men, and that the exposure of either parent may cause health problems in the offspring. Therefore, the risk control strategy should aim to lower the exposure levels rather than try to protect individuals who plan to have children. Adverse effects on reproduction should be used as critical health effects when setting occupational exposure limits. Such a development would in the long run diminish the need for separate work environment standards for workers of different age and sex. For the time being, however, it may be wise to use extra safety margins for pregnant women, but that should not lead to discrimination against female workers.

References

1. Lindbohm, M.-L. Effects of styrene on the reproductive health of women: a review. In *Butadiene and Styrene: Assessment of Health Hazards* (eds M. Sorsa, K. Peltonen, H. Vainio and K. Hemminki), IARC Scientific Publications No. 127. International Agency for Research on Cancer (1993)
2. Baranski, B. Effects of the work place on fertility and related reproductive outcomes. *Environmental Health Perspectives*, **101** (Suppl. 2), 81–90 (1993)
3. Gold, E.B. and Tomich, E. Occupational hazards to fertility and pregnancy outcome. *Occupational Medicine: State of the Art Reviews*, **9**, 436–469 (1994)
4. Ogilvy-Stuart, A.L. and Shalet, S.M. Effect of radiation on the human reproductive system. *Environmental Health Perspectives*, **101** (Suppl. 2), 109–116 (1993)
5. Vermeulen, A. Environment, human reproduction, menopause and andropause. *Environmental Health Perspectives*, **101** (Suppl. 2), 91–100 (1993)
6. Mattison, D.R., Plowchalk, D.R., Meadows, M.J. *et al.* The effects of smoking on oogenesis, fertilization, and implantation. *Seminars in Reproductive Endocrinology*, **7**, 291–304 (1989)
7. Nordic Criteria for Reproductive Toxicity *Nordic Council of Ministers*. Nord 1992:16. AKA-PRINT APS (1992)
8. Lindbohm, M.-L., Hietanen, M., Kyyrönen, P. *et al.* Magnetic fields of video display terminals and spontaneous abortion. *American Journal of Epidemiology*, **136**, 1041–1051 (1992)
9. O'Leary, L.M., Hicks, A.M., Peters, J.M. *et al.* Parental occupational exposures and risk of childhood cancer: a review. *American Journal of Industrial Medicine*, **20**, 17–35 (1991)
10. Lindbohm, M.-L. Effects of parental exposure to solvents on pregnancy outcome. *Journal of Occupational and Environmental Medicine*, **37**, 908–914 (1995)
11a. Sallmén, M., Lindbohm, M.-L., Kyyrönen, P. *et al.* Reduced fertility among women exposed to organic solvents. *American Journal of Industrial Medicine*, **27**, 699–713
11b. Sallmén, M., Anttila, A., Lindbohm, M.-L. *et al.* Time to pregnancy among women occupationally exposed to lead. *Journal of Occupational and Environmental Medicine*, **37**, 931–934 (1995)
12. Taskinen, H., Kyyrönen, P., Hemminki, K. *et al.* Laboratory work and pregnancy outcome. *Journal of Occupational Medicine*, **36**, 311–319 (1994)
13. Schaumburg, I. and Olsen, J. Congenital malformations and death among the offspring of Danish pharmacy assistants. *American Journal of Industrial Medicine*, **18**, 555–564 (1990)
14. Cordier, S., Ha, M-C., Ayme, S. *et al.* Maternal occupational exposure and congenital malformations. *Scandinavian Journal of Work and Environmental Health*, **18**, 11–17 (1992)
15. Laumon, B., Martin, J.L., Bertucat, I. *et al.* Exposure to organic solvents during pregnancy and oral clefts: a case-control study. *Reproductive Toxicology*, **10**, 15–19 (1996)
16. Donald, J.M., Hooper, K. and Hopenhayn-Rich, C. Reproductive and developmental toxicity of toluene: a review. *Environmental Health Perspectives*, **94**, 237–244 (1991)
17. Brown, N.A. Reproductive and developmental toxicity of styrene. *Reproductive Toxicology*, **5**, 3–29 (1991)
18. Lemasters, G.K., Samuels, S.J., Morrison, J.A. *et al.* Reproductive outcomes of pregnant workers employed at 36 reinforced plastics companies. II. Lowered birth weight. *Journal of Occupational Medicine*, **31**, 115–120 (1989)
19. Swan, S.H., Beaumont, J.J., Hammond, K. *et al.* Historical cohort study of spontaneous abortion among fabrication workers in the semiconductor health study: agent-level analysis. *American Journal of Industrial Medicine*, **28**, 751–769 (1995)
20. Correa, A., Gray, R.H., Cohen, R. *et al.* Ethylene glycol ethers and risks of spontaneous abortion and subfertility. *American Journal of Epidemiology*, **143**, 707–717 (1996)
21. Taskinen, H., Lindbohm, M.-L. and Hemminki, K. Spontaneous abortions among women working in the pharmaceutical industry. *British Journal of Industrial Medicine*, **43**, 199–205 (1986)
22. McDonald, A.D., McDonald, J.C., Armstrong, B. *et al.* Fetal death and work in pregnancy. *British Journal of Industrial Medicine*, **45**, 148–157 (1988)
23. Lindbohm, M.-L., Taskinen, H., Sallmén, M. *et al.* Spontaneous abortions among women exposed to

organic solvents. *American Journal of Industrial Medicine*, **17**, 449–463 (1990)

24. Taskinen, H. Prevention of reproductive health hazards at work. *Scandinavian Journal of Work and Environmental Health*, **18** (Suppl. 2), 27–29 (1992)

25. Baker, S.R. and Wilkinson, C.F. (eds) The effect of pesticides on human health. In *Advances in Modern Environmental Toxicity*, Vol. 18. Princeton Scientific Publishing Co., Princeton, New Jersey (1990)

26. Cock, J. de, Westveer, K., Heedrick, D. *et al.* Time to pregnancy and occupational exposure to pesticides in fruit growers in The Netherlands. *Occupational and Environmental Medicine*, **51**, 693–699 (1994)

27. Cock, J. de, Heedrick, D., Tielemans, E. *et al.* Authors reply. *Occupational and Environmental Medicine*, **52**, 429–430 (1995)

28. Taskinen, H.K., Kyyrönen, P., Liesivuori, J. *et al.* Greenhouse work, pesticides and pregnancy outcome. In: *Abstracts of 11th International Symposium, Epidemiology in Occupational Health*, 5–8 Sep. Nordwijkerhout, The Netherlands. *Epidemiology*, **6** (Suppl. 109) (1995)

29. James, W.H. Offspring sex ratio as an indicator of reproductive hazards associated with pesticides. *Occupational and Environmental Medicine*, **52**, 429–430 (1995)

30. Nurminen, T. Maternal pesticide exposure and pregnancy outcome. *Journal of Occupational and Environmental Medicine*, **37**, 935–940 (1995)

31. McDonald, A.D., McDonald, J.C., Armstrong, B. *et al.* Occupation and pregnancy outcome. *British Journal of Industrial Medicine*, **44**, 521–526 (1987)

32. Gold, E. and Sever, L.E. Childhood cancers associated with parental occupational exposures. *Occupational Medicine: State of the Art Reviews*, **9**, 495–539 (1994)

33. Kristensen, P., Andersen, A., Irgens, L.M. *et al.* Cancer in offspring of parents engaged in agricultural activities in Norway: incidence and risk factors in the farm environment. *International Journal of Cancer*, **65**, 39–50 (1996)

34. Taskinen, H. Effects of parental occupational exposures on spontaneous abortion and congenital malformation. *Scandinavian Journal of Work and Environmental Health*, **16**, 297–314 (1990)

35. Anttila, A. and Sallmén, M. Effects of parental occupational exposure to lead and other metals on spontaneous abortion. *Journal of Occupational and Environmental Medicine*, **37**, 915–921 (1995)

36. Wulff, M., Högberg, U. and Sandström, A.I.M. Perinatal outcome among the offspring of employees and people living around a Swedish smelter. *Scandinavian Journal of Work and Environmental Health*, **21**, 277–282 (1995)

37. Bellinger, D., Leviton, A., Waternaux, C. *et al.* Longitudinal analyses of prenatal and postnatal lead exposure and early cognitive development. *New England Journal of Medicine*, **316**, 1037–1043 (1987)

38. Dietrich, K.N., Kraft, K.M., Bier, M. *et al.* Early effects of fetal lead exposure: Neurobehavioral findings at 6

months. *International Journal of Biosociological Research*, **8**, 151–168 (1986)

39. Taskinen, H., Olsen, J. and Bach, B. Experiences on legislation protecting reproductive health. *Journal of Occupational and Environmental Medicine*, **37**, 974–979 (1995)

40. Sikorski, R., Juszkiewicz, T., Pazkowski, T. *et al.* Women in dental surgeries: reproductive hazards in occupational exposure to metallic mercury. *International Archives of Occupational and Environmental Health*, **59**, 551–557 (1987)

41. Louik, C. and Mitchell, A.A. Occupational exposures and birth defects: final performance report, Grant 1 RO1OH02598-O1A1. NIOSH, USA (1992)

42. Ericson, A. and Källen, B. Pregnancy outcome in women working as dentists, dental assistants or dental technicians. *International Archives of Occupational and Environmental Health*, **61**, 329–333 (1989)

43. De Rosis, F., Anastasio, S.P., Selvaggi, L. *et al.* Female reproductive health in two lamp factories: effects of exposure to inorganic mercury vapour and stress factors. *British Journal of Industrial Medicine*, **42**, 488–494 (1985)

44. Stijkel, A. and Reijnders, L. Implementation of the precautionary principle in standards for the workplace. *Occupational and Environmental Medicine*, **52**, 304–312 (1995)

45. Taskinen, H. Prevention of reproductive health hazards at work. *Scandinavian Journal of Work and Environmental Health*, **18** (Suppl. 2), 27–29 (1992)

46. Chashischin, V.P., Artunina, G.P. and Norseth, T. Congenital defects, abortion and other health effects in nickel refinery workers. *Science of the Total Enviroment*, **148**, 287–291 (1994)

47. Barlow, S. M. and Sullivan, F.M. *Reproductive Hazards of Industrial Chemicals*. Academic Press, New York (1984)

48. Tannenbaum, T.N. and Goldberg, R.J. Exposure to anesthetic gases and reproductive outcome. *Journal of Occupational Medicine*, **27**, 659–668 (1985)

49. Ahlborg, G. Jr. and Hemminki, K. Reproductive effects of chemical exposures in health professions. *Journal of Occupational and Environmental Medicine*, **37**, 957–961 (1995)

50. Borm, P.J.A., Kant, I., Houben, G. *et al.* Monitoring of nitrous oxide in operating rooms: identification of sources and estimation of occupational exposure. *Journal of Occupational Medicine*, **32**, 1112–1116 (1990)

51. Rowland, A.S., Baird, D.D., Weinberg, C.R. *et al.* Reduced fertility among women employed as dental assistants exposed to high levels of nitrous oxide. *New England Journal of Medicine*, **327**, 993–997 (1992)

52. Skov, T., Maarup, B., Olsen, J. *et al.* Leukaemia and reproductive outcome among nurses handling antineoplastic drugs. *British Journal of Industrial Medicine*, **49**, 855–861 (1992)

53. McDevitt, J.J., Lees, P.S.J. and McDiarmid, M.A. Exposure of hospital pharmacists and nurses to anti-

neoplastic agents. *Journal of Occupational Medicine*, **35**, 57–60 (1993)

54. Valanis, B., Vollmer, W.M., Labuhn, K. *et al.* Antineoplastic drug handling protection after OSHA guidelines. *Journal of Occupational Medicine*, **34**, 149–155 (1992)

55. Florack, E.I.M. and Zielhuis, G.A. Occupational ethylene oxide exposure and reproduction. *International Archives of Occupational and Environmental Health*, **62**, 273–277 (1990)

56. Hemminki, K., Mutanen, P., Saloniemi, I. *et al.* Spontaneous abortions in hospital staff engaged in sterilising instruments with chemical agents. *British Medical Journal*, **285**, 1461–1463 (1982)

57. Rytömaa, T. Ionizing radiation (in Finnish) In: *Työperäiset Sairaudet* (ed. M. Antti-Poika) Työterveyslaitos (Finnish Institute of Occupational Health), Helsinki (1994)

58. Lione, A. Ionizing radiation and human reproduction. *Reproductive Toxicology*, **1**, 3–16 (1987)

59. Bengtsson, G. Introduction: present knowledge on the effects of radioactive contamination on pregnancy outcome. *Biomedical and Pharmacotherapy*, **45**, 221–223 (1991)

60. Bound, J.P., Francis, B. J. and Harvey, P.W. Downs syndrome – prevalence and ionising radiation in an area of North West England 1957–91. *Journal of Epidemiology and Community Health*, **49**, 164–170 (1995)

61. Hemminki, K., Hemminki, E., Lindbohm, M.-L. *et al.* Exogenous causes of spontaneous abortion. In *Early Pregnancy Failure* (eds H.J. Huisjes and T. Lind). Churchill Livingstone, New York (1990)

62. IRCP. *1990 Recommendations of the International Commission of Radiological Protection.* IRCP Publications 60, Pergamon Press, New York (1991)

63. Taskinen, H., Kyyrönen, P. and Hemminki, K. Effects of ultrasound, shortwaves, and physical exertion on the pregnancy outcome in physiotherapists. *Journal of Epidemiology and Community Health*, **44**, 196–201 (1990)

64. Quellet-Hellstrom, R. and Stewart, W.F. Miscarriages among female physical therapists who report using radio- and microwave-frequency electromagnetic radiation. *American Journal of Epidemiology*, **138**, 775–786 (1993)

65. Larsen, A.I., Olsen, J. and Svane, O. Gender-specific reproductive outcome and exposure to high-frequency electromagnetic radiation among physiotherapists. *Scandinavian Journal of Work and Environmental Health*, **17**, 324–329 (1991)

66. Evans, J.A., Savitz, D.A., Kanal, E. *et al.* Infertility and pregnancy outcome among magnetic resonance imaging workers. *Journal of Occupational Medicine*, **35**, 1191–1195 (1993)

67. Mevissen, M., Buntenkotter, S. and Loscher, W. Effects of static and time-varying (50 Hz) magnetic fields on reproduction and fetal development in rats. *Teratology*, **50**, 229–237 (1994)

68. Delpizzo, V. Epidemiological studies of work with video display terminals and adverse pregnancy outcomes (1984–1992). *American Journal of Industrial Medicine*, **26**, 465–480 (1994)

69. Schnorr, T.M., Grajewski, B.A., Hornung, R.W. *et al.* Video display terminals and the risk of spontaneous abortion. *New England Journal of Medicine*, **324**, 727–733 (1991)

70. Touitou, Y., Motohashi, Y., Reinberg, A. *et al.* Effect of shift work on the night-time secretory patterns of melatonin, prolactin, cortisol and testosterone. *European Journal of Applied Physiology*, **60**, 288–292 (1990)

71. Nurminen, T. Female noise exposure, shift work, and reproduction. *Journal of Occupational and Environmental Medicine*, **37**, 945–950 (1995)

72. Bisanti, L., Olsen, J., Basso, O. *et al.* Shift work and subfecundity: a European multicenter study. *Journal of Occupational and Environmental Medicine*, **38**, 352–358 (1996)

73. Lalande, N.M., Hétu, R. and Lambert, J. Is occupational noise exposure during pregnancy a risk factor of damage to the auditory system of the fetus? *American Journal of Industrial Medicine*, **10**, 427–435 (1986)

74. Nurminen, T. Fetal development and pregnancy complications in working mothers. *Thesis*, University of Tampere, Finland (1990)

75. Hartikainen, A-L., Sorri, M., Anttonen, H. *et al.* Effect of occupational noise on the course and outcome of pregnancy. *Scandinavian Journal of Occupational and Environmental Health*, **20**, 444–450 (1994)

76. Ahlborg, G. Physical work load and pregnancy outcome. *Journal of Occupational and Environmental Medicine*, **37**, 941–944 (1995)

77. Ekblad, U. Biological agents and pregnancy. *Journal of Occupational and Environmental Medicine*, **37**, 962–965 (1995)

78. Somogyi, A. and Beck, H. Nurturing and breastfeeding: exposure to chemicals in breast milk. *Environmental Health Perspectives*, **101** (Suppl. 2), 45–52 (1993)

79. Jensen, A.A. and Slorach, S.A. *Chemical Contaminants in Human Milk.* CRC Press, Boca Raton, Florida (1990)

80. Taskinen, H. and Ahlborg, G. Jr. Assessment of reproductive risk at work. *International Journal of Occupational and Environmental Health*, **2**, 59–63 (1996)

81. Stijkel, A. and van Dijk, F.J.H. Developments in reproductive risk management. *Occupational and Environmental Medicine*, **52**, 294–303 (1995)

82. Council Directive 92/32/EEC, of 30 April 1992, amending for the 7th time Directive 67/548/EEC. *Official Journal of the European Communities*, L-154/1, June 5 (1992)

83. Sullivan, F.M. The European Community directive on the classification and labeling of chemicals for reproductive toxicity. *Journal of Occupational and Environmental Medicine*, **37**, 966–969 (1995)

Chapter 15

The management of occupational asthma and hyperreactive airways disease in the workplace

P Sherwood Burge

Introduction

Occupational asthma is the commonest occupational lung disease, at least as recognized in the UK [1]. Since the disease occurs at the time of exposure, this allows the exposures that actually caused the disease to be investigated. This is very different from the pneumoconioses and malignant diseases which are due to work, where there is a long latent interval between exposure and disease. It is also possible to identify certain work as causative of occupational asthma with confidence, unlike the situation for instance with occupational lung cancer where the increased risk of a particular occupation becomes apparent only from epidemiological studies. Occupational asthma is a largely preventable disease and the identification of a case in a workplace requires action by the occupational health department and the employer (and perhaps the insurance company).

Definitions

Asthma

Asthma is defined, in terms of physiology, as widespread narrowing of the intrathoracic airways, which is reversible, at least in part, over short periods of time, either spontaneously or under treatment [2]. The degree of reversibility has not been defined – the short period of time is usually taken as less than 24 hours. Measures of reversibility are either absolute changes in lung function or are expressed as a percentage of a denominator. The best denominator is the predicted normal lung function value (rather than the observed value), as low absolute pre-bronchodilator values can otherwise result in large percentage changes, when they are used as the denominator. For instance a forced expiratory volume in 1 second (FEV_1) of 0.5 litres pre-bronchodilator and 0.6 litres afterwards can be expressed as $0.6 - 0.5/0.5 \times 100 = 20\%$, the 100 ml improvement being within the short-term variability of this measure [3]. Asthma can be defined as a reversibility of FEV_1 (expressed as per cent predicted) of $\geq 15\%$ (i.e. in the example above with a predicted FEV_1 of 3.0 litres, reversibility $= 0.6 - 0.5/3 \times 100 = 3.3\%$.

Asthma can also be defined from diurnal variation in peak expiratory flow (PEF). By coincidence, the percentage change in PEF happens to be very similar to the percentage change in FEV_1. A diurnal variation (as per cent predicted) $\geq 15\%$ can be used to define asthma. About 60% of diagnosed asthmatics have a mean diurnal variation over 17.6% [4]. As asthma can be an intermittent disease, the increased diurnal variation does not have to be present all the time.

Occupational asthma

Occupational asthma is asthma caused by exposure at work. There are different views about qualifications of this statement, relating to whether there should be evidence of (a) an allergic mechanism, (b) the absence of pre-existing asthma, and (c) a latent interval from first exposure to the onset of symptoms. The mechanism for occupational asthma is often difficult to define; in one study the mechanism was thought to be allergic in 56%, irritant in 18%, pharmacological in 2% and unknown in the remaining 24% [5]. The prognosis has been shown to be independent of the perceived mechanism, at least in one study [6]. The situation is much clearer from an occupational health point of view, where the employer should take all reasonable and practicable steps to protect the health of the worker. If the worker shows consistent asthmatic reactions to the work exposure, the worker should no longer be exposed, whatever the mechanism. If the mechanism is truly irritant, it should be easier to reduce the work exposures and leave the original worker in the same job. It is often difficult to reduce exposures sufficiently in a sensitized worker to allow continuation in the same job [7].

Allergic occupational asthma

The mechanism for occupational asthma can be classed as allergic when IgE antibodies to a relevant occupational allergen can be detected. IgE antibodies are generally found when the antigen is a large molecular weight protein of biological origin, such as urinary proteins in rodents or enzymes in detergent workers and bakers. Even in these circumstances individuals with occupational rhinitis with similar exposures have IgE antibodies with far less frequency than their colleagues with occupational asthma [8]. Antibodies are not formed against small molecular weight chemicals on their own, but can sometimes be detected when the chemical is conjugated to a protein, such as human albumin. The antibody formed may have some determinants from the carrier protein itself, as well as the small molecular weight hapten (carrier specificity). The commonest cause for occupational asthma is isocyanate exposure, where isocyanate/human serum albumin IgE antibodies can be detected in about 20% of cases. The disease in those with and without IgE antibodies is similar, with a latent interval between first exposure and first symptom, reactions elicited by exposures that previously caused no reactions, and affecting only a (usually small) proportion of those with similar levels of exposure. Some would use these three additional qualifications to define an allergic mechanism in the absence of

specific IgE [9]. Isocyanate asthma is, however, described after a single large exposure which may affect a large proportion of the exposed workers [10].

The requirement for no pre-existing asthma is also problematical. Most would accept that an individual with pollen asthma can in addition develop asthma to a cat, and that the asthma is likely to improve if exposure to the cat ceases. In exactly the same way, occupational asthma can develop in a worker with pre-existing asthma. Before developing sensitization to the occupational allergen (e.g. glutaraldehyde in a health care worker), such a worker would be able to work normally. After sensitization, their usual work would no longer be possible.

Irritant-induced occupational asthma

The most difficulty arises when the mechanism is generally regarded as being irritant, for instance with sulphur dioxide or chlorine. There is a clear distinction between a single large exposure to such an irritant followed by persisting asthma which is not precipitated by minor exposure to the same agent (irritant-induced asthma, see below) and individuals who subsequently react to the same material with very low exposures (perhaps irritant-induced occupational asthma). Many definitions are made for legal compensation, where the situation is different [9]. There is clearly no justification for the employer to compensate a worker with occupational asthma for pre-existing disability.

Irritant-induced asthma

A single large exposure to an irritant can cause asthma for the first time, which can persist long after the cause has been removed and the acute attack resolved. Such reactions have been known for a long time [11–13] and were given some respectability when called reactive airways dysfunction syndrome (RADS) [14], but are now generally called irritant-induced asthma. The proposed definition required a single large exposure resulting in airflow obstruction usually immediately, with associated increased non-specific reactivity which persisted for more than 3 months. Unfortunately there are many workers with similar asthma dating from a single exposure whose reactivity is within the range found in the normal population, who nevertheless have continuing symptoms and an increased diurnal variation in PEF (i.e. asthma). Most such workers are treated with inhaled steroids to control the asthma, which can result in improvement of non-specific reactivity, which relapses when they are stopped.

In this chapter the term 'occupational asthma' will be used irrespective of the perceived mechanism if continuing low-level exposures result in repeated falls in lung function. Irritant-induced asthma will be confined to asthma caused by a single large exposure, where subsequent low-level exposures are tolerated without any measurable detriment.

Epidemiology

The incidence of occupational asthma can be estimated from surveillance registers. The interpretation of surveillance register data is very dependent on the criteria for entry to the register. There are a number of registers of incidence data in the UK which include occupational asthma.

RIDDOR

Cases always arise in a workplace, so it seems logical to make the employer responsible for notifying cases. Such a scheme is in operation in the UK, where the employer is required to notify cases under the Reporting of Injuries, Diseases and Dangerous Occurrences Regulations (RIDDOR). The reports go to the Employment Medical Advisory Service, the group of government doctors who advise on health in the workplace. A notification usually results in a visit, and can result in prosecution. Not surprisingly there are few reports (an average of 62 per year from 1986 to 1992) (Health and Safety Commission, Annual Report 1992/3, statistical supplement). The scheme was confined to seven principal causes, including isocyanates, colophony, grains and flour and laboratory animals, but has recently been extended to any cause.

Industrial injury benefit

Occupational asthma has been a prescribed disease with no-fault compensation from the government since 1981. The initial scheme included the same seven causes only, which was expanded by a further seven agents in 1986. The addition of wood dusts was the only one that had an appreciable impact on the number of cases (the average annual cases increasing from 163 to 220). In 1991 an open category was introduced requiring greater proof of cause and effect. There were 532 cases per year in the first two years. Both these sources exclude the self-employed, who form about 12% of the workforce. At the same time, the insurance industry was compensating around 800 cases a year, but does not publish any details.

Shield and SWORD

An alternative approach is to set up a confidential reporting scheme, which cannot lead to prosecution or direct action. Such schemes are very dependent on the enthusiasm and appropriateness of those who report. Shield is a voluntary scheme in the West Midlands region of the UK, run by the regional Midland Thoracic Society, to which all chest physicians and government compensation doctors, and some occupational physicians, report. A report leads to information as to whether other cases have been reported from the same employer (but not their names), and the suspected cause; i.e. is of some benefit to the reporter. The area covered is around 10% of the UK, and averaged 90 reports per year from 1989 to 1992 [5]. Shield does not specify any particular agent or test necessary for reporting, merely that the diagnosis is the most likely one in the opinion of the reporter. Only 38% of the cases had a cause among the 14 available for government compensation at the time, and of these only 27% were reported from the government compensation board, implying that both groups were seeing largely distinct subsets of those with occupational asthma.

Similar diagnostic criteria are required for SWORD, a national voluntary reporting scheme run jointly by the national societies of occupational and thoracic medicine, covering a total population of about 55 million (and recently extended to Eire). For the first 3 years (1989–92) there were 509 notifications per year [1], increasing to an estimated 977 per year for 1993–94 when a sampling system was used and the numbers multiplied by the sample proportion [15]. Occupational physicians report about 19% of the cases. The effects on the approximate number of reports per year for a population of 55 million is shown in *Table 15.1*.

Table 15.1   Effects of constraints on notification on the reported incidence of occupational asthma in the UK (population 55 million). Average number of reports per year (1989–92)

RIDDOR (employer notification +/− regulatory visit)	Government compensation; limited list (14)	Government compensation; open list	Shield (local voluntary scheme; mainly chest physicians)	SWORD (national voluntary scheme, occupational and chest physicians)
62	220	532	900	977

SENSOR

In the USA the Sentinel Events Notification System for Occupational Risks (SENSOR) operates in six states [16]. The numbers reported are very low, the diagnostic criteria stricter than SWORD or Shield. The system is designed to lead to investigation of the workplace following each notification, similar to the RIDDOR scheme in the UK.

Finland

The best register is in Finland, where occupational diseases are notifiable by law, and a register has been in place since 1964. The register includes all cases notified by clinicians, all claims settled by insurance companies and all cases diagnosed by the Institute of Occupational Health. There was a large increase in notifications after 1982, when compensation was opened to self-employed farmers, the self-employed being otherwise excluded [17].

These registers show a common group of agents responsible for most occupational asthma, particularly isocyanates which head all but the Finnish register; other commonly reported agents include flour and grain, colophony, laboratory animals and wood dusts (*Table 15.2*). There are also regional differences likely to be due to the particular local exposures, especially cows in Finland, coolant oil aerosols in Shield, and Western Red Cedar in British Columbia. The incidence by occupation can be calculated from the SWORD, Shield and Finnish data. Spray painters usually head the list, with an incidence per 100 000 per year between 729 and 3111. Bakers, farmers and plastic makers all top the $1000/10^6$ in some registers. Some examples are shown in *Table 15.3*.

The incidence of irritant-induced asthmas is much less well defined, as reactions are often short lived, and contact with a respiratory physician only likely for the more severe reactions. The SWORD surveillance scheme in the UK has inhalation accidents as one of its categories. The reactions are not necessarily asthmatic, although most probably have an asthmatic element. Many more are reported by occupational physicians than chest physicians. An estimated 1180 cases were reported over 5 years, about 10% of all occupational lung diseases. Men were affected five times more often than women, reflecting the preponderance of men in the chemical and engineering industries where the incidence was highest (*Table 15.4*). Chlorine was the commonest agent responsible in 12% of reports, followed by nitrogen oxides in 9%. Other common causes are shown in *Table 15.5*.

Risk assessment

It is likely that peak exposures are more relevant than cumulative exposure in the development of respiratory sensitization. There is little evidence that cumulative exposure is a relevant risk factor. The exposure needed to sensitize a worker (the sensitizing dose) is likely to be much greater than the exposure needed to elicit an asthmatic reaction in a previously sensitized individual (the eliciting dose). Although sensitization is generally related to the level of exposure, there is little evidence for a no-effect level for the common causes of occupational asthma, such as isocyanates. As such, exposure standards are usually set as maximal allowable concentrations, which should be reduced below this level by all reasonable and practicable methods. Working with occupational sensitizers implies a risk of sensitization in the workplace. The only safe way of determining minimal risk is to have implemented good surveillance (including leavers), for a reasonable period of time, and to have detected no cases.

Table 15.2   Common causes of occupational asthma. Percentages of total reports

Agent	Shield (1989–91)	SWORD (1989–91)	Finland (1992)	Quebec (1986–88)	Michigan and New Jersey (1988–92)
Isocyanates	20	22	3	25	19
Animals	2	10	45	15	1
Flour/grain	10	7	25	14	2
Woods	6	4	2	13	1
Solder	8	6		2	1
Resins	5	5	2		7
Aldehydes	2	3	2	1	5
Welding	2	2	5		2
Drugs/pesticides	<1	2		5	2
Coolant oils	7	1			10
Co/Cr	5	1	1		4
Unknown		8	4	15	20

Table 15.3   Incidence of occupational asthma from reporting schemes

Occupation	Finland (1990)		Shield (1989–91)		SWORD (1989–91)	
	Cases	Rate/10^6/year	Cases	Rate/10^6/year	Cases	Rate/10^6/year
Baker	32	4000	20	445	64	285
Spray painter	14	3111	22	1833	108	729
Farmer	180	1401	8	44	43	34
Solderer/welder	30	1035	26	112	106	158
Plastic maker			38	1054	81	387
Chemical			3	143	77	346
Woodworker			18	130	65	45
Other	119	52	149	25	984	13
Total	375	152	284	42	1528	19

Table 15.4   Incidence of inhalation injuries by occupation. (Data from the UK SWORD surveillance scheme, 1990–93)

Occupational group	Cases	Rate/million/year
Chemical processor	156	164
Engineering/electrical	343	32
Other manufacturing	163	15
Transportation/construction	100	10
Health and science professionals	59	9
Sales and services	163	6
Others	121	3

There is a long list of possible causes of occupational asthma [18], with varying degrees of risk. With some agents the risk can be very high (e.g. over 30%), such as with complex salts of platinum [19,20], some enzymes [21] and castor beans [21]. A high level of risk (around 5%) is seen with isocyanates [22], colophony [23], wood dusts [24], baking

flour and enzymes [25], latex [26], hairdressing [27], laboratory animals and insects [28] and many others. There are a very large number of agents where the risks are generally less, such as formaldehyde [29], glutaraldehyde [30], acid anhydrides [31,32], coolant oils [33] and nickel [34]. All sensitizers should be labelled and data sheets made

Table 15.5 Incidence of inhalation injuries by agent. (Data from the UK SWORD surveillance scheme, 1990–93)

Agent	%
Gases	36
Organic chemicals	22
Inorganic chemicals	14
Combustion products	10
Metals	5
Others	6
Total no.	869

available to the workforce, together with the company policy for exposure control, surveillance and action following sensitization [35].

Surveillance

Where the risk is not negligible, surveillance of exposed workers is indicated [36]. The aim of surveillance is to identify cases at an early stage, as the long-term prognosis is worse if exposure continues for more than 6–12 months after first symptoms [37–42]. It is important to identify the workforce to be included, as occupational asthma is often as common in those with indirect exposure as in those directly exposed to respiratory sensitizers [23,43]. The level of surveillance should be related to the risk assessment. Before starting surveillance, the exposures should be confined to the minimum number of workers possible, and plans agreed for the management of the first case. Suitable agreements should include the continuation of normal employment during investigation, and the identification of equivalent jobs without exposure for sensitized individuals. With these arrangements in place, the difficult diagnosis of occupational asthma becomes more manageable, as a worker can be relocated without loss on a firm suspicion of a diagnosis. If the workers is to be dismissed because no suitable alternative work is possible (e.g. a paint sprayer in a small garage), the diagnosis should be secure before dismissal, as the financial consequences of an incorrect diagnosis are severe [40].

Surveillance can be by questionnaire, lung function or immunological tests.

Questionnaires

Questionnaires are the most appropriate instrument for respiratory surveillance. There is a choice between a short screening questionnaire designed to be sensitive but non-specific, and a long questionnaire which attempts to separate occupational asthma from other causes of lung disease. Unfortunately, none of the longer questionnaires is sufficiently sensitive for routine use. It is better to use a brief screening questionnaire such as the one in *Figure 15.1*. It can be administered by a responsible person in the workplace without medical training, or by computer. A negative response to all questions makes occupational asthma unlikely. A positive response to any question should be followed by investigation by a clinician competent in the diagnosis of occupational asthma and other lung diseases.

The screening questionnaire will pick out those with smoking-related lung diseases, who also warrant education and assessment in the occupational health department to minimize work loss. Smokers are at increased risk of developing occupational asthma to a number of agents such as laboratory animals [44,45], green coffee beans [46,47], acid anhydrides [31], platinum salts [20] and colophony [48]. Help with smoking cessation is an important part of the work of an occupational health department, which may also help to reduce the incidence of occupational asthma.

Lung function

Lung function testing is also an important part of respiratory surveillance. FEV_1 and forced vital capacity (FVC) are the most appropriate measurements to make. Peak flow is not a suitable alternative for intermittent measurements as it is insensitive for measuring long-term decline [49]. Spirometry is conceptually easy to perform in the occupational health setting, but is often performed with poor quality control. It is very important to set up proper quality-control systems, as the most common cause for changes in measurement is faulty technique [50]. Although lung function testing is an important part of respiratory surveillance, the results in individuals are difficult to interpret [51]. The average worker has an annual decline in FEV_1 and FVC of around 30 ml/year [49]; this is about one-quarter of the short-term measurement error [3]. Quite large

Since your last medical
(or in the last 12 months for new starters):

Have you had any episodes of wheeze or chest tightness?	Yes	No
Have you taken any treatment for your chest?	Yes	No
Have you woken from sleep with cough or chest tightness?	Yes	No
Have you had any episodes of breathlessness?	Yes	No
Have you had any time off work with chest illness?	Yes	No
Have you developed chest tightness or breathlessness after exercise?	Yes	No
Have you developed any difficulty breathing?	Yes	No

The following additional questions maybe added:

Have you had irritation or watering of the eyes?	Yes	No
Have you had a stuffy nose?	Yes	No
Have you had soreness of the nose, lips or mouth?	Yes	No
Have you had itching or irritation of the skin?	Yes	No

Figure 15.1 Screening questionnaire for the detection of occupational asthma. Any positive response should lead to a full history and investigation by a health professional with expertise in the diaganosis of occupational asthma. The questionnaire has been designed to be sensitive rather than specific

changes in FEV_1 are observed when measured during surveillance, without obvious explanation; occupational asthma can also develop without changes in FEV_1. The main use of FEV_1 measurement is as a baseline for detecting accelerated loss of FEV_1 in individuals (several years' readings are usually required) (*Figure 15.2*) and for investigating the mean change in a group of workers with similar exposure, for which it is particularly appropriate.

IgE antibodies

Most non-occupational asthma is due to the development in childhood of specific IgE antibodies to environmental allergens, such as house dust mites, pollens and animals. Specific IgE antibodies can be measured in blood, for instance using the RAST technique, or estimated by skin prick testing. About 30% of the adult population have specific IgE to common environmental antigens, and

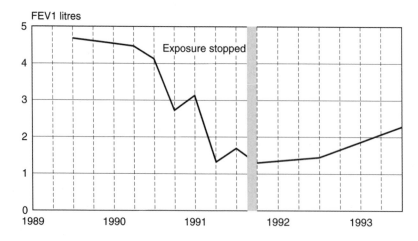

Figure 15.2 Serial surveillance measures of FEV_1 in a worker exposed to isocyanates, who did not demonstrate either asthma or any acute reactions to work exposure. The fall in FEV_1 stopped after removal from isocyanate exposure

are therefore atopic. A much smaller percentage have any disease related to the sensitization, i.e. it is possible to be sensitized without disease. Very large exposures to environmental allergens are, however, more likely to cause an asthmatic attack in a previously normal person who has prior IgE antibodies to that antigen, than in a person without IgE antibodies [52]. Specific IgE sensitization is thought to underlie occupational asthma due to large molecular weight antigens, such as laboratory animals, latex, flour, enzymes, insects, green coffee beans, soya, cow epithelium and biotechnology bacterial and fungal antigens among others. Small molecular weight chemicals are unable to act as antigens on their own, but may do so when conjugated to body proteins, such as serum albumin, where they form a hapten. The specific IgE may be directed to the hapten alone, but may also be directed at part of the binding molecule, whose tertiary structure may be altered by the hapten (carrier specificity). Small molecular weight chemicals to which specific IgE can be directed include ammonium hexachlorplatinate (skin prick testing only) and acid anhydrides (with albumin conjugation). Isocyanates can also bind to albumin, but isocyanate-specific IgE antibodies are only found in about 20% of cases of isocyanate asthma [10]. Testing for specific IgE antibodies can either be by skin prick testing or by measurement in the blood, for instance by RAST. For most antigens the skin prick test method is more sensitive, it is appropriate for use in the occupational health setting, and does not cause sensitization or systemic reactions when appropriate concentrations are used (intradermal testing is less specific and carries the risk of both sensitization and systemic reaction). There is a variable relationship between sensitization, as measured immunologically, and disease. Control of sensitization, however, will precede control of disease. Repeated skin prick testing is an important outcome measure for process control, and has been particularly well documented in the control of small mammal allergy [53,54] and detergent enzyme allergy [55].

The frequency of surveillance depends on the agent. Pre-exposure assessment is always indicated. For agents with a high risk of sensitization in the first year of exposure, 3-monthly assessment is indicated for the first year, usually followed by annual assessments. In addition to routine assessments, all individuals should be seen following sickness absence which might have been due to respiratory disease. All exposed workers should be asked to report any symptoms which could be due to occupational asthma.

Surveillance failures

Respiratory symptoms picked up on a surveillance questionnaire may be due to occupational or other causes. As the surveillance will have been carried out because of a perceived risk, each individual should be carefully investigated to confirm or exclude occupational asthma.

History

A full history of the symptom in relation to exposure is needed, with the date of onset, any improvement on days away from work or on holiday/sick leave, and the timing of the symptom in relation to onset on workdays, and the effects of successive daily exposure. If the symptom improves on days away from work or holiday/ sick leave, the worker should be further investigated for occupational asthma, whatever is found from lung function measurements and smoking history. Workers with occupational asthma often have symptoms starting after leaving work, causing nocturnal waking with cough and breathlessness. Most are also at their worst on waking the following morning. It is therefore not helpful to screen workers by asking whether the symptoms occur at work. Other workers do, however, have symptoms which start after variable periods of work exposure, the interval often shortening as the work week progresses and as the disease becomes more severe. If recovery is complete before the next day's exposure, the asthma is usually similarly severe each workday. If recovery is incomplete, symptoms usually increase towards the end of the work week [56,57]. There are a few individuals whose symptoms are maximal on the first workday and improve with subsequent daily exposures. Such a pattern is similar to that seen with cotton exposure (byssinosis) [58], but also occurs in other situations where endotoxin exposure occurs, such as exposures to contaminated coolant oils [33], swine confinement and poultry breeding buildings and perhaps sewage works.

Serial measurements of lung function

Lung function should start with spirometry and reversibility to a standard beta agonist such as salbutamol or terbutaline. The physiological confirmation of occupational asthma requires serial measures of peak expiratory flow (or FEV_1). After instruction and the demonstration of successful meter reading, the worker should be asked to record the best of at least three measurements every 2 hours from waking to sleeping. The best two readings of peak expiratory flow on each occasion should be within 20 l/min; if not, further readings should be made so that the maximum true peak flow is recorded on each occasion. There is no need to be exact in the timing. Workers who have difficulty of making measurements while working (e.g. they may be wearing personal respiratory protection) should be asked to make measurements on waking, on arrival at work, during each formal work break, at the end of work, mid-evening and at bedtime (with suitable adjustment for shift workers). Similar readings should be made on days away from work, taking care to make the first reading on waking rather than getting up, which may be much later when the 'morning dip' has worn off. The worker should be visited within a week of starting the record, to check compliance and technique. The usual first analysis of the record should be after 2 weeks.

The best method of analysis involves calculating the daily maximum, mean and minimum peak flow, and the daily diurnal variation [59]. The OASYS computer program achieves this, as well as correcting for meter non-linearity, adjusting the daily readings to start with the first reading at work and stopping at the last reading before work on the next day, and making an assessment of the likelihood of a work-related effect being present (*Figure 15.3*) [60]. A normal 2-week record has a diurnal variation less than 15% throughout, has a normal mean peak flow (from predicted tables), and has no difference between rest days and workdays. If the record is normal the worker should continue at work and rejoin the surveillance programme, with reinforced instructions to come again if work-related symptoms recur. A few workers will return records with obvious asthma; the remainder should keep a further 2-week record, providing 4 weeks for analysis. If the record is still equivocal, the worker should be removed from exposure for 2 weeks, while further records are kept, followed by a return to the ori-

ginal job for a further 2 weeks [51]. It is very important to make the peak flow measurements while the worker is still exposed, as these often provide the only objective confirmation of occupational asthma. If IgE antibodies to the occupational antigen are available, they should also be measured. If no definite work-related changes are shown, occupational asthma is unlikely.

It is reasonable for exposure to continue in workers with positive IgE antibodies to an occupational allergen, who are asymptomatic and have normal peak flow records. It is wise to increase surveillance and check occupational controls in such individuals, who should be reminded of the early symptoms of occupational asthma. If the occupational health service does not have a clinician competent to do these investigations, they should be referred to a suitable specialist.

Action following detection of occupational asthma

The first step is to remove the affected worker from exposure, and to repeat the peak flow monitoring in the relocated job to make sure that the occupational asthma is controlled. Continuing exposure can result from incidental exposure while reaching the new workplace or visiting the canteen, etc. The exposure in the workplace of the affected worker should be checked to make sure that control measures were working properly. If the worker was not on regular surveillance, the group requiring surveillance should be reassessed and the risk assessment re-evaluated. If specific IgE has been detected, it should be measured serially after relocation. It may have a half-life of around a year [61]. If the levels do not fall, it is likely that continuing exposure is occurring.

Action following irritant asthma

Irritant asthma almost always implies a failure of exposure control. Exposure may occur for a number of reasons, such as cleaning up after an accident, when appropriate respiratory protection was not used. The emergency plans should be reassessed and improved.

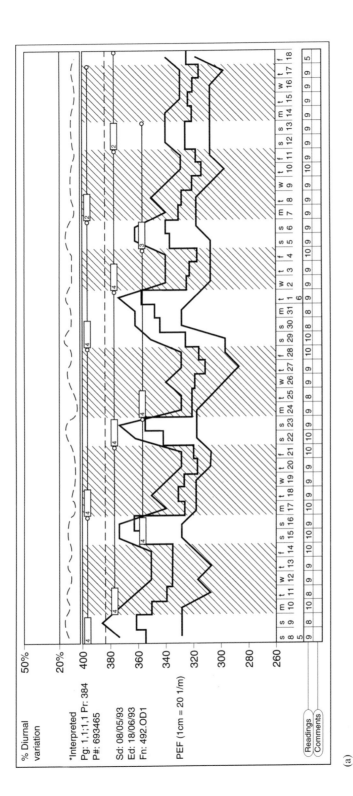

Figure 15.3 (a) Serial plot of peak expiratory flow in a laboratory technician exposed to glutaraldehyde, used for cleaning work surfaces, and latex in gloves. Sensitization to glutaraldehyde was confirmed by specific provocation testing. The plot shows diurnal variation in PEF, expressed as per cent, predicted in the top panel. The middle section shows the daily maximum PEF (upper continuous line), mean (middle bars) and minimum (lower continuous line). Days at work have a shaded background; days away from work a clear background. The small numbers in boxes show the score allotted by OASYS-2 [60], ranging from 4 (definite occupational effect) to 1 (no occupational effect). The overall weighted score for the record is 3.29 in the definite occupational effect category. The bottom panel shows the date and the number of readings each day from which the record is made.

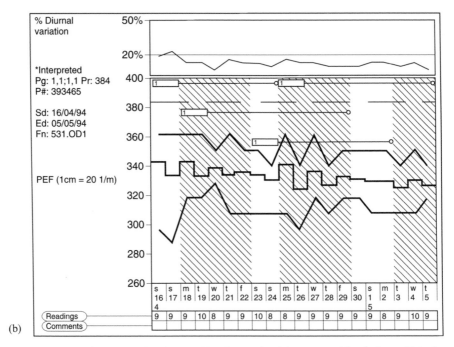

Figure 15.3 (*continued*) (b) The same technician working in another laboratory without glutaraldehyde exposure, but still exposed to latex. There is now no occupational effect (score 1), showing successful relocation

Prognosis

Once occupational asthma has developed, asthma is likely to be precipitated by non-specific factors such as respiratory infection, cold air, perfumes, indoor and outdoor pollution and exercise, in the same way as in non-occupational asthma [62]. Removal from workplace exposure will abolish the occupational asthma (i.e. the asthma due to coming to work each day), but frequently leaves a worker with asthma exacerbated by the non-specific factors. Workers are likely to need more time off work with respiratory infections than they would have needed before developing occupational asthma, and will be disadvantaged in the open labour market. In particular, they should not work with any of the high-risk causes of occupational asthma, as well as the material to which they are sensitized. Overall, around 50% of affected workers make a complete recovery. Recovery can continue for about 2 years following last exposure [63]. The likelihood of complete recovery is dependent on whether exposure continues after first symptoms, being generally worse if exposure continues for more than a year (*Figure 15.4*) [37–40,42,64]. Recovery is also dependent on the causative agent, being worse for wood dusts, isocyanates, flour and colophony, compared to laboratory animals and platinum salts [37].

Continuing exposure outside the workplace is likely for many agents such as flour and colophony, which may contribute to continuing symptoms. The situation with platinum salts is interesting, as exposure outside the workplace is very unlikely. Two refineries of the same company have different policies for sensitized workers. In one, 3-monthly surveillance identifies sensitized workers at an early stage; they are then removed completely from exposure. Follow-up studies have shown complete resolution of the asthma in all (Newman Taylor, pers. comm.). The second refinery has less regular surveillance and reduces rather than eliminates exposure. The follow-up data show much more continuing asthma [65].

Prognosis in general has not been shown to be related to the perceived mechanism, those thought to be due to irritant mechanisms having a similar prognosis to those with an allergic mechanism [6].

Irritant-induced asthma (without occupational sensitization) is more likely to result in complete recovery, which can be complete within days or last several years. Repeat testing of non-specific

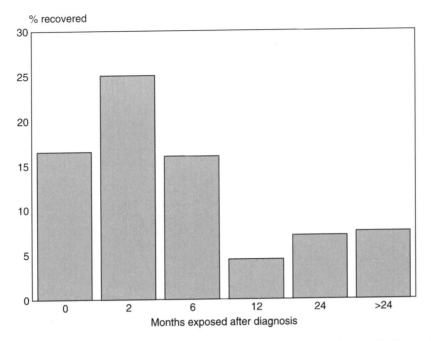

Figure 15.4 Prognosis of occupational asthma for workers reported by chest physicians to SWORD, relating to the time between first symptoms of occupational asthma and the time that the worker was removed from exposure to the causative agent (from Ross and McDonald [37,42])

bronchial reactivity with histamine or metacholine is particularly appropriate in this group; recovery of responsiveness may occur some time after lung function has returned to normal. Symptoms may persist even after responsiveness has returned to values within the normal range. There are several studies showing complete recovery following very severe irritant asthma, even when requiring ventilation for the acute attack [66]. There are other individuals who are left with asthma long-term. The protracted course of compensation claims can also delay recovery.

Rehabilitation or compensation

Compensation is often seen as a negative aspect of occupational asthma by occupational physicians. The problems of compensation deter many physicians from making the diagnosis of occupational asthma. The worker with disability often wants compensation for the financial losses incurred, and does not understand why compensation should depend on whether the workplace or other factors are the causes of the disability and

whether negligence has occurred (no-fault compensation versus compensation for negligence). Most societies believe that disability due to factors in the workplace should result in some sort of compensation. Who should pay differs greatly between different countries (*Table 15.6*). Compensation is not a substitute for rehabilitation, which should be centred on returning a worker with occupational asthma to a fulfilling and useful employment with hope for the future. This will often involve retraining, and is likely to be much more cost effective, particularly for a younger worker precluded from following his chosen career. The most appropriate place for the rehabilitation to occur is in the workplace where the disease started. It is often also the cheapest solution. In a hospital where the author works, a number of nurses have developed occupational asthma due to the wearing of latex gloves, in accordance with the agreed work practice, and have had to give up their jobs because of their disease. None use latex as an essential part of their jobs. There is sufficient latex in the air of ordinary ward environments to precipitate their asthma. In the author's opinion, the most appropriate action would be to create latex-free areas

Table 15.6 Source of compensation of occupational asthma in Europe

Country	Employer	Insurance	General tax
Austria	+		
Belgium	+		
Bulgaria	+		
Denmark	+		
Finland	+		
France	+		
Germany	+		
Italy	+		
Norway	+	+	
Portugal	+		
Romania	+		
Holland	+	worker	
Spain		+	+
Sweden		+	+
UK			+

and retrain those nurses for work there, rather than expect them to sue their employer for loss of earnings.

The insurance companies may help, particularly if the premiums paid by the employer reflect the risks being taken. If a premium is reduced (or increased) by substantial amounts depending on the degree of risk in the workplace, there can be a cost advantage for safety improvements at the time when the disease occurs. If several years elapse before a claim is settled and premiums raised, the cost is unlikely to be borne by the actual working unit where the problem arose. Insurance premiums can be used as a help to the occupational health department in their attempt to reduce the risks of the workplace.

References

1. Meredith, S.K. and McDonald, J.C. Work-related respiratory disease in the United Kingdom, 1989–1992: report of the SWORD project. *Occupational Medicine*, **44**, 183–189 (1994)
2. Ciba Foundation Study Group No 38 (eds R. Porter and J. Birch) *Identification of asthma*. Churchill Livingstone, Edinburgh (1971)
3. Tweeddale, P.M., Alexander, F. and McHardy, G.J.R. Short term variability in FEV1 and bronchodilator responsiveness in patients with obstructive ventilatory defects. *Thorax*, **42**, 487–490 (1987)
4. Higgins, B.G., Britton, J.R., Chinn, S. *et al.* Comparison of bronchial reactivity and peak expiratory flow variability measurements for epidemiologic studies.

American Review of Respiratory Diseases, **145**, 588–593 (1992)
5. Gannon, P.F. and Burge, P.S. The SHIELD scheme in the West Midlands Region, United Kingdom. Midland Thoracic Society Research Group. *British Journal of Industrial Medicine*, **50**, 791–796 (1993)
6. Cannon, J., Cullinan, P. and Newman Taylor, A.J. Consequences of occupational asthma. *British Medical Journal*, **311**, 602–603 (1995)
7. Slovak, A.J.M., Orr, R.G. and Teasdale, E.L. Efficacy of the helmet respirator in occupational asthma due to laboratory animal allergy (LAA). *American Industrial Hygiene Association*, **46**, 411–415 (1985)
8. Slovak, A.J.M. and Hill, R.N. Laboratory animal allergy: a clinical survey of an exposed population. *British Journal of Industrial Medicine*, **38**, 38–41 (1981)
9. Department of Social Security. *Occupational Asthma*, Cmd 1244. HMSO, London (1990)
10. Pezzini, A., Riviera, A., Paggiaro, P.L. *et al.* Specific IgE antibodies in 28 workers with diisocyanate-induced bronchial asthma. *Clinical Allergy*, **14**, 453–461 (1984)
11. Kaufman, J. and Burkons, D. Clinical, roentgenologic and physiologic effects of acute chlorine exposure. *Archives of Environmental Health*, **23**, 29–34 (1971)
12. LeQuesne, P.M., Axford, A.T., McKerrow, C.B. *et al.* Neurological complications after a single severe exposure to toluene diisocyanate. *British Journal of Industrial Medicine*, **33**, 72–78 (1976)
13. Weiner, A. Bronchial asthma due to organic phosphate insecticides. *Annals of Allergy*, **19**, 397–401 (1961)
14. Brooks, S.M., Weiss, M.A. and Bernstein, I.L. Reactive airways dysfunction syndrome (RADS). Persistent asthma syndrome after high level irritant exposure. *Chest*, **88**, 376–384 (1985)
15. Ross, D.J., Sallie, B.A. and McDonald, J.C. SWORD '94: surveillance of work-related and occupational respiratory disease in the UK. *Occupational Medicine*, **45**, 175–178 (1995)
16. Reilly, M.J., Rosenman, K.D., Watt, F.C. *et al.* Surveillance for occupational asthma – Michigan and New Jersey, 1988–1992. *MMWR CDC Surveillance Summaries*, **43**, 9–17 (1994)
17. Meredith, S. and Nordman, H. Occupational asthma; measures of frequency from four countries. *Thorax* (1996)
18. Burge, P.S. Occupational asthma. In *Respiratory Medicine*, 2nd edn (eds R.A.L. Brewis, B. Corrin, D.M. Geddes and D.J. Gibson). W.B. Saunders, London (1995)
19. Hunter, D., Milton, R. and Perry, K.M.A. Asthma caused by the complex salts of platinum. *British Journal of Industrial Medicine*, **2**, 92–98 (1945)
20. Venables, K.M., Dally, M.B., Nunn, A.J. *et al.* Smoking and occupational allergy in workers in a platinum refinery. *British Medical Journal*, **299**, 939–942 (1989)
21. Figley, K.D. and Elrod, R.M. Endemic asthma due to castor bean dust. *Journal of the American Medical Association*, **90**, 79–82 (1928)

22. Diem, J.E., Jones, R.N., Hendrick, D.J. *et al.* Five year longitudinal study of workers employed in a new toluene diisocyanate manufacturing plant. *American Review of Respiratory Diseases*, **126**, 420–428 (1982)

23. Burge, P.S., Perks, W., O'Brien, I.M. *et al.* Occupational asthma in an electronics factory. *Thorax*, **34**, 13–18 (1979)

24. Vedal, S., Chan-Yeung, M., Enarson, D. *et al.* Symptoms and pulmonary function in Western Red Cedar workers related to duration of employment and dust exposure. *Archives of Environmental Health*, **41**, 179–183 (1986)

25. Musk, A.W., Venables, K.M., Crook, B. *et al.* Respiratory symptoms, lung function, and sensitisation to flour in a British bakery. *British Journal of Industrial Medicine*, **46**, 636–642 (1989)

26. Jaeger, D., Kleinhans, D., Czuppon, A.B. *et al.* Latex-specific proteins causing immediate-type cutaneous, nasal, bronchial, and systemic reactions. *Journal of Allergy and Clinical Immunology*, **89**, 759–768 (1992)

27. Blainey, A.D., Ollier, S., Cundell, D. *et al.* Occupational asthma in a hairdressing salon. *Thorax*, **41**, 42–50 (1986)

28. Burge, P.S., Edge, G., O'Brien, I.M. *et al.* Occupational asthma in a research centre breeding locusts. *Clinical Allergy*, **10**, 355–363 (1980)

29. Burge, P.S., Harries, M.G., Lam, W.K. *et al.* Occupational asthma due to formaldehyde. *Thorax*, **40**, 255–260 (1985)

30. Gannon, P.F.G., Bright, P., Campbell, M. *et al.* Occupational asthma due to glutaraldehyde and formaldehyde in endoscopy and X-ray departments. *Thorax*, **50**, 156–159 (1995)

31. Venables, K.M., Topping, M.D., Howe, W. *et al.* Interaction of smoking and atopy in producing specific IgE antibody against a hapten protein conjugate. *British Medical Journal*, **290**, 201–204 (1985)

32. Barker, R.D., Harris, J.M., van Tongeren, M. *et al.* The determinants of bronchial hyperresponsiveness in a cohort of workers exposed to acid anhydrides. *European Respiratory Journal*, **8**, 193s (Abstract) (1995)

33. Robertson, A.S., Weir, D.C. and Burge, P.S. Occupational asthma due to oil mists. *Thorax*, **43**, 200–205 (1988)

34. Shirakawa, T., Kusaka, Y. and Morimoto, K. Specific IgE antibodies to nickel in workers with known reactivity to cobalt. *Clinical and Experimental Allergy*, **22**, 213–218 (1992)

35. Baranski, B. *Anonymous Criteria for the Classification of Skin and Airway Sensitising Substances in the Work and General Environments*. WHO, Copenhagen (1996)

36. Health and Safety Executive. *Medical Aspects of Occupational Asthma*, MS25. HMSO, London (1990)

37. Ross, D.J. and McDonald, J.C. Health and employment after a diagnosis of occupational asthma. *European Respiratory Journal*, (1997) in press

38. Malo, J.-L., Cartier, A., Ghezzo, H. *et al.* Patterns of improvement in spirometry, bronchial hyperresponsiveness, and specific IgE antibody levels after cessation of exposure in occupational asthma caused by snow-crab processing. *American Review of Respiratory Diseases*, **138**, 807–812 (1988)

39. Weir, D.C., Robertson, A.S., Jones, S. *et al.* The economic consequences of developing occupational asthma. *Thorax*, **42**, 209 (1987)

40. Gannon, P.F., Weir, D.C., Robertson, A.S. *et al.* Health, employment, and financial outcomes in workers with occupational asthma. *British Journal of Industrial Medicine*, **50**, 491–496 (1993)

41. Chan-Yeung, M., MacLean, L. and Paggiaro, P.L. Follow-up study of 232 patients with occupational asthma caused by western red cedar (*Thuja plicata*). *Journal of Allergy and Clinical Immunology*, **79**, 792–796 (1987)

42. Ross, D.J. and McDonald, J.C. The outcome of occupational asthma in the UK. *European Respiratory Journal*, **8**, 301s (1995)

43. Boran, A.M. Prevalence of occupational asthma in the electroplating industry. *PhD thesis*, University of Birmingham (1993)

44. Cullinan, P., Lowson, D., Nieuwenhuijsen, M.J. *et al.* Work related symptoms, sensitisation, and estimated exposure in workers not previously exposed to laboratory rats. *Occupational and Environmental Medicine*, **51**, 589–592 (1994)

45. Venables, K.M., Upton, J.L., Hawkins, E.R. *et al.* Smoking, atopy, and laboratory animal allergy. *British Journal of Industrial Medicine*, **45**, 667–671 (1988)

46. Thomas, K.E., Trigg, C.J., Baxter, P.J. *et al.* Factors relating to the development of respiratory symptoms in coffee process workers. *British Journal of Industrial Medicine*, **48**, 314–322 (1991)

47. Zetterstrom, O., Osterman, K., Machado, L. *et al.* Another smoking hazard: raised serum IgE concentration and increased risk of occupational allergy. *British Medical Journal*, **283**, 1215–1217 (1981)

48. Burge, P.S., Perks, W.H., O'Brien, I.M. *et al.* Occupational asthma in an electronics factory; a case control study to evaluate aetiological factors. *Thorax*, **34**, 300–307 (1979)

49. Quanjer, P.H., Tammeling, G.J., Cotes, J.E. *et al.* Lung volumes and forced ventilatory flows. Report of Working Party on Standardization of Lung Function Tests, European Community for Steel and Coal. Official Statement of the European Respiratory Society. *European Respiratory Journal*, **16** (Suppl.), 5–40 (1993)

50. Enright, P.L., Johnson, L.R., Connett, J.E. *et al.* Spirometry in the Lung Health Study. 1. Methods and quality control. *American Review of Respiratory Disease*, **143**, 1215–1223 (1991)

51. Burge, P.S. Single and serial measurements of lung function in the diagnosis of occupational asthma. *European Journal of Respiratory Disease*, **63** (Suppl. 123), 47–59 (1982)

52. Bryant, D.H. and Burns, M.W. Bronchial histamine reactivity: its relationship to the reactivity of the bronchi to allergens. *Clinical Allergy*, **6**, 523–532 (1976)

53. Davies, G.E., Thompson, A.V., Niewola, Z. *et al.* Allergy to laboratory animals: a retrospective and a prospective study. *British Journal of Industrial Medicine*, **40**, 442–449 (1983)

54. Botham, P.A., Davies, G.E. and Teasdale, E.L. Allergy to laboratory animals: a prospective study of its incidence and the influence of atopy on its development. *British Journal of Industrial Medicine*, **44**, 627–632 (1987)

55. Juniper, C.P., How, M.J., Goodwin, B.F.J. *et al. Bacillus subtilis* enzymes: a 7 year clinical, epidemiological and immunological study of an industrial allergen. *Journal of the Society of Occupational Medicine*, **27**, 3–12 (1977)

56. Burge, P.S., O'Brien, I.M. and Harries, M.G. Peak flow rate records in the diagnosis of occupational asthma due to isocyanates. *Thorax*, **34**, 317–323 (1979)

57. Burge, P.S., O'Brien, I.M. and Harries, M.G. Peak flow rate records in the diagnosis of occupational asthma due to colophony. *Thorax*, **34**, 308–316 (1979)

58. McKerrow, C.B., McDermott, M., Gilson, J.C. *et al.* Respiratory function during the day in cotton workers – a study in byssinosis. *British Journal of Industrial Medicine*, **15**, 75–83 (1958)

59. Lenfant, C. and Khaltaev, N. Global strategy for asthma management and prevention. NHLBI/WHO workshop. NIH USA95-3659 (1995)

60. Gannon, P.F.G., Newton, D.T., Belcher, J. *et al.* The development of OASYS-2, a system for the analysis of measurements of peak expiratory flow in workers with suspected occupational asthma. *Thorax*, **51**, 484–489 (1996)

61. Venables, K.M., Topping, M.D., Nunn, A.J. *et al.* Immunologic and functional consequences of chemical (tetrachlorphthalic anhydride)-induced asthma after four years of avoidance of exposure. *Journal of Allergy and Clinical Immunology*, **80**, 212–218 (1987)

62. Burge, P.S. Occupational asthma in electronics workers caused by colophony fumes: follow-up of affected workers. *Thorax*, **37**, 348–353 (1982)

63. Hudson, P., Cartier, A., Pineau, L. *et al.* Follow-up of occupational asthma caused by crab and various agents. *Journal of Allergy and Clinical Immunology*, **76**, 682–688 (1985)

64. Chan-Yeung, M., Chan, H., Salari, H. *et al.* Grain-dust extract induced direct release of mediators from human lung tissue. *Journal of Allergy and Clinical Immunology*, **80**, 279–284 (1987)

65. Baker, D.B., Gann, P.H., Brooks, S.M. *et al.* Cross-sectional study of platinum salts sensitization among precious metals refinery workers. *American Journal of Industrial Medicine*, **18**, 653–664 (1990)

66. Weil, H., George, R., Schwarz, M. *et al.* Late evaluation of pulmonary function after acute exposure to chlorine gas. *American Review of Respiratory Disease*, **99**, 374–379 (1969)

Chapter 16

Occupational skin diseases

P-J Coenraads and C Timmer

Introduction

Many occupational physicians will acknowledge that skin disorders are among the most frequently encountered diseases related to occupational activities. Publications based on analyses of national statistics are scarce, and suffer from deficiencies, but from these papers emerges a pattern that indicates that skin disorders may comprise more than 40% of the total number of cases registered as occupational in origin. Most publications dealing with aspects of occupational skin diseases are not written by occupational physicians, but by dermatologists based in clinical centres, which explains the trend to be biased towards selected clinical material. This statement is by no means meant to discredit the work of dermatologists; on the contrary, this speciality can be regarded as quite outstanding in devoting a considerable effort towards occupational aspects through various occupational dermatology clinics and (inter)national working parties.

One aspect of this bias towards clinical material instead of the factory population was pointed out in a review of all publications in a leading journal on occupational and environmental dermatitis. It showed that 88% of the articles dealt with allergic contact dermatitis, in contrast to the real situation at the workplace, where other forms of dermatitis, in particular irritant contact dermatitis, dominate.

Many countries have occupational skin disease registers in some form or another. However, there are not many publications based on an analysis of these government or social insurance statistics,

and one wonders in how many countries these statistics are accessible and accurate. It can be assumed that even the best statistics are an underestimate of the true size of the problem, since many cases go unreported. Some publications are based on cases for which compensation is claimed, and thus represent only the top end of the spectrum of severity. Many occupational dermatology clinics have published their numbers, but in addition to selection bias, many of these papers suffer from the deficiency that denominators (size of the source population, the working population at risk) are not given.

A brief summary of the major branches of industry as a source of occupational skin disease cases in some countries is given in *Table 16.1*. (For a full discussion and references see the chapter on epidemiology in [1].)

Virtually all publications concern developed, industrialized countries. There is evidence to suggest that occupational skin diseases are common

Table 16.1 Some reported incidences of occupational skin disease per 1000 workers per year

Country	Industry	
USA	Construction	0.7
	Metal	1.8
	Agriculture	2.8
Finland	Metal and machinery	1.0
	Sanitary services	1.3
Germany	Construction	0.7
	Health service	2.8

in developing countries. 'Contact dermatitis', which includes non-occupational cases, accounted for the majority of cases seen in clinics in Mexico and Central America. Contact dermatitis was common in rural areas in Kenya; the majority due to chemical sprays in agriculture. In general, more specific knowledge on the occurrence of occupational skin diseases in developing countries is lacking.

Classification

As a response to exposure to various external agents, the skin can show various reaction patterns leading to disease. The range of 'true' occupational skin diseases is in practice rather limited. It should be kept in mind that there is often a combination of exposure at work and in the home environment; therefore the term 'occupational and environmental skin disease' is perhaps more appropriate.

Typical occupational skin diseases are as follows:

- subtypes of contact eczema/dermatitis
- contact acne and folliculitis
- depigmentations and hyperpigmentations
- infections
- benign and malignant tumours – various rare diseases e.g. lichenoid reactions.

It is generally accepted that, in industrialized countries, about 90% of all forms of occupational skin disease is confined to the hands and forearms, less frequently to the face, while sometimes other parts of the body are involved. Most cases are diagnosed as contact eczema or dermatitis. Thus, occupational dermatology is often a matter of hand eczema.

Clinical dermatologists recognize various subtypes of eczema/dermatitis. The problem is that most existing classifications of eczema/dermatitis are not based on a single characteristic: on the contrary, they are based on combinations of morphological, aetiological, constitutional or other features, and do not always seem to be logical. Not all types are caused by occupational factors: some are to a certain degree work related and only the irritant and the allergic type can be regarded as wholly occupational or environmental. Despite its common use for over a century, the term 'eczema' has given rise to confusion. In dermatological literature, eczema and 'dermatitis' are commonly

applied to the same morphological pattern. However, in the Anglo-Saxon literature, eczema is used less often and skin conditions of this kind are often referred to as dermatitis.

The majority of occupational skin diseases are formed by subtypes of contact dermatitis, of which a classification is as follows:

- allergic contact dermatitis
- irritant contact dermatitis
- photoallergic and phototoxic reactions
- contact urticaria.

Although contact urticaria should in a strict sense not be part of this list, it is included because repeated contact urticarial reactions of the hands tend to progress to eczema.

Common skin disorders can be aggravated by work or can be provoked in a predisposed person. Since these diseases are often a form of eczema, their distinction from occupational eczema/dermatitis can sometimes be difficult. In atopic dermatitis particularly, there is considerable interaction. Examples of these common work-related diseases are as follows:

- atopic dermatitis
- stasis dermatitis
- seborrhoeic dermatitis
- psoriasis
- mycosis and mycotic eczema
- urticaria.

Hand eczema

Hand eczema/dermatitis is one of the most common manifestations of occupational skin disease. Because different casual and aggravating factors interact, it is often a difficult problem. Manual tasks cannot be performed and healing is often slow. There is a tendency towards a chronic relapsing course. This relatively unfavourable prognosis urges the occupational physician to undertake action as soon as possible and to establish prevention programmes.

The clinical appearance may vary: in the acute stages vesicles are visible, whereas the chronic stage shows a scabby, chapped, sometimes thickened skin. Vesicles are often found at the sides of the fingers and the palms. On clinical appearance it is difficult to distinguish between allergic and contact dermatitis, and atopic dermatitis also may be solely confined to the hands. Usually both hands are involved. Histopathology is unhelpful in distinguishing between the different types of eczema.

As shown in *Figure 16.1*, hand eczema is an inflammation, starting at the interface of dermis and epidermis. The term eczema stems from a Greek word with the meaning 'boiling over', which is in fact an appropriate description of this inflammatory process with blistering. The very early events leading to this inflammation may be different, but ultimately the process is similar for all major causes. Often there is considerable interaction between these causes. Skin atopy, for example, carries an increased risk for irritant contact dermatitis (not for contact allergy), and irritant contact dermatitis may enhance the risk of contact sensitization.

Recent epidemiological studies challenge the primary role of common allergies to metals, especially nickel, and to a lesser extent chromate. It seems that a history of atopic dermatitis or current symptoms pointing towards skin atopy is a major cause of recurrent hand eczema. Metal sensitivity is also associated with skin atopy. (For a further discussion on the interplay between exposure factors, metal sensitivity and skin atopy see [5].)

Some key points concerning hand eczema are as follows:

- act quickly to prevent a chronic relapsing course
- make sure it is eczema, not something else (e.g. psoriasis)
- suspect mycosis if only one hand is involved
- irritant contact dermatitis is more common than allergic contact dermatitis
- skin atopy is a major causal or contributing factor
- thorough history-taking is as important as patch testing
- do not overestimate the role of nickel and chromate allergy
- stop contact with liquids, soaps, cleansers, occlusive gloves
- do not only rely on corticosteroid creams
- monitor the compliance with therapy.

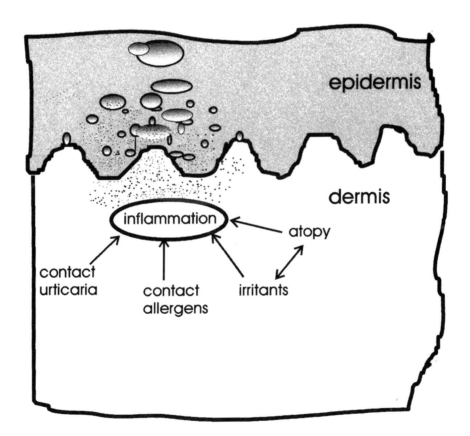

Figure 16.1 Eczema of the hands: inflammation at the interface of dermis and epidermis may be caused by different factors. In the acute phase, tiny blisters are visible; later, scaling and chapping dominate

Treatment requires frequent contact with the patient. Regular adjustment of the therapy is necessary because the manifestation of hand eczema changes – from acute vesicular to dry scaling and chapping. Regular application of emollients is as important as the corticosteroid-containing creams. Corticosteroids help reduce the inflammation, whereas the emollients are essential in restoring the skin barrier function, in reducing chapping and in overcoming dryness and scaling.

Examples

A physician training to be a gynaecologist became severely handicapped by eczema of his hands. It started after his full-time posting to the operating centre and he concluded that he became allergic to surgical gloves, and requested special (expensive) allergenic gloves.
  Further examination and history-taking revealed that he had an 'atopic background': his brother and sister have asthma, and he had dermatitis on his arms and legs during childhood. Patch tests showed allergy to inhalation allergens such as pollen and house-dust mite, but not to latex; patch testing showed no allergy to components of his latex rubber gloves.

Conclusion A flare-up of atopic dermatitis combined with irritant contact dermatitis: his hand eczema was provoked by occlusion, frequent hand-washing and disinfection. He should seriously reconsider his career plans, as his atopic constitution increases the risk to developing latex allergy.

A young lady applies for a part-time job as a cleaner in a large restaurant kitchen. She says that she has a 'dry' skin and that she had childhood eczema in the folds of knees and elbows. Cheap earrings cause severe itching and redness of her earlobes.

Conclusion. Her 'dry' skin is probably a manifestation of her skin atopy. Her childhood eczema was probably atopic dermatitis, which is a risk factor in her proposed job. Wet work and skin atopy increase the risk to develop hand eczema. Her contact allergy to nickel causes no problems now, but may become relevant when the damaged skin of her hands is in contact with metal kitchen utensils under wet circumstances. A careful assessment of her new job (see Risk inventories, below) is necessary and proper advice on skin care and skin protection is mandatory. She should avoid an additional burden on her skin from housekeeping activities at home: dishwashing should be done by her partner.

A laboratory technician in an agrochemicals factory gets severe hand eczema every time he takes samples from a particular reactor. Although he avoids this procedure as much as possible, his hand eczema does not clear completely. After a period off work there is some improvement, but the eczema slowly but gradually returns in the course of two weeks when he resumes his work.
  Patch tests reveal a contact allergy to a trimethyl ammonium compound, which is used in the reactor. There is no 'contamination' with this chemical on the instruments or glassware in his laboratory. In this lab, he works with a multitude of inorganic chemicals (e.g. HCl, NaOH, H_2O_2 etc), wears occlusive gloves and washes his hands more than 10 times daily.

Conclusion. Although he has a relevant contact allergy, the persistence of his problem is irritant contact dermatitis. The acute flares of his hand eczema can be ascribed to allergic contact dermatitis from a particular chemical after working at the reactor. His irritant contact dermatitis may have facilitated the induction of the contact allergy to the trimethyl ammonium compound, which is known to be a weak sensitizer.

Contact dermatitis

For a brief description of the entity eczema see the section on hand eczema (above). It is clear that for diagnosing this condition regular experience with patients is more effective than a description on paper. The next paragraphs deal with a summary of some basic principles. (For further documentation see major textbooks [1–3].)

Allergic contact eczema

Allergic contact eczema is based on an immunological phenomenon in which the skin reacts hyperergically to a substance after previous contact with that substance. An allergen must be present and the worker has to be sensitized to that allergen. After interaction of the allergen with the individual's immune system, a state of delayed type hypersensitivity may be induced. The process of sensitization can be divided into two phases. In the first or inductive phase, sensitization takes place and, in the second or eliciting phase, the hypersensitivity becomes clinically manifest. The minimum interval between these two phases ranges from 5 to 7 days, but in practice it is much longer and can take years. Once sensitized, the period between contact and an eczematous reaction is about 48 h.

A contact allergy implies involvement of the whole individual. This means that an eczematous reaction can develop on any part of the skin after contact with the allergen, that is, also at those parts which have never previously been in contact with the allergen. Once established, an allergy to a certain substance may persist for years, although clinical signs may be absent. Renewed exposure to an allergen, even after long periods without contact with it, may cause an acute eczematous reaction with fierce redness and vesicles. In situations where the allergy is not recognized and the worker continues contact with the allergen, the clinical picture of a chronic eczema is induced. This shows as dull red or grey, with thickening of the skin, while vesicles are absent. It may not be recognized as a possible allergic contact dermatitis.

Most commonly affected by allergic contact eczema are the hands, forearms and face. It is impossible to predict which worker may become sensitized. However, several factors influence the induction of contact allergy:

1. The nature of the allergen (sensitization potential). Largely depending on the chemical structure, some substances frequently cause contact sensitization; others are virtually non-allergenic. Therefore, allergic contact eczema is more common in some industries than others.
2. Age. Allergic contact dermatitis in individuals under 15 years of age is rare. In elderly individuals, allergic skin reactivity appears to decrease. Age is strongly associated with duration of exposure at the workplace; therefore, age as such is not important during the years of employment.
3. The condition of the surface of the skin. A damaged surface may increase the possibility of penetration. Contact sensitization to chromate and rubber chemicals, for instance, occurs more readily after the damaging effect of the very alkaline cement. Therefore, irritant contact dermatitis is a predisposing factor.
4. Concentration of the allergen. Contact with higher concentrations increases the chance of inducing sensitization. Even contact with very low concentrations may cause sensitiza-

tion under appropriate circumstances (e.g. chromate in cement).
5. The nature of the vehicle or solvent influences the biovailability of the allergen.
6. Surface-active agents. Their presence may result in enhanced contact with and penetration of the allergen. An example is the contact allergy to biocides in metalworking fluids, which is enhanced by the emulsifiers in these oils.
7. Frequency, duration and intensity of exposure. Occlusion increases penetration; therefore, a faulty glove is worse than no glove.

There are many individuals with a proven and relevant sensitization to ubiquitous allergens (e.g. nickel, chromate), who do not suffer from eczematous reactions. Apparently, the quality of their epidermis prevents sufficient penetration. These individuals may get skin problems when given 'wet' work. Generally speaking, a worker sensitized to a rare, industry-specific allergen (e.g. methacrylate) is at an advantage, since such an allergen is easier to avoid than the ubiquitous ones such as nickel or chromate.

Irritant (contact) dermatitis

Irritant contact dermatitis is also referred to as traumiterative dermatitis. The damage to the skin develops after the action of irritant or toxic substances (as opposed to allergenic substances in allergic contact eczema) and is dependent on the chemical characteristics and concentration of the substance, the properties of the epidermis, etc. Three types are distinguished, of which the third is the most relevant in the present context.

1. Acute type. There is one overwhelming exposure of short duration, followed by a sensation of stinging, burning or pain. The symptoms gradually decrease and may be accompanied by itching. The dermis and epidermis respond quickly to repair the damage. Healing starts early and follows a straightforward course. In severe cases, scarring may result. It is perhaps better to classify this 'chemical burn' under the heading of 'accidents'.
2. A type appearing after a few hours to days has also been described.
3. Subacute/chronic irritant dermatitis. Generally, none of the minor damaging factors is in itself strong enough to produce overt disease; accumulation is necessary. Thus, it is the summa-

tion of a number of subliminal damages during a period of time: a 'cumulative insult dermatitis'. It is the most common type of all occupational skin diseases.

Most workers are not exposed to strong irritants in daily life, but mild ones are omnipresent in the domestic and work environments. Mild irritant factors to which almost everyone is exposed are, for example, soaps, shampoos, detergents, polishes, solvents and vegetable juices. Even more difficult to recognize is the weak but definite irritant effect of ambient air, such as dry wind, central heating, blow-heaters in washrooms. The effects of these factors vary from person to person, from site to site and depend on age, pre-existing resistance and repair capacity. The mild exposures are not usually followed by clinically perceptible skin changes. In most cases without visible alterations, adaptation has taken place. This phenomenon, also called hardening, is probably based on a slight thickening of the epidermis which is sufficient to inhibit penetration of a damaging substance.

Repeated harmful exposures decrease the resistance of the skin. The repair capacity of the skin becomes exhausted, especially if re-exposure occurs too soon and at a time when repair from the previous exposure has not yet been completed. After a number of such exposures, the skin damage may become clinically evident. When the adaptation is insufficient, the first effects of the irritant substance are usually dryness and erythema, causing scaling and fissuring. This may be followed by a typical acute eczematous reaction. The process is shown in *Figure 16.2*.

Irritant dermatitis is often induced by the action of several substances that contaminate the skin at the workplace. Once established, skin damage can be maintained by a number of factors that would normally not be strong enough to produce visible skin changes. This explains the fact that chronic irritant dermatitis sometimes requires months to heal completely. Also when the dermatitis seems to be healed on clinical inspection, the function of the skin can still be impaired and relapses are common. Extensive information must be provided to the worker in order to avoid an excessively long recovery period or frequent relapses of the dermatitis.

The classic example of chronic irritant hand dermatitis is found in housewives and professions with similar types of exposure (e.g. cleaning personnel, caterers, etc.). Moisture and remnants of soap (often accumulating under rings) cumulatively damage the skin and lead to the development of a slowly spreading eczematous process on the skin of the hands. Also, insufficient rinsing causes accumulation of soap residues on the skin.

It is obvious that irritant contact dermatitis is usually located on the hands and arms, as these are the sites where exposure normally takes place. Clinically it is often indistinguishable from allergic contact ezcema. It should be emphasized that patch testing is only suitable to reproduce an allergic reaction in order to confirm or exclude the diagnosis of allergic contact eczema. Patch testing cannot detect certain irritants as the cause of a worker's dermatitis; a problem is the fact that there are no routinely available techniques to evaluate irritant dermatitis. (For a concise review, see the text on cutaneous irritation in [1].) In general, the pathophysiological process leading to irritant contact dermatitis is insufficiently understood.

Some common irritants are as follows:

● soaps and detergents
● metalworking fluids
● solvents
● fruit juices and vegetable juices
● machine oils.

There is interaction between allergic and irritant contact eczema. In some professions, allergic contact eczema prevails, whereas other occupations lead to relatively more chronic irritant dermatitis. Combinations are also common. Occupations with a relatively high incidence of irritant dermatitis are, for instance, barkeepers, dishwashers, cooks, dentists, nurses, hairdressers and hospital cleaning personnel. A secondary contact allergy can of course develop. Bricklayers, for example, can develop a chronic irritant dermatitis followed by an allergy to chromate and cobalt in cement and possibly complicated by an allergy to rubber chemicals in gloves.

Some key points with regard to irritant contact dermatitis are as follows:

● long induction period and slow healing
● prolonged skin vulnerability after healing
● cumulative effect of different agents
● eliciting agent is often 'the last drop'
● contact allergy may be secondary.

Exposure to small, sharp man-made or natural fibres may cause a clinical picture that resembles mild eczema. It is small-papular in appearance and vesicles are absent. It usually occurs on the dorsal sides of the hands and the forearms, but some-

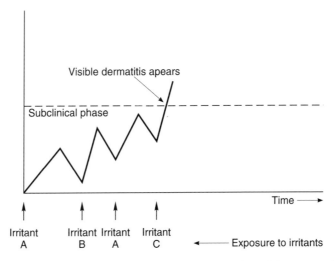

Figure 16.2 Process leading to irritant contact dermatitis – a free interpretation of the concept by Malten [4]. Cumulative insults to the skin, resulting in visible dermatitis after some time. The dermal repair mechanism fails to comply when the re-exposure to the same or another irritant occurs too soon.

times areas covered by loose clothing are involved. The cause is direct physical trauma from the sharp ends of the fibres. It is a matter of definition to distinguish this entity, also called glassfibre dermatitis, from irritant contact dermatitis.

Photoallergic and phototoxic eczema

The action of ultraviolet or visible light is essential for the induction of this type of eczema, thus it usually appears on parts of the body exposed to sunlight. The phototoxic reaction is based on a non-immunological phenomenon and can be elicited in almost everyone. After skin contact with a chemical substance (also vapours and aerosols), absorbed light transforms this chemical, whereupon the activated product causes a series of reactions in the tissue. Phototoxic agents may act topically, i.e. when applied to the skin, or systemically. Well documented are phototoxic reactions after exposure to tars (containing anthracene, benzopyrene, phenanthrene, etc.), for example in roofers. Other topical phototoxic agents are plants (umbelliferae containing furocoumarines and psoralene), drugs and dyes.

Like allergic contact eczema, photoallergy is immunologically mediated: it only appears in those who have been sensitized previously. The incriminated substance can only act as an allergen after exposure to light. Absorption of photons of specific energy by the sensitizer leads to the formation of an excited molecule, which can interact with other components in the skin to form an active allergen (hapten). As in allergic contact eczema, cross- and group sensitization may occur. The clinical picture of a photoallergic reaction may be indistinguishable from ordinary contact eczema, but it manifests itself only at skin areas exposed to light (e.g. face, V of neck, hands and forearms).

The most common photocontact allergens are halogenated phenols, phenothiazines and sulphonamines. Some substances act also as ordinary allergens, and some are both phototoxic and photoallergic. Caution must be exerted when assessing a worker who gives a history of skin reactions to (sun)light; there are various other photodermatoses and one of these, the polymorphic light eruption (PMLE), which is not occupation related, appears to be more common than phototoxic or photoallergic eczema.

Contact urticaria

Recurrent eczema of the hands may also result from repeated immediate (type I, IgE mediated) immunological reactions after exposure to certain substances. Therefore, this entity is dealt with here under contact dermatitis. Although urticaria is not really a type of eczema/dermatitis, it may lead to eczema. Well documented is 'protein contact dermatitis', found in workers handling food: within 30 min a variety of symptoms, ranging from itching and burning to eczematous vesicles, emerge after contact with chicken, seafood, vegetables and spices. It is also the cause of occupational contact eczema in veterinarians handling cows. One should keep in mind that 'ordinary' urticaria, for which often no cause is detected, is much more common.

The clinical picture of contact urticaria is represented by itching, burning and wheal formation at the site of the contact. Generalized urticaria and anaphylaxis may sometimes occur. It can be distinguished from allergic and irritant contact eczema by the fact that symptoms occur almost immediately after exposure. Contact urticaria may be immunological or non-immunological. Immunologically mediated contact urticaria has, besides the already mentioned food proteins, been documented as resulting from a wide range of agents. It is potentially more dangerous than non-immunological contact urticaria. Contact urticaria to latex proteins in surgical gloves is an increasing problem.

In several instances it is not known whether the reaction is immunologically mediated or non-immunological. The mechanism of non-immunological contact urticaria is a direct histamine-liberating action of a number of chemicals, for example, products from plants (nettles), jellyfish, thurfyl nicotinate and DMSO.

Patch testing

Patch testing is an elegant and relatively safe and simple procedure by which to detect a contact allergy. However, it is full of pitfalls. The advantage is that the test is performed directly on the body structure to be tested: a small amount of the suspected allergen is applied to the skin in order to reproduce a small area of contact dermatitis. The suspected allergen has to be properly diluted and is usually left on the skin for 48 h. The major textbooks give the appropriate dilutions for many known allergens [1–3].

The reading and interpretation of patch test results has to be done by an experienced person: false-positive reactions or irrelevant reactions occur easily and wrong advice based on a false positive reaction can have grave consequences.

Occupational physicians can master the technique of patch testing only if they do it often. In practice, most occupational physicians are not in a position to perform patch testing frequently enough to maintain their expertise and to maintain a stock of test materials. It is far more practical and cost-effective to seek cooperation from a dermatologist who has an interest in this topic. Normally, (standard) series are applied on the skin of the back. Typical series may vary locally. The European standard series, and its equivalents, such as the Japanese or the American standard series, has been agreed upon by international committees and is updated regularly. The standard series is remarkably efficient in detecting the relevant contact allergen in the majority of patients. It consists of about 20 common occupational and environmental allergens, which can be divided into a few major groups. *Table 16.2* gives the allergens used in the standard patch test series.

It should be emphasized that patch testing is only suitable for detecting a delayed-type contact allergy in a sensitized individual.

Occasionally a 20-minute patch test may help in detecting a (IgE mediated) contact urticaria. Irritant reactions cannot be evaluated by patch testing. Patch testing is also unsuitable to predict allergies in future.

Some key points concerning patch testing are as follows:

- reading patch test results requires experience
- false-positive or irrelevant reactions occur frequently

Table 16.2   Allergens in the standard patch test series

Metals	nickel
	chromate
	cobalt
Rubber additives	mercaptobenzathiazole and related compounds
	thiuram and related compounds
	paraphenylenediamine
Preservatives	quaternium 15
	cl-, m-isothiazolinone
	formaldehyde
	parahydroxybenzoates
Plastics, glues	epoxy resin
	p-tert-butylphenolformaldehyde resin
Botanical products	balsam of Peru
	colophony
	sesquiterpene lactones
Other	perfume mix
	medicaments, wool alcohols

- avoid testing mixtures
- do not test substances of unknown composition
- do not test a patient with active dermatitis
- do not perform 'predictive' testing
- always collaborate with a dermatologist
- do not use patch tests to study irritancy.

Work-related aspects of common skin diseases

The appearance of occupational eczema is not always characteristic, and several other disease entities may mimic contact eczema. Their similarity may even go as far as an apparent relationship with occupational exposure. These disease entities are not primarily caused by occupational (exposure) factors: rather their precipitation or course is in a number of instances work related to various degrees. The following paragraphs contain a brief review of the occupational aspects of the most common differential diagnostic entities of contact eczema. Most of these diseases can be found on the hands, arms and face, but some may be confined to other parts of the body (e.g. seborrhoeic eczema and stasis eczema). The most common and perhaps the most problematic disease within this context is atopic dermatitis.

Atopic dermatitis

This type of eczema belongs with hay fever, allergic asthma and CNSLD to the group of diseases in which atopic 'allergy' is involved. Depending on the criteria used, about 10–20% of the population may be assumed to have an atopic constitution. The majority (about 80%) of patients with atopic dermatitis have an IgE mediated allergy to inhalation allergens such as, for example, house dust mite, pollen and animal dander. It is not unusual to have this skin disease without such an allergy: 20% have normal IgE levels without detectable IgE reactivity. Direct skin contact with the above-mentioned allergens is normally not the cause of atopic skin lesions.

Atopic dermatitis in children manifests itself characteristically in the flexures of knees and elbows. In adults the hands, wrists, the side of the neck and the face are also frequently involved. Sometimes, only the hands are affected. This should always be kept in mind in a worker with a chronic eczematous process of the hands. The feet may be involved too, leading to an erroneous suspicion of contact allergy to shoe (often the rather occlusive safety shoes) materials.

Many patients say that they have a 'dry' skin. This is probably a reflection of changes in epidermal lipids and reduced hydration of the horny layer of the epidermis. A characteristic feature is severe itch provoked by woollen garments. Criteria to diagnose atopic dermatitis have been published and a scoring system to grade an atopic skin diathesis is described by Diepgen (for references, see his text in [5]).

A history of atopic dermatitis is relatively frequent among persons with irritant dermatitis and should be regarded as a risk factor. In many professions that affect the skin of the hands in the same way, such as nurses, hairdressers and cleaning personnel, atopic dermatitis promotes the development of irritant dermatitis. Conversely, one could also argue that atopic dermatitis is aggravated or provoked by exposure to irritants. Several epidemiological studies demonstrated clearly that a history of atopic dermatitis is a major risk factor for occupational hand eczema (see also the section on hand eczema, above). A history of atopic dermatitis should play a role in job counselling.

Examples of occupations where persons with a history of atopic dermatitis may get problems are as follows:

- hairdressing
- metalworking
- tiling and bricklaying
- baking
- nursing
- catering.

There seems to be no increased risk of developing a delayed type contact allergy in persons with atopic dermatitis. The study of the International Contact Dermatitis Research Group demonstrated no evidence of increased risk of developing an allergic contact eczema in patients with atopic dermatitis as compared with patients with other types of eczema such as seborrhoeic or nummular eczema.

Some key points concerning atopic dermatitis are as follows:

- may be confined to hand and feet only
- should always be considered when eczema is chronic
- is a major risk factor for irritant contact dermatitis
- prick tests with inhalation allergens may be negative

● false-positive patch tests occur frequently.

There are occupational exposures to inhalation allergens that may cause a manifestation of atopic symptoms, including atopic dermatitis. This was observed in occupations with, for example, exposure to animal dander among laboratory animal handlers, workers in fur preparation, etc. Another typical example is baker's eczema: in addition to the exposure to irritants, allergy to amylase in dough and possibly other wheat proteins plays a role. In general, an atopic person is at risk when he becomes a baker.

Contact urticaria is also more commonly seen among atopics: see the earlier mentioned immediate-type (IgE mediated) reactions to latex proteins in surgical gloves and to food proteins in the fish processing and catering industry.

Dyshidrotic eczema

This type of hand eczema is also referred to as acrovesicular eczema, pompholyx or cheiropompholyx, and is a controversial entity. It is a descriptive term for an eruption of tiny to pea-sized vesicles in the palms of the hands and along the fingers. The process is almost always symmetrical. In many cases this dermatosis is not accompanied by redness, except in those cases where the vesicles are eroded and the skin is macerated. The eruptions may show spontaneous remissions and flare-ups, the sun or heat possibly having a provocative effect. A seasonal rhythm may sometimes be detected. The eruptions can be regarded as a cutaneous reaction to a number of possible aetiological factors, in which the thick horny layer prevents exudation, resulting in deep-seated vesicles.

Several theories concerning the origin of dyshidrotic eczema have been proposed, but none is satisfactory. Assumed causal factors are as follows (it is obvious that these factors can be occupational):

● allergic reactions to fungi and bacteria
● allergic contact eczema
● an allergic contact eczema elsewhere on the body (e.g. feet) may be accompanied by a dyshidrotic eruption of the hands
● delayed type hypersensitivity to an orally or parenterally administered or inhaled substance
● particular form of atopic dermatitis
● physical fatigue and nervous stress.

The aetiological agent is often difficult to assess, as none of these factors offers an entirely satisfactory explanation. In nickel-sensitive individuals this eczema can be provoked by a high oral dose of nickel. There is a tendency to classify all cases of recurring vesicular eczematous eruptions localized on the sides of the fingers, a rather common phenomenon, as dyshidrotic eczema. Apparently, the sides of the fingers are 'crossroads' for different types of eczema. 'True' cases of dyshidrotic eczema, however, are rare. Perhaps it is better to avoid the term and to name the eruption after the incriminated causal factor (e.g. allergic contact eczema, atopic eczema, etc.). It still remains to be seen whether dyshidrotic eczema is a clinical entity. For further details see the text by Menne [5] and by Schwanitz in [5].

Nummular eczema

The name is derived from the latin word for a coin. This type of eczema often starts on the anterior sides of the hands, forearms and legs, but may appear on all sites of the body surface. Characteristic are the round, coin-sized lesions which are red, scaly and often with vesicles. Itching is usually present. The lesions may spread centrifugally and reach a diameter of more than 10 cm; large confluent plaques can develop. The aetiology is still unclear; a number of theories has been suggested and it is questionable whether this disease can be regarded as an aetiological entity. Nummular eczema is often quite resistant to treatment.

From an occupational point of view it is important to keep in mind that an allergic contact eczema may mimic a nummular eczema both clinically and histologically. This has been observed particularly in cement eczema (chromate allergy) and allergic contact eczema due to epoxy resins.

Psoriasis

This common skin disease occurs in about 1–2% of the population. Psoriasis localized on the palms of the hands can be difficult to diagnose and can easily be confused with chronic eczema. Diagnosis may be easier when the process is localized to the dorsal surfaces of the hands, although confusion with other dermatoses may readily occur. The diagnosis is often suspected or established when the characteristic lesions of psoriasis are present at the typical sites such as the elbows, knees, scalp and lower back. Inspection of the nails for pitting and subunqual hyperkeratosis is also helpful. Psoriasis of the nails is often confused with a mycotic infection.

Occupational factors are not the cause of psoriasis, but they are capable of aggravating or precipitating this disease. These factors include almost every chemical or mechanical insult to the skin. The intensity of these insults may be well below the level that would cause skin changes in normal subjects. The emergence of psoriasis at the site of minor traumata (e.g. scratch wounds or cuts) is known as the Koebner phenomenon.

Factors known to provoke psoriasis are as follows:

- acids and alkalines (e.g. in cement)
- mechanical friction (e.g. by a hammer, screwdriver)
- wounds
- medicines (e.g. beta-blockers, lithium)
- upper airway infections.

Opinions differ as to whether pustulosis palmoplantaris is a single entity or should be regarded as a form of pustular psoriasis. The pustules are sterile and should not be confused with those that may occur in secondary infected eczema and mycosis. The disease is relatively rare.

Mycosis

A mycotic infection of the palms of the hands can be difficult to distinguish from chronic eczema. When such an eczematous process is not symmetrical but localized on one hand only, a mycosis should always be suspected. When the diagnosis is overlooked and treatment with local corticosteroid has been applied, the clinical picture becomes impossible to recognize. This is has been described as 'tinea incognita'; the local inflammatory reaction responsible for the clinical manifestations is suppressed by the steroids. Candidiasis, which is actually a yeast infection, has a predilection for the interdigital webs and the nailfolds.

Damp and warm conditions may enhance a mycotic infection and complicate healing. Such conditions can be encountered in 'wet' work (e.g. catering, cleaning services, food industry). Also the wearing of rubber or plastic gloves or boots creates such circumstances.

Seborrhoeic eczema

This eczema is located at the face and trunk. It is characterized by redness and scaling; in adults, vesicles are virtually never present. Often the scales have a 'fatty' appearance.

Characteristic is its confinement to certain skin areas; nasolabial folds, scalp and preauricular areas, eyelashes, the area between the eyebrows and the presternal area. Usually a diagnosis is easy to make. However, the eczema may spread to anywhere in the body. Its name reflects the association with areas densely packed with sebaceous glands. The cause is unknown. The disease may flare up under aspecific stimuli such as change in weather (in temperate climates exacerbations are often seen in autumn and spring), or physical and emotional stress.

Because of this sometimes erratic course an occupational contact factor may be suggested, especially when there is predominant involvement of the face. Sometimes a contact allergic reaction to epoxy resins is a dermatitis on the face that resembles seborrhoeic eczema.

Stasis dermatitis

This type of eczema is located at the lower part of the leg, often at the medial side of the ankle. It is a result of venous insufficiency due to incompetence of the valves. Often, varicose veins are also present at the affected lower leg, and ankle oedema as well as a characteristic pigmentation may be an accompanying sign. The condition is constitutional or acquired (e.g. after deep vein thrombosis). Stasis eczema may spread secondarily beyond the ankle or lower leg. Contact eczema caused by boots or socks may erroneously be suspected. Persons whose occupation involves a lot of standing are at risk of early manifestation or aggravation of this condition. Prevention is often easy to achieve by fitting compressive elastic stockings.

Occupational acne and folliculitis

Chloracne

Chloracne may be defined as an acneiform eruption caused by exposure to certain halogenated aromatic hydrocarbons. Since bromine compounds cause acne more readily than chlorinated compounds, the term 'halogen acne' is preferred. Compounds that can cause halogen acne in humans are polychlorbifenyl (PCB), polychlordibenzofuranes (PCDF) and polychlordibenzodioxins (dioxins).

It should be emphasized that halogen acne is a symptom of systemic intoxication (percutaneous, orally or by inhalation). Halogen acne is the most sensitive indicator for this intoxication, since blood or tissue contamination levels are often too low to affect other organs in the acute stage. The primary lesion of halogen acne is the blackhead; in mild cases this can be the only symptom. The characteristic clinical picture of acne consists of multiple small cysts, and when larger areas are affected it resembles 'ordinary' acne cystica, although with fewer inflammatory reactions. The distribution of halogen acne lesions has a predilection for areas below and lateral to the eyes and behind the ears and the scrotum.

Reasons to suspect halogen acne are as follows:

● unusual localization of acneiform lesions
● predominance of cysts with little inflammation
● no history of acne vulgaris in puberty
● more persons in the working environment affected.

Oil/tar acne

Oil acne is caused by direct contamination by mineral oils and its derivatives, grease or liquid petroleum, but also by soot and tar. This form of acne appears at exposed skin areas, including those areas that are covered by greasy, unclean working clothes. Characteristic for this acne is the fact that it appears at sites that are not sites for acne vulgaris. Oil acne usually disappears after improvement of hygienic conditions at the workplace.

The following are reasons to suspect oil or tar acne:

● monomorphous clinical picture, many comedones
● occupational exposure to greasy or tar-like product
● exposed body areas affected
● localization unusual for acne vulgaris
● more persons in the working environment affected.

Folliculitis

Physical or chemical injury to the skin may produce an inflammation of the hair follicles. Although this folliculitis is not primarily of infective origin, pustules containing staphylococci may be present. The process can be caused by blocking of the follicle openings or by chemical irritation of the follicle. It is encountered in occupations with exposure to mineral oils and soluble oils in the metal industry. Apart from the absence of blackheads, the distinction between this condition and oil acne is not clear.

Pigment changes

Depigmentation

Depigmentation or leucoderma indicates loss of skin pigment that was present before. A variety of clinical pictures can represent this phenomenon: localized or generalized, sharply or vaguely demarcated. The generalized forms belong mostly to congenital syndromes. The majority of the localized forms can be classified under vitiligo, which is defined as a disease of unknown cause with hereditary elements, characterized by white (pigment-free) patches. The disease occurs in about 1% of the general population, with an equal sex distribution. Favoured sites are hands, elbows, knees and anogenital region. Several theories about its pathogenesis have been developed; in general terms it is ascribed to an autoimmune process directed against melanocytes.

Several physical and chemical agents can cause depigmentations that may be almost identical to vitiligo. To distinguish from vitiligo, it can be helpful to check the anogenital region. The depigmentations by external agents may also appear at non-exposed sites. In particular, a small patchy type has to be suspected of being chemically induced depigmentation. The mechanism is a direct interaction with melanin production in the pigment cells.

The depigmenting agent monobenzyl ether of hydroquinone (in some countries sold illegally) is notorious for causing irreversible depigmentation.

Chemicals causing depigmentation are as follows:

● hydroquinone and its monobenzyl ether
● phenol and phenol derivatives

● arsenic and mercury compounds
● other: mercaptoethylamines, sulphhydryl compounds and isopropylcatechol.

Physical agents that produce depigmentation are ionizing and ultraviolet (UV) radiation, and thermal and physical trauma.

Hyperpigmentation

Hyperpigmentation, which is an accumulation of normal skin pigment, can be induced by several chemicals and drugs:

● mineral oils
● halogenated hydrocarbons
● photodynamic action of psoralenes and tar products
● arsenic (may also cause depigmentation)
● medicines.

Subcutaneous deposits of substances may also cause colouring of the skin, i.e. without melanocyte-mediated pigment. Examples of such substances are carbon, mercury, silver compounds and iron compounds.

Occupational skin cancer

Although epidemiological data are lacking, it can be assumed that occupational factors play a role in a sizeable proportion of all skin cancers, which is the most common form of cancer in the USA. Three main types can be distinguished: basal cell epithelioma, squamous cell carcinoma and melanoma. Only melanoma contributes to mortality.

Factors causing occupational skin cancer are as follows:

● ultraviolet light: this can be artificial UV or UV exposure in outdoor work; light-skinned persons especially are at risk
● phototoxic chemicals may play an additional role
● ionizing radiation
● arsenic: by ingestion/inhalation, not by skin contact
● polycyclic aromatic hydrocarbons.

The most common offenders are tar and tar products, and also contaminants of oil distillation products. A well-known example from the past are

roofers, who were exposed to coal tar vapours in combination with sunlight.

Prevention

The general approach is not essentially different from any other occupational disease prevention programme: first should come a close look at the work process, while personal protection is offered as a last resort. Unfortunately, many doctors start with the last option by prescribing gloves.

Measures at the source

This approach to the problem should have the highest priority. For the prevention of skin problems, the following points should be considered:

Changing the production process or work methods:
● if possible, 'wet' work should be 'dry'
● reduce frequency of hand washing
● no skin contact with biocides
● avoid the prolonged wearing of gloves
● change standing work to walking/sitting.

Replacing problematic chemicals by substances with lower skin risk:
● replace low molecular epoxy resin by high molecular epoxy resin
● replace amines in two-component resins by amides
● use glassfibres with a diameter that is non-irritant
● replace GMTG in permanent wave hairdressing solutions
● replace impure 'natural' substances (e.g. balsam of Peru, colophony) by synthetic compounds
● change to plastic if there is prolonged skin contact with rubber.

Elimination of non-essential additives or impurities:
● ferrosulphate eliminates hexavalent chromate in cement (mandatory in Scandinavia)
● eliminate perfume and dyes from metalworking fluids
● metal objects that are in prolonged contact with the skin should not leak nickel
● eliminate abrasives from hand cleansers.

Ventilation and exhaust

This measure is important, but its role in preventing skin disorders is rather limited. Local exhaust can be effective in situations where airborne contact dermatitis may arise.

The following are situations where local exhaust may be effective:

- mixing and application of epoxy resins
- working with tropical woods
- welding and soldering
- working with glassfibre.

Separation of man and source

In a number of situations this can be a very complex organizational procedure. Enclosing the production process may require a major engineering effort. In the chemical industry this has had a major impact, although the problem may shift to the maintenance and repair crews, who are often contractors from outside.

In a metal factory, enclosing was only moderately successful, because objects that were wet from metalworking fluids had to be removed by hand.

Reduction of frequency and duration of exposure is particularly important in preventing irritant contact dermatitis. In hairdressers shops the problem usually occurs among junior personnel who do most of the shampooing and permanent waving. In the health care sector, a closer look at the infection prevention protocols may reduce the frequency and the amounts of soaps and disinfectants used to clean the hands: often just water or the less irritant isopropylalcohol may be sufficient.

Gloves

Personal protection devices, which in practice usually means gloves, should have the lowest priority. The ideal glove does not exist. In terms of impermeability to chemicals there are many types of glove on the market. The problem is often the occlusive effect on the skin. Also, the glove material itself can give rise to skin problems: a well-known example is the emergence of latex allergy in the health care sector. (For a full discussion on gloves see [6].)

The following are general points regarding gloves:

- prolonged wearing of gloves is almost certain to cause skin problems
- a leaking glove is worse than no glove at all
- wear cotton gloves as inner gloves
- avoid rubber on the skin, use PVC whenever possible
- elastyrene (styrene–butadiene) is a good alternative for rubber in surgical gloves when there is a contact allergy to glove materials
- most thin gloves do not protect against epoxy resin and methacrylate
- too often the way gloves are put on or taken off is wrong, and leads to contamination of the skin
- occlusive gloves are useless when the hand eczema has an atopy component
- latex gloves are permeable for nickel.

Barrier creams

The application of a barrier cream as an 'invisible glove' has a theoretical logic. Managers often claim a beneficial effect after the introduction of such a product, but often do not realize that this is also accompanied by a series of other measures and changes of attitudes (e.g. skin awareness) that may have caused the desired effect. Unfortunately, the effect of barrier creams alone has never been documented by the publication of a proper intervention study.

There are various types of barrier creams on the market, often for specific purposes, such as for exposure to metalworking fluids (which are often oil-in-water emulsions), or exposure to solvents or mineral oils. Some barrier creams contain chemicals that specifically bind or chelate allergens (e.g. ascorbic acid or EDTA to bind chromate). Prevention of allergic contact dermatitis by these creams has not been convincingly demonstrated. The amount of allergen that is capable of eliciting a reaction in a sensitized person is so small that it is unlikely that any specific barrier cream can trap enough molecules of the allergen to prevent an inflammatory response.

Barrier creams that are highly effective are the sun creams.

After-work emollients

The idea to apply a bland emollient (ointment or fatty cream) after hand cleansing at the end of the work shift, or in between, stems from dermatological practice: slightly irritated skin tends towards dryness and chapping, and this effect can be counteracted by the application of emollients. The beneficial effects of such measures may also be due to a greater awareness of skin care and protection in general. It is possible that the claimed beneficial effects of barrier creams are largely due to this emollient effect: a bland emollient may therefore be as effective as a specific barrier cream.

Risk inventories

Whether stipulated by law or not, factories or enterprises may require *some* kind of assessment of occupational hazards. Approaches may vary according to law or custom. A practical approach, structured as a checklist, aimed at the hazards for the skin is outlined below. It is designed as a step-wise or cascade approach, from general to specific. Only if any item scores positive does one proceed to the next step.

For example, it is obvious that the procedure can be closed after Step 1 in an administrative department where documents are processed. In a department where these documents are printed by offset machines, and where inks, solvents, etc., are used, the procedure may go to more specific steps.

Step 1

1.1 Is there wet work:
- any liquid substances in use other than regular handwashing? ☐
- special hand cleansers in use? ☐
- occlusive gloves in use? ☐

1.2 Are there any hazardous chemicals in use? ☐

1.3 Is there visible soiling of the skin? ☐

1.4 Are there physical agents:
- radiation/UV? ☐
- heat/cold? ☐
- dust? ☐
- fibres, particles? ☐

In Step 2 the criteria for 'wet work' may be somewhat arbitrary: exact epidemiological data to support these criteria are lacking. It is mainly derived from a preliminary version on 'wet work' of the German Technical Guidelines for Hazardous Substances. In general, the risk-

intervention procedure is based on the notion that skin contact with liquids is the most common cause of problems. Item 2.2 may require some elementary dermatological knowledge.

Step 2

2.1 Wet work:
- skin contact with water/liquids > 2 h daily? ☐
- handwashing > 20 times daily? ☐
- handwashing with aggressive detergents? ☐
- impermeable gloves > 2 h daily? ☐

2.2 Is there skin contact with hazardous substances:
- allergens? ☐
- irritants? ☐
- solvent vapours? ☐
- physical agents? ☐

2.3 Is there contamination of tools and working clothes? ☐

2.4 Is there microtrauma caused by
- abrasion? ☐
- metal chips? ☐
- fibres? ☐

Steps 3 and 4 are more difficult to formalize: here the assessor should equip him/herself with an elementary knowledge of occupational dermatology and occupational hygiene. In very specific instances, a dermatologist with an interest in the topic may have to be consulted.

Step 3

Specify frequency and intensity of above-mentioned items

Step 4

Obtain specific information, formulations, etc.

The exit step is most useful to gain some insight into the size of the problem, especially in large factories. It will also force the enterprise to have a close look at its sickness monitoring and registration programme. According to specific findings, the above-mentioned procedure may have to be modified.

```
                 Exit step
           Review suspected cases
           over the past 12 months
```

References

1. Rycroft, R.J.G., Menné, T. and Frosch, P.J. (eds) *Textbook of Contact Dermatitis*, 2nd edn. Springer Verlag, Berlin (1995)
2. Rietschel, R.L. and Fowler, J.F. *Fisher's Contact Dermatitis*, 4th edn. Williams and Wilkins, Baltimore, Maryland (1995)
3. Adams, R. *Occupational Skin Disease*, 2nd edn. Grune and Stratton, New York (1990)
4. Malten, K.E. Thoughts on irritant contact dermatitis. *Contact Dermatitis*, **7**, 238–247 (1981)
5. Menné, T. and Maibach, H.I. (eds) *Hand Eczema*. CRC Press, Boca Raton, Florida (1994)
6. Mellström, G.A., Wahlberg, J.E. and Maibach, H.I. *Protective Gloves for Occupational Use*. CRC Press, Boca Raton, Florida (1994)

Chapter 17

Musculoskeletal disorders

E-P Takala

Introduction

Pain in the lower back, neck, shoulders or upper limbs is an increasing cause of absence from work in most industrialized countries. During a two-year period in a large forest industry company in Finland, musculoskeletal diseases formed the largest disease group leading to sick leave, comprising 34% of all lost days. By comparison, about 10% of all lost days were due to acute respiratory infections.

Although all occupational health practitioners encounter patients with musculoskeletal disorders, only a small number of the disorders are occupational diseases. According to the WHO, the definition of the concept 'occupational disease' includes diseases in which work is the main causal factor. The agreements of national compensation systems finally define what is termed an 'occupational disease' in each country. In most cases of musculoskeletal disorder seen in occupational health care practice, the cause of the disease is multifactorial, work being only one of the several factors in the causal network. Therefore, according to the WHO definition, such diseases are more properly called 'work-related diseases'.

It has been estimated that a biomedical explanation can be found for less than 20% of the patients with low back pain, even with the most sophisticated diagnostic tools. For other body areas the medical diagnosis remains more or less uncertain for most patients with musculoskeletal disorders, too. However, modelling the pathological process of a disease can help us in the prevention and treatment, even when the diagnosis is uncertain (*Figure 17.1*).

Musculoskeletal disorders can be conceptualized as individual responses to external loads. The most important external loading factors are biomechanical forces affecting the body at work and during leisure time. Gravity is the most common force and affects us even in static postures. Other forces are those needed for the performance of work tasks. Depending on individual factors such as age, gender, constitution of the connective tissue, anatomical structure and anthropometrics or general health, the external loads will create different mechanical doses on the tissues. In the worst case the dose will be harmful, resulting in microscopic or visible injuries. The responses to the mechanical dose can be directly mechanical or metabolic. The human body has, however, the capacity to adapt to the different loads by recovering from the state of fatigue, by regeneration of the injured tissues, or by strengthening the structures. The long-term effects of loading with insufficient adaptation are harmful, and will be manifested as musculoskeletal disorders. On the other hand, the benefits of loading will be seen as increased resistance to the loads after systematic training or rehabilitation.

These twofold effects are dependent on the dose imposed on the body. If the loading is too high with respect to the capacity, the result will be a disorder or disease. Adaptation to too low loads means a reduction in capacity; a well-known example is osteoporosis after long-term immobilization. Even 'normal' loads in work life may be too high for the body with reduced capacity,

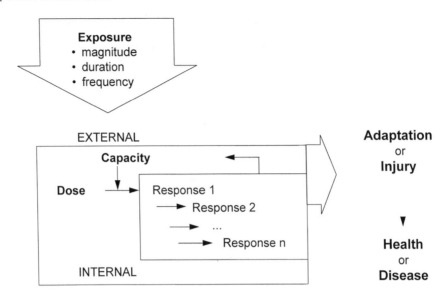

Figure 17.1 A conceptual model for work-related musculoskeletal disorders (after Armstrong *et al.* [1])

resulting in injuries and disorders. The quantity of the external load as well as the internal dose has two dimensions: its magnitude, which can be expressed in mechanical terms as newtons or newton-metres and time, which has two important aspects: duration and frequency.

This model can be applied in the prevention and treatment of workers with musculoskeletal disorders. The basic principles of prevention and treatment are twofold: (a) reduce harmful factors (risk factors), and (b) enhance individual resistance against these harmful factors. Successful practice is based on a thorough analysis of both of these aspects, i.e. analysis of work and of individual health status.

Assessment of workers with musculoskeletal disorders

The assessment of health status has different roles depending on our purpose. In occupational health care practice, several goals can be identified:

1. *Verification and classification of musculoskeletal diseases.* This is the traditional approach in clinical practice, aiming at the correct diagnosis and treatment.

2. *Description of the course of a disease or follow-up of treatment.* For this goal, assessment methods giving numerical measurements are most suitable.

3. *Assessment of the ability to work* means matching the individual functional capacity to the demands of the work. A medical diagnosis tells very little about the worker's ability to do his/her job. The ability to work is a continuum from total disability to perfect health, although the social security and compensation systems in many countries handle it as though it were an on–off phenomenon. Assessment methods describing function are essential for this purpose.

4. *Screening of diseases* is sensible in the case of diseases in which an early diagnosis leads to an improved clinical outcome in terms of survival, function or quality of life. The natural course of most work-related musculoskeletal disorders is undulant and dependent on the work. A cost-effective screening method should be valid and simple to use.

5. *Health promotion.* It has been claimed that demonstration of the reduced functional capacity of the musculoskeletal system of people will motivate them to positive health behaviour, i.e. actively to improve their health. This statement may be true for some workers, but the effects have generally not been shown.

Alternative promoting manoeuvres should be considered before starting a health programme in a company.

6. *Epidemiological purposes*, i.e. estimating the magnitude of musculoskeletal problems in a working population.

The general rules presented in *Table 17.1* may help the practitioner in his/her selection of the most suitable assessment strategy and tools. The text expounds on these guidelines.

Keep the goals in mind

The assessment methods should be selected with the goals in mind. A battery of tests suitable for one purpose will usually not be cost-effective for other purposes.

Do no harm

The benefits and harm of the assessment methods should be weighed. 'Do no harm' is the old rule of medical practice that we have to keep in mind with regard to treatment as well as to diagnostic procedures. Invasive methods should be reserved for special clinics. Iatrogenic diseases are common. Therefore, avoid medicalization of phenomena that are normal physiological responses, such as pain after prolonged static postures.

Use systematic approaches

The results of measurements or assessment have several potential biases. Examinations of the same patient by different examiners or at different times may give different results. The disagreement of results may have its aetiology in the examiners, the examined subject or in the performance of the examination. A systematic approach will

Table 17.1. General rules for selection of strategy and tools for assessment of workers with musculoskeletal disorders

1. Keep the goals in mind
2. Do no harm
3. Use systematic approaches
4. Remember danger signals ('red flags')
5. Remember economy when selecting tests – ask 'So what?'
6. Remember the demands and resources of society
7. Try to find out harmful and health-promoting factors

usually reduce this kind of disagreement and lessen the bias. Checklists of items to be asked about the medical history and standardized clinical assessment will help in the diagnosing as well as in the follow-up of the patient. The selection of items for the standard protocols should be based on research to guarantee the validity of the assessment.

Unfortunately, the repeatability and validity of many generally used clinical manoeuvres in respect of the above-mentioned goals has been studied insufficiently. In the selection of items that have not been tested in a scientific manner, the practitioner can well use his/her common sense. If he/she has a good rationale to use some tests, they can be added to the test battery and systematically tested in practice. If the test seems to be useful in practice, it can be used until the rationale for using it or the validity of the test has been disproved by scientific research.

The clinical history usually gives the most important information on the patient's status. The use of checklists or standard questions guarantees that the essential questions will be asked. Standard questionnaires, visual analogue scales or pain drawings can be used to compile numerical data for the follow-up of health status.

Symptoms may appear only during specific work tasks or movements. Therefore, manoeuvres simulating these tasks or movements may provoke the symptoms and give hints of these conditions (e.g. straight leg raising in sciatica or isometric muscle tests for tendinitis). However, a short physical examination test does not always provoke the symptoms in the early phase of a musculoskeletal disease, especially if the symptoms appear after several hours of work. Functional tests may give additional information on the pathology.

Functional tests may either test a complicated motor performance (e.g. work simulation) or single parts of this performance (muscle force and endurance, joint mobility and stability, muscle coordination). Most functional tests give a numerical output and can therefore be applied to several goals. Unfortunately we know little about the validity of most functional tests. Wide normal variation hinders interpretation of the results.

Remember danger signals ('red flags')

The nature of musculoskeletal diseases is usually more harmful than dangerous. There are, however, some conditions in which direct actions are needed. In the Clinical Practice Guideline of Acute Low Back Problems in Adults [2], these conditions have been called 'red flags'. These three red flags – fracture or dislocation, tumour or infection, and severe neural compression – can be applied to the other anatomical regions as well. Rheumatoid arthritis is the fourth condition that should be remembered with neck and upper limb pain, because it can cause rupture of the transverse ligament of the first cervical vertebra, leading to risk of compression of the spinal cord or rupture of tendons in the upper limbs.

Medical history will give essential clues for these conditions. Intensive permanent pain not relieved by rest should raise suspicion of these red flags. A major accident or even minor accidents in patients with a history of weakened structures (osteoporosis, rheumatoid arthritis, treatments with corticosteroids) should be further examined as if there were a fracture or dislocation. The red flags for cancer or infection are: history of cancer, unexplained weight loss, immunosuppression, urinary infection, intravenous drug use, prolonged use of corticosteroids, pain not improved with rest, and age of the patient over 50 years. Neural compression gives symptoms and signs of cauda equina syndrome (acute urinary retention or overflow incontinence, loss of anal sphincter tone or faecal incontinence, saddle anaesthesia) or global or progressive motor weakness in the extremities.

Remember economy, and the demands and resources of society

Economy in the selection of tests means that we should select only useful tests and avoid useless ones. The demands and resources of the society affect this economical approach. For example, expensive sophisticated imaging may be used only if we have such resources, and if the results of these assessments will influence further action. Therefore, most such techniques will be useful only in special clinics. On the other hand, legal aspects, such as compensation systems or even fear of litigation, can lead us to use methods that may be useless from the medical point of view.

The simple question 'So what?' will help in many decisions in selecting clinical assessment methods. If the practitioner cannot answer this question, the proposed method is useless.

Try to find out harmful and health-promoting factors

There are two basic rules for action in medical practice: reduce harmful factors or risk factors, and optimize or reinforce health-promoting factors. Looking for these two items will target the treatment and prevention of musculoskeletal problems. These questions may lead to a thorough assessment of work and leisure time.

Table 17.2 gives some examples of possible combinations of tests to assess the functional status of the musculoskeletal system with different goals.

Work assessment

The basic function of the musculoskeletal system is movement. The 'work' of our ancestors was

Table 17.2.   Examples of possible combinations of tests to assess functional status of the musculoskeletal system for different goals

1. *Verification and classification of musculoskeletal diseases*
   - description of disability due to symptoms
   - clinical examination relevant to anatomical area of symptoms
   - tests of mobility and muscular function guided by anatomical area and disability

2. *Description of course of disease or follow-up of treatment*
   - assessment of disability (e.g. standard questions or visual analogue scales)
   - measurement of mobility if restrictions have been detected
   - tests of muscle force and endurance if goal is to improve these functions

3. *Assessment of ability to work*
   - description of disability due to symptoms in different work tasks; what the worker can and cannot do
   - thorough assessment of the work
   - functional tests that simulate movements and postures essential for performing the work

4. *Screening for diseases*
   - questionnaire survey of musculoskeletal disorders
   - further investigation of workers with positive answers in survey; see points 1 and 3

5. *Health promotion*
   - questionnaire survey of health behaviour (smoking, diet, alcohol consumption, physical activity)
   - simple functional exercising tests in groups of workers (i.e. number of repetitions of standard movements in standard time, walking distance in standard time, etc.)

almost continuous movement in search of nourishment. Sometimes short periods of heavy physical exertion were necessary in fighting or fleeing. These heavy exertions were followed by long periods of rest. Work has constrained the human body into static postures or repeated physical exertions during some tens of generations. There has not, however, been any biological evolutionary adaptation to the demands of modern work. Our body is structurally and functionally similar to that of our ancestors.

The assessment of work is an essential part in the prevention and treatment of musculoskeletal disorders in occupational health practice. The aim of the assessment is to identify risk factors and describe the extent of each risk factor in terms of magnitude, duration and frequency. *Table 17.3* describes the common work-related risk factors of musculoskeletal disorders in different anatomical areas.

Information on the relevant risk factors can be obtained from the workers, foremen and employers, or it can be collected with different methods by the occupational safety or health personnel. A general view of the existence of the risk factors is easy to get by asking workers about them. Positive answers should be examined further, to estimate the extent of each risk factor. Important questions are 'when?' and 'where?' for exact location of the risk factors in time and place of the work process. After this orientation the extent of the risks can be estimated by different informal or formal measuring methods of the work. Verbal descriptions by the worker or foreman may sometimes be sufficient. Visual observation gives additional understanding of the problems. Video-recording of the problematic work tasks provides good documentation and serves as a reference for ergonomic change. Formal measurements by observational or other methods are needed only if it is necessary to express the exact extent of the problem, or if the aim is to measure exactly the effects of ergonomic change.

Understanding of the work is essential in order to be able to make suggestions for ergonomic improvements. The spectrum of work tasks is wide, and it is impossible for one person to have a deep understanding of them all. Information obtained by a systematic walk-through visit of the different workplaces should be the minimum requirement for the occupational health practitioners treating workers with musculoskeletal problems. Examples of different means to assess work systematically will be found in [3].

Each workplace has its own culture and language. Health care professionals will therefore have difficulties in understanding the technical terms of the other workplaces. Conversely, workers seldom understand medical jargon. A good occupational health care team will have someone with basic knowledge of work assessment methods and ergonomics as well as with understanding of the technical language, in order to be able to communicate with the workers and engineers.

Table 17.3. Work-related risk factors of musculoskeletal disorders

Low back	Heavy physical work
	Manual material handling: lifting, carrying, pulling and pushing
	Twisting, bending and other non-neutral trunk postures
	Motor vehicle driving, whole body vibration
	Prolonged sitting
	Monotonous work, job dissatisfaction
Neck and shoulder	High mechanical forces (sudden acceleration–deceleration of the body; heavy helmets or other protective headgear)
	Non-neutral postures of the head
	Working with arms elevated
	Repetitive shoulder flexion or abduction
	Prolonged static working postures
	Heavy physical work, manual material handling
	Monotonous work, job dissatisfaction, haste
Elbow, forearm, wrist and hand	Repetitive movements of the hands
	Gripping with high forces
	Non-neutral postures of the wrist
Knees	Kneeling postures
All body areas	Prolonged monotonous work in constrained postures
	Sharp edges of surfaces or tools compressing the body parts
	Accidents

Prevention and treatment

As mentioned earlier, the basic principles of prevention and treatment are twofold: (a) reduce harmful factors, and (b) enhance factors that improve resistance against harmful factors, or in the case of treatment, enhance factors that improve recovery. *Table 17.4* lists methods for the prevention and treatment of musculoskeletal

Table 17.4. Methods for the prevention and treatment of musculoskeletal disorders

- Ergonomics:
  Optimization of working methods, environment, and/or tools
  Optimization of organization of work – quantity and contents of work; work/rest schedules
- Prevention of accidents
- Maintenance of general health and especially functioning of musculoskeletal system
- Improvement of health care and rehabilitation practices; adequate medical treatment
- Supporting workers with musculoskeletal problems
- Education of employers, workers and society about the topics related to musculoskeletal disorders

disorders, while the text deals with each one in detail.

Ergonomics

According to Grandjean, 'the primary aim of ergonomics is to optimize the functioning of a system by adapting it to human capacities and needs'. Ergonomic principles can be applied to the relationships between the worker and work as well as between the human being and leisure activities. A good ergonomic solution will not only reduce the harmful risk factors but change the external load so that the responses of the body will be beneficial; a good solution will improve the reduced functional capacity or maintain the good functional capacity of the body. In addition to these human aspects, a good ergonomic solution will increase productivity and also benefit the employer.

Traditional ergonomics emphasized the local environment, the workstation, tools and working methods. The modern approach regards the local or individual situation as a part of the whole production system. Changing one part of the system will result in changes in some other parts, and these uncontrolled changes will not necessarily be improvements. For example, changing the process in one part of the production line may reduce the harmful load of the workers in this workstation. However, the increased productivity may be seen as an increase of the harmful load in some other workstation distal to the original change on the line.

According to the system approach, ergonomics considers at least four identifiable major aspects.

The orientation of the first three approaches is the relationship between the individual worker and the work (microergonomics). The fourth aspect focuses on the whole production system (macroergonomics):

1. Human–machine interface technology (hardware ergonomics) studies the human physical and perceptual characteristics and applies these data to the design of controls, displays, tools, seating, work surfaces and workspace arrangements.
2. Human–environment interface technology (environmental ergonomics) concerns the effect of factors such as noise, vibration, lighting and other physical agents on human performance and health.
3. User–system interface technology (software ergonomics) considers primarily the cognitive aspects of human performance. It has important applications in computer-based work systems and controlling of complicated work processes. A poorly designed computer interface may be harmful to the musculoskeletal system by increasing the prolonged static components or psychological stress of the work.
4. Organization–machine interface technology (macroergonomics) mainly focuses on the overall organization and design of the work. The solutions on the organizational level affect the quantity and contents of the individual worker's work. The scheduling of activity and rest periods is one quantitative aspect of work organization. Monotony and meaningfulness of work are qualitative aspects that can be changed by designing its contents.

Because ergonomics is a multidisciplinary task the occupational health station should have good contacts with the management and safety personnel of the company. Participation of the workers in the design and implementation of the ergonomic changes will bring the users' point of view into the process and ensure its success.

Prevention of accidents

Major accidents may result in permanent changes and decreased function of the musculoskeletal organs. Even minor accidents or so-called 'near accidents' may cause microscopic injuries to the tissues, and launch the process leading to musculoskeletal disorders.

Maintaining good health

Several individual risk factors of general health, such as smoking, obesity, sedentary lifestyle or alcohol abuse, have adverse effects on musculo-skeletal health as well. Good physical fitness will keep the doses of sudden instantaneous loads of work or daily living within the tolerance capacity of the body and prevent injuries. The accident risks of various sport activities should be kept in mind when physical exercises are recommended.

Improvement of health care and rehabilitation practices

Adequate medical treatment will reduce the dis-ability and other consequences due to disease. For most musculoskeletal disorders there are no specific treatments. The effectiveness of many commonly used treatments has been disproved in controlled clinical trials. Intensive treatment with ineffective passive methods will prompt the patient to take an inactive role and slow down the recov-ery. In addition, unnecessary examinations and treatments will reduce the resources of the health care system, and decelerate the treatment of patients who really need action (see 'red flags', above). For most patients, non-medical treatment (temporary reduction of the exposure and ergo-nomic actions for preventing new episodes) is the treatment of choice. Health care practitioners often have, however, to reassure the patient about the benign natural course of the disease and about the uselessness and hazards of passive treatments.

Supporting the workers with musculoskeletal problems

Musculoskeletal disorders will seldom result in total disability. Usually the discomforting symp-toms will appear only during some work man-oeuvres. Reducing the mechanical load for some weeks by reorganizing the work enables the patient to work while waiting for recovery. Unfortunately, the flexibility needed for short-term reorganizations is often resisted by the management or co-workers.

Like most diseases, musculoskeletal disorders can awaken fears of malignity or permanent inva-lidity in the patient. Health practitioners can reduce these fears by adequate support and information.

Education

Relevant information to the employers, workers and the society about the topics related to musculo-skeletal disorders will enhance the implementation of prevention and treatment, and reduce resistance against the needed actions. The needed informa-tion can be disseminated in well-organized public programmes or in local health promotion pro-grammes within the company.

Types of musculoskeletal disorder

Low back

For persons under the age of 45, low back prob-lems are the most frequent cause of disability in many industrialized countries. Despite the advances of scientific research during the past dec-ades, the exact anatomical and physiological cause of pain can be shown in only a small number of patients, even with the most sophisticated meth-ods. Fortunately, the course of low back disorders is usually benign, and most patients recover within a few weeks.

Patients with low back disorders have been labelled with dozens of different diagnostic names. Due to the uncertainty of diagnosis, most have very limited use in medical practice. Based on scientific literature and experiences from different medical disciplines, the following rules have been recommended [2]:

1. The initial assessment of patients with acute low back problems focuses on the detection of 'red flags'. These red flags are indicators of potentially serious spinal pathology, such as a fracture or dislocation, a tumour or infection, severe neural compression, or other non-spinal pathology. If the clinical history and examina-tion including neurological screening and straight leg raising gives indication of these harmful conditions, further examinations should be conducted to target these diseases (e.g. imaging, laboratory tests or consultations of specialists).

2. In the absence of red flags, imaging studies and further testing are usually not helpful during the first four weeks of low back symptoms.

3. Symptom control methods can be used to keep the patient as active as possible while awaiting spontaneous recovery, and may later be needed to overcome a specific activity intolerance. Acetaminophenon (paracetamol) is a safe and usually sufficient drug for pain control. Non-steroidal anti-inflammatory drugs including aspirin may be used, but the potential side-effects of these drugs should be kept in mind. Patients may be taught self-application of heat or cold to the back at home. Spinal manipulation may be helpful for patients with acute low back problems without radiculopathy when used within the first month of symptoms.

4. Some activity modification may be necessary during the acute phase. However, bed rest for longer than a couple of days may debilitate the patient. Patients should be encouraged to return to work and to their normal daily activities as soon as possible. Low-stress aerobic activities can safely be started in the first two weeks of symptoms to help avoid debilitation. Exercises of trunk muscles can later be added to the rehabilitation programme.

5. If low back symptoms persist, further evaluation may be indicated. Patients with sciatica may recover more slowly, but further evaluation can also safely be delayed. Psychological or socioeconomic problems may affect the recovery. Therefore, a multidisciplinary approach is needed for rehabilitation of prolonged problems.

The aim of the treatment should be to have the patient return to work as soon as possible. An ergonomic work analysis is essential to find out the risk factors at work that should be modified. Sometimes the modifications needed can be done so that no sick leave is taken. Usually the implementation of ergonomic changes takes time, especially if the solution involves rebuilding of the workstation or changing the whole production process. Previous low back problems highly predict problems in the future. Therefore, the ergonomic actions should be started and changes undertaken even if the worker has fully recovered from his/her first attack of low back pain and returned to work after sick leave.

Neck and shoulder

Work-related disorders of the neck, shoulder and upper limbs have been named after the proven or hypothetical causal component with different names, including 'repetitive strain injury' (RSI), 'cumulative trauma disorders' (CTD), 'occupational cervicobrachial disease' (OCD), 'occupational overuse syndrome' (OOS) and others. Diagnostic labels such as *'cervical spondylosis'* or *'tension neck'* have described the suspected pathology of the cervical spine or muscles of the neck and shoulder area. There is no 'gold standard' for the diagnosis of the disorders of this body area.

The symptoms of the patient are of little help in pinpointing exactly the pathology into spinal or muscular structures of the neck and shoulder. Experimental studies have shown that irritation of spinal structures can cause pain sensation in the area of the large shoulder muscles. Vice versa, tension of the muscles increases biomechanical load on the cervical spine. Therefore, prolonged biomechanical stress, although of muscular origin, could be one cause of spinal degeneration. Mechanical compression of neural structures by the structures of the spine, as well as by contracted muscles, will cause neural irritation and pain, and the pain will further increase the contraction of the muscles. The result is a complicated system of several potential vicious circles.

Controlled trials of the common neck and shoulder disorders among the working population are scanty. None of the commonly used treatments has been shown to be superior over others. Soft cervical collars may even be harmful and slow down the recovery. Exercising the shoulder muscles has been shown to be as effective as the traditional treatment with massage or physical modalities.

Symptoms of the shoulder joint have been mostly associated with *tendinous pathology of the rotator cuff* or *osteoarthritis of the acromioclavicular joint*. Mechanical impingement of the rotator cuff on the undersurface of the anterior acromion during the elevation of the humerus between 60° and 120° is the probable cause of the injury of the tendons. Pain during resisted movements or isometric contractions of the shoulder muscles are major signs of tendinitis. Treatment is conservative and symptomatic. Local corticosteroid injections may help some patients. Surgical intervention should be considered in cases resistant to conservative treatment.

'*Frozen shoulder*' or capsulitis is an inflammatory lesion of the glenohumeral joint capsule that leads to its thickening and contraction, resulting in painful stiffness of the active and passive shoulder movements. The aetiology of the capsulitis is unknown. It is important to know the long but benign course of the disease, and that none of the proposed treatments has been shown beneficial over the placebos.

One rational approach in the treatment of neck and shoulder problems is similar to that recommended for low back disorders. The initial investigation focuses on 'red flags'. If no indicators of serious diseases are seen, imaging or laboratory examinations can wait. Symptomatic medication can be used and dynamic physical exercises are probably more beneficial than harmful. Isometric stabilization of the shoulder joints is one basic requirement for all manual tasks. Because even very low levels of continuous static contraction of the muscles may be harmful and start the pathological vicious circles, static loading of the shoulders should be avoided.

Workstations should be investigated and adjusted according to the anthropometry of the workers. In sedentary work, there should be enough space on the table to give mechanical support to the arms. In some cases, armrests on the chair can be used for this purpose. Sometimes extra supports or arm suspensions may be useful. In any case, the worker should be allowed to select the most suitable way to rest his/her arms from several possible solutions. For this selection the worker should be allowed to try out the alternatives in his/her actual work for several hours. Reorganizing of the work is one way to avoid static postures and to bring more variability to the work. Working with elevated arms, or supporting of tools, can be reduced by redesigning the work process, work stations or suspension of the tools.

Elbow, forearm, wrist and hand

The most common disorders of this body area are *epicondylitis, tendinous disorders of the wrist* and the *carpal tunnel syndrome*. Common external risk factors are repetitive movements of the hands, gripping with large force and non-neutral postures of the wrists. In the assessment of patients with carpal tunnel syndrome, the possible

conditions with accumulated fluid in the tissues should be kept in mind (thyroid diseases, pregnancy, hormonal disorders).

The basic treatment of these disorders is rest. Avoidance of the repetitive work for a week or two is usually sufficient. For some patients, immobilization with a splint for a few days may be necessary. Sometimes functional splints may be used at work, especially if the quantity of the above-mentioned risk factors is low.

Sharp edges of surfaces or tools compressing the forearms or hands may give acute or slowly appearing symptoms. Identification of the cause, and its avoidance, are usually sufficient treatment.

Again the preventive actions should be focused on the work. The repetition of movements can be reduced by changing the process or by reorganizing the work. The use of too large or too small hand tools produces high internal forces in the structures of the forearm. Therefore, hand tools should fit into the hand of the users. Redesign of the tools may change the mechanical properties of the tools and reduce the need for muscular force. Tools using pneumatics or electrical engines reduce the need for dynamic muscular force, and increase productivity of the work. Sometimes the new tools may increase the static load of the work and thus bring new risks. Neutral postures of the wrist can often be reached by reshaping the tools or by changing the workstation or working methods.

Rounding and moulding of sharp edges and handles reduces the risks of local compression. Sometimes personal protection by moulding sleeves or gloves may be necessary.

Lower limbs

Kneeling has been shown to increase the risk of *osteoarthritis of the knee*, especially in heavy physical work. Other common conditions are *bursitis of the knees*. Kneeling postures can often be avoided by changing the work methods. If this is not possible, moulding of knees reduces the risk of bursitis.

Acknowledgement

I acknowledge Dr Eira Viikari-Juntura for discussions in preparing the manuscript. The contents of *Table 17.4* were originally presented by her (in Finnish).

References

1. Armstrong, T.J., Buckle, P., Fine, L.J. *et al.* A conceptual model for work-related neck and upper-limb musculoskeletal disorders. *Scandinavian Journal of Work and Environmental Health*, **19**, 73–84 (1993)
2. Bigos, S.J., Bowyer, O.R., Braen, G.R. *et al.* Acute low back problems in adults. *Clinical Practice Guideline No 14.* US Department of Health and Human Services, Rockville, MD (1994)
3. Wilson, J.R. and Corlett, E.N. *Evaluation of Human Work. A Practical Ergonomics Methodology.* Taylor and Francis, London (1990)

Further reading

Grandjean, E. *Fitting the Task to the Man. A Textbook of Occupational Ergonomics*, 4th edn. Taylor and Francis, London (1988)

Kuorinka, I. and Forcier, L. (eds). *Work Related Musculoskeletal Disorders (WMSDs): A Reference Book for Prevention.* Taylor and Francis, London (1995)

Riihimäki, H. Low-back pain, its origin and risk indicators. *Scandinavian Journal of Work and Environmental Health*, **17**, 81–90 (1991)

Sackett, D.L., Haynes, R.B. and Tugwell, P. *Clinical Epidemiology. A Basic Science for Clinical Medicine.* Little, Brown, Boston (1985)

Chapter 18

Noise

A Kjellberg

This chapter deals with the effects of occupational noise exposure, but does not cover the technical aspects of noise and noise control. For these latter issues the reader is referred to Chapter 7 in the previous edition of this handbook [1]. The basic characteristics of noise-induced hearing loss (NIHL) are described in textbooks of occupational medicine, and two consensus documents have recently been published [2,3]. Many aspects of NIHL are therefore treated rather briefly here. The emphasis is instead on non-auditory effects of noise at work and other psychological aspects of the noise problem. When dealing with these aspects it is important to keep in mind the conventional definition of noise as unwanted sounds. Noise, thus, is subjectively defined and may include faint sounds and meaningful sounds like conversations and music.

Different noise effects

Hearing loss is the most obvious and serious consequence of noise exposure at work. Noise may, however, have other undesired effects, which sometimes occur at levels below the one that constitutes a risk for hearing damage:

- non-auditory physiological and health effects
- annoyance and other subjective reactions
- interference with the perception of speech and other auditory signals
- interference with the performance of non-auditory tasks
- interference with sleep.

These effects, with the exception of sleep disturbances, are treated in the above order after a section on hearing loss and problems related to the use of hearing protectors. Interference with sleep will not be treated since it very seldom is a problem in occupational settings (for a recent review of noise and sleep, see [4]).

Noise-induced hearing impairment

Hearing loss is one of the most common of all physical impairments and occupational noise exposure is one of its major causes. The NIHL is irreversible and may have a profound influence on the person's life quality because of the deteriorated communication ability. It is also, in most cases, possible to prevent the development of NIHL. The implementation of preventive measures, including both noise control and individual protection, is thus the central issue.

Acoustic trauma

Short exposures to high-level sounds may cause structural damage to the ear and an immediate permanent hearing loss (*acoustic trauma*). Apart from accidents, such levels are rarely found in workplaces outside military contexts.

Temporary threshold shift

Moderate noise exposure may cause a temporary elevation of the hearing threshold, a temporary threshold shift (TTS). TTS is seldom more than 40 dB and is a joint function of sound level, duration and frequency. Regardless of exposure time, no TTS is likely for sound levels below 70 dB. The fastest increase of TTS occurs during the first 2 h of exposure and recovery from TTS is also fastest during the first hours after exposure. After exposure to a broad-band noise, the maximum TTS is found in the 3–6 kHz frequency region, with a maximum generally at 4 kHz [5]. High-frequency noise causes a TTS in high frequencies, whereas low-frequency noise has an effect both on low and mid-frequency thresholds.

There is evidence that a negative subjective evaluation of the noise increases the TTS [6].

Noise exposures that do not cause a TTS are not likely to lead to a permanent threshold shift, a NIHL. However, the size of TTS is not a valid predictor of the individual risk for developing a NIHL.

Permanent threshold shift, noise-induced hearing loss

The development of a permanent threshold shift, NIHL, is typically a slow process over many years of noise exposure. This hearing loss is the result of degeneration of sensory cells in the cochlea and the first sign of a damage is typically changes of the stereocilia. This degeneration of sensory cells may, in turn, lead to a degeneration of the nerve fibres to the damaged region. Vasoconstriction in the cochlea due to noise and a resulting reduced capacity for exchange of nutrients has been suggested as a mechanism behind the cell degeneration. The empirical evidence for such an effect of noise is, however, equivocal [7].

Development of NIHL

NIHL is typically first seen as an elevation of the hearing threshold at 6 kHz. As the damage progresses the 4, 3 and 8 kHz thresholds are raised and, eventually, the impairment is spread to the lower frequencies. In later stages the largest threshold shift is usually found for 4 kHz.

The damage is usually symmetric, but some exposure situations, e.g. rifle shooting, may cause asymmetric hearing loss. After 10–15 years the threshold elevation at higher frequencies levels off and the further development of the NIHL primarily affects the lower frequencies.

For most people the primary problem caused by NIHL is its effects on speech communication. Certainly most of the energy in the speech signal is found in the low-frequency bands, where the hearing capacity is least affected by the NIHL. The information is, however, carried by the 0.5–4 kHz frequency band and the higher frequencies are critical for the perception of many consonants. Since consonants generally carry more information than vowels, the result of the hearing impairment is often a feeling of hearing but not understanding. The mean audiometric threshold in the 1–4 kHz range is a rough indicator of the person's speech comprehension level.

Critical noise exposure factors

Sound level and exposure time

Sound levels below 75 dB(A) do not seem to constitute a risk for hearing damage. The exposure limit of 85 dB(A) adopted by many countries therefore is no guarantee against NIHL.

The risk for NIHL is, in Europe and in the ISO Standard 1999-1990 [8], assumed to be a direct function of the total sound energy, which is doubled with each increase of 3 dB. This implies that the permitted exposure time is halved when the level is raised by 3 dB (in the USA this so-called *Q* factor is 5 dB). The equal energy rule is thought to be valid up to a sound level of 140 dB; the risk for NIHL, thus, should be more or less independent of the temporal exposure pattern below this level.

Frequency

The sensitivity of the ear is highly frequency dependent. The lowest hearing thresholds are found around 3 kHz and the thresholds rise rapidly below 400 Hz and less rapidly above 5 kHz. Corresponding differences in subjective sensitivity also exist at levels above the hearing threshold. In most noise regulations, consideration is taken to this differential sensitivity by using A-weighted sound levels units [dB(A)], which means that the level is measured through the A filter of the sound-level meter. This means that only the part of the sound falling in the 0.02–20 kHz frequency range affects the sound-level value, and that the lowest frequencies have a very small influence. The A filter is based on subjective sensitivity data, but these correspond rather well with frequency differences in the energy transmission in the outer and middle ear. In most cases the A-weighted sound-level therefore seems to be a fairly good predictor of the risk for NIHL.

Impulse noise

An impulse noise is a sudden, short-lasting increase of the sound level, e.g. the sound of a hammer blow or a rifle shot. There are several reasons to treat these sounds separately from continuous noise. The short duration means that these sounds generally add very little to the exposure dose also when the level is high. Obviously there must exist an intensity limit above which the sound damages the ear irrespective of its duration. As mentioned above, 140 dB has been adopted by most countries as an absolute limit for impulse sounds. The empirical basis for this limit is, however, rather weak.

The subjective intensity of a sound, its *loudness*, is built up gradually by a summation of energy, *temporal summation*, during the initial 0.1–0.5 s. A 0.05 s impulse sound thus sounds weaker than the same sound presented for 0.5 s. This temporal summation of the sensation level is a central nervous system phenomenon; the integration time in the sensory organs of the inner ear, which is critical for the damaging effects, is only about 35 ms [9]. An impulse sound therefore may constitute a risk for NIHL without being very strong subjectively.

Tinnitus

Tinnitus, a ringing or buzzing in the ear, is a common consequence of NIHL. The character of the perceived sound varies regarding loudness, pitch, bandwidth, localization and temporal pattern. The incidence, but not the severity, of tinnitus increases with deteriorating hearing thresholds. For a minority, tinnitus causes severe and handicapping distress [10].

Other factors contributing to NIHL

Age

In groups that are not exposed to high-level noise, the hearing gradually deteriorates with increasing age. The impairment decreases with decreasing frequency down to 1 kHz. ISO 1999 gives curves for the normal age decrement and a method for estimation of the expected combined effects of noise exposure and ageing [8]. It has been suggested that very young and very old people are more susceptible to noise than others. However, no firm evidence for such an interaction exists [11].

Drugs and other chemicals

Several types of ototoxic drugs have been identified: aminoglycoside antibiotics, antineoplastic agents, loop-inhibiting diuretics, salicylates and quinine compounds. Two of these drug types, aminoglycoside antibiotics and antineoplastic agents, can interact with noise, resulting in a greater noise effect on hearing than would be obtained with noise or the drug alone. There is also evidence indicating that the NIHL is strengthened by simultaneous exposure to toluene, carbon monoxide and carbon disulphide [11,12].

Other factors

Some studies indicate an interaction between noise and whole-body vibration. The effects have been small and no human data of NIHL have been reported [12].

Individual susceptibility to NIHL

There are large differences in sensitivity to noise. Rather little, however, is known about what factors determine this susceptibility to NIHL. There is some evidence that persons with a low degree of pigmentation and smokers are more susceptible than persons with a dark complexion and non-smokers. However, these and other suggested non-auditory determining factors can only explain a very small part of the individual differences.

Another line of research has been to relate susceptibility to differences in the functioning of the auditory system, primarily the stapedius reflex.

The stapedius muscle of the middle ear is contracted when the sound exceeds a threshold level. The effect is a substantially reduced transmission and a protection of the inner ear against loud noise. The reflex threshold varies widely, with a mean around 85 dB for a 1000 Hz tone. There are data suggesting that individual differences in reflex characteristics may explain part of the individual susceptibility to NIHL [13].

The individual exposure history may also affect susceptibility. Thus a series of animal studies indicate that prior exposure to lower level sounds may protect against the effects of subsequent high-level noise exposure.

Hearing protection

NIHL is generally preventable, and legislation, regulations and guidelines exist which, if enforced, should reduce the problem dramatically. A central question therefore is why the problem still exists to such a large extent.

The main strategy against noise problems in the workplace should be to reduce the noise to a level that does not constitute a risk for NIHL, i.e. at least to below 85 dB(A) or, preferably, below 75 dB(A). In many work environments such a reduction is clearly not possible; hearing protectors must then be used to avoid NIHL. However, free access to hearing protectors in the workplace has repeatedly been found not to give any guarantee against problems of NIHL. One reason for this might be that the protectors are inadequate for the levels and frequency composition of the noise. In the choice of protectors it should be noted that the real protection generally lies well below the noise reduction rating based on laboratory tests given by the manufacturer. Another reason is that they do not fit or are not used in a proper way. Each user therefore must carefully be instructed and the fit must be checked for each ear. The attenuating capacity of the protector also deteriorates with age.

Perhaps the most important reason for failure is that hearing protectors are not used consistently enough to provide an effective protection. There are two main reasons for not using protectors. One is that hearing protectors create problems, the other that the risk for hearing impairment is underestimated.

Problems created by hearing protectors

Discomfort

A large minority report discomfort from using hearing protectors. Earmuff users most often complain of heat and damp, whereas itching seems to be the main complaint among earplug users. Sensitive persons may develop inflammation in the skin of the auditory canal, often as a result of using dirty earplugs.

Communication problems

Hearing protectors do not only attenuate noise but also speech and other acoustic signals. Provided that the noise and the speech are equally attenuated, the signal-to-noise ratio remains unaffected by the hearing protector. Therefore hearing protectors often have little or no degrading effect on speech comprehension; they might even improve speech discrimination by reducing the distortion from very high sound levels. However, in fact, hearing protectors may impair speech communication and generally do so for a person with a hearing impairment.

One reason is that the speech signal may be attenuated to a level below the hearing threshold. Since the threshold is elevated among the hearing impaired, this is more likely to happen in this group. This threshold elevation is most pronounced in the mid- and high-frequency region, which is the region most critical for speech comprehension and the region most effectively attenuated by hearing protectors. This frequency-dependent attenuation may also impair speech comprehension in another way; the masking by low-frequency sounds of high-frequency sounds is much more effective than masking in the opposite direction. The high-frequency sound components are also more important than the low-frequency components for localization of a sound source; sound localization therefore may be impaired by hearing protectors.

Speech comprehension may also be impaired as a result of the speaker wearing hearing protectors. Normally the effect of a raised noise level is at least partly compensated by a strengthening of the voice. This regulation of speech level is disturbed by hearing protectors; when the effective noise level is lowered by the protectors, the voice is not raised as much as would have been the case without the protectors.

Underestimation of the risk for hearing impairment

The gradual onset of NIHL

The development of NIHL is rather slow and speech comprehension and the impairment therefore might develop rather far before it is recognized by the person.

Conflict subjective–objective risk assessment

The common exposure limit of 85 dB(A) is the level of the traffic noise found in an average city street. Obviously, people in general put up with this level without wearing hearing protectors. The highest level deemed acceptable by the legislation, thus, does not cause immediate subjective reactions that motivate hearing protection.

The loudness of a sound, its subjective intensity, is doubled with approximately each 10 dB increase of the sound. This could be compared to the assumed sound-level duration trade-off mentioned above, implying that the permitted exposure time is halved with each 3 dB increase of the sound. Changes in loudness probably determine the subjective need for hearing protection, which, thus, may correspond badly with the actually increased risk for NIHL.

Furthermore, if the risk for NIHL below 140 dB is independent of the temporal exposure pattern, the effect of a whole day of work in 85 dB could also be reached by 15 1-min periods with a slightly more than trebled loudness (100 dB). Obviously, this relation does not correspond to the spontaneous subjective risk judgement.

As mentioned above, the subjective impression of an impulse noise is another case where the subjective impression does not constitute an adequate warning for the risk of hearing impairment.

Conclusions

For effective protection, it is essential that ear protectors are always worn when the noise constitutes a risk for hearing damage. The protectors therefore must be comfortable. There is no pro-

tector that fits everybody and the discomfort problems can, therefore, only be solved by keeping alternative hearing protectors available. Discomfort problems may also be reduced by not using the same hearing protector the whole day. Individual fitting of hearing protectors and careful instruction of how they should be used is, of course, also essential for optimal protection. Comfort must be given priority in the selection of protector, since the only effective protector is the one always worn when needed. It is also important that the protectors (or the sensitive parts of them) are regularly replaced on a schedule appropriate for the particular type of hearing protector.

The potential communication problems must be considered in jobs where the apprehension of speech and other verbal signals is essential for security. The preferred solution would of course be to remove the need for hearing protectors by lowering the noise level. Where this is impossible, the choice of hearing protector must be based on a careful matching of type of protector, workplace noise, critical auditory signals and the individual hearing capacity, and on-site testing of the protector. In this way it may be possible to find a protector that gives adequate protection without impairing the perception of auditory signals.

In the past decade new types of hearing protector technology have been developed which may reduce some of the problems mentioned above [14]. In hearing protectors with active noise reduction, the noise is cancelled by a signal that is exactly out of phase with the noise. This technique is especially effective for low frequencies, which are least attenuated by conventional hearing protectors. Another line of development has been the amplitude-sensitive protectors, which prevents the sound level from exceeding a predetermined level and which may amplify the signal at lower levels. This type of protector provides for good attenuation when levels are high, without impairing communication at lower noise levels. They therefore provide a good alternative in work environments with high intermittent noise.

The conflict between spontaneous subjective risk perception and the actual long-term risks for hearing impairment accentuates the need for teaching workers and their foremen about NIHL and its prevention and for active enforcement of protector use. Feedback from regular audiometry is another important feature of a hearing conservation programme [15].

Non-auditory health and physiological effects of noise

Research on the physiological non-auditory effects of noise have dealt with, for example, neuro-endocrine, gastrointestinal and immunological and neoplastic effects [16]. Fatigue, headaches, irritability and other symptoms have also often been reported as over-represented among groups exposed to noise. However, the control for the effects of confounding factors has generally been unsatisfactory. Two possible health effects, namely cardiovascular and psychiatric effects, have attracted particularly great interest. For general coverage of the area, see reviews in [17–23].

Cardiovascular effects

In laboratory studies, noise has rather consistently been shown to produce increases in diastolic blood pressure [21]. Most studies on non-auditory long-term health effects of noise have also dealt with the noise as a risk factor for hypertension. No clear picture emerges from the epidemiological studies which have reported both positive and negative findings. This may partly be the result of methodological flaws. Another reason may be that the hypertensive effect is the result of an inter-action between noise and other factors, e.g. work task characteristics [20,21].

Psychiatric effects

Reports in the 1970s of higher mental hospital admission rates among the noise exposed attracted much attention. Some studies of psychiatric symptoms in the community also indicated an association between noise exposure or noise annoyance and symptom frequency. Later and more controlled studies have questioned the causal role of noise. There seems to be better support for noise sensitivity as an indicator of vulnerability to minor psychiatric disorder, as well as for stronger annoyance responses among persons with a psychiatric disorder [22].

Interference with perception of speech and other auditory signals

The average voice level is about 55 dB(A) in ambient noise levels up to 48 dB(A) at a distance of 1 m, with large individual variations. The voice level also varies much between situations; the voice is, for example, raised when communication is critical, or when talking to an audience or into a microphone. For each increase of 10 dB of the noise level the speaker automatically raises his voice by 3–6 dB. The signal-to-noise ratio is thus normally lowered in noise. A full compensation for the noise requires a conscious effort, and shouting above 78 dB(A) does not lead to any further improvement of intelligibility.

Sentences are normally comprehended even when the voice level is 5 dB below the noise level, whereas single words require a level of 10 dB above the noise level.

Wholly satisfactory communication at a distance of 2.5 m between speaker and listener requires a noise level of, at most, 45 dB(A). In rooms where it is important to have perfect communication using normal voice levels, it is thus necessary to have an even lower ambient noise level.

The expected speech interference effect can be estimated from a frequency analysis of the noise by calculating the articulation index or the speech interference level [24,25].

Noise may cause problems also by interfering with the perception of other auditory signals than speech. It is, for example, important to take consideration of the ambient noise in the design of auditory signals. The level, frequency and temporal pattern of the warning signal should be chosen with regard taken to ambient noise characteristics [26].

The effects of noise on speech comprehension are aggravated by a hearing loss; the difference in speech comprehension between a person with normal hearing and one with a hearing impairment is thus strengthened in noise (e.g. when several persons talk simultaneously).

For a more comprehensive review of speech communication in noise and methods for assessment of speech interference see [27].

Annoyance and other subjective reactions to noise

Noise is not only a problem in workplaces where it constitutes a risk of developing hearing damage; it may also cause serious problems at levels far below those at which such damage may occur. However, systematic research on other problems than hearing damage has been sparse in workplaces. Therefore, most knowledge of the adverse effects of noise at lower levels emanates from research that has dealt with problems in residential areas and from laboratory studies.

Subjective responses

Different subjective qualities

Loudness is a non-evaluative noise characteristic only referring to the subjective intensity of the sound. Loudness can with good accuracy be predicted from the physical sound qualities of the sound. The evaluative response to the sound, *annoyance*, is also partly determined by the physical characteristics of the noise, but also by many other aspects of the noise, the situation and the individual.

Figure 18.1 shows the relation between four classes of variables which affect loudness and annoyance. The figure shows that loudness to a very high degree is determined by the physical noise characteristics. Furthermore, loudness is a major determinant of annoyance. However, the effects of the physical characteristics on annoyance are not wholly mediated by their effects on loudness; it may, for example, also be a result of a particularly disharmonic combination of frequencies. The influence of the different factors affecting annoyance will vary from one case to another, and nothing general, therefore, may be said of their relative importance.

The following four sections treat these different classes of variables affecting the subjective response to noise. For more comprehensive reviews, see [28,29].

Effects of physical noise characteristics on subjective response to noise

The basic relations between the physical qualities of the noise and the subjective response are common knowledge and have been summarized by many authors [30]. Therefore, these relations are only treated briefly.

Sound level

The loudness of a sound is in most cases doubled with each 10 dB increase of the sound pressure level. The most important exception to this rule

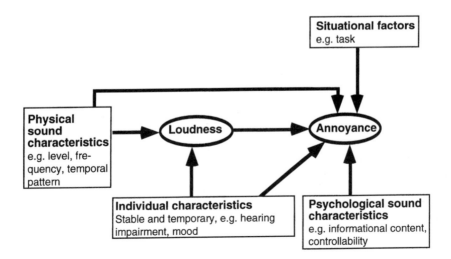

Figure 18.1 Relation between two subjective responses to noise, loudness and annoyance and four classes of determining factors.

is low-frequency noise. A 100 Hz tone that is raised by 10 dB is experienced as 4–5 times louder. Other things being equal, annoyance is closely-associated with loudness and, thereby, to sound level. However, when annoyance judgements by different persons from different workplaces are compared, sound level generally has been found to explain a very small part of the individual differences. This is particularly true for workplaces with a moderate sound level, where other factors beside the sound level will be of greater importance.

Studies of community noise have shown that total annoyance is equal to the maximum annoyance caused by a separate source of noise when the other sources cause considerably less annoyance. Therefore a lowering of the overall sound level will not reduce annoyance if it is accomplished without an attenuation of the critical noise. In other cases, where the separate sources are about equally annoying, a certain summation of annoyance takes place, which makes the overall level a more relevant criterion for evaluating the measures taken against the noise.

In reports of noise surveys in residential areas, the effect of noise level is often not described in terms of degree of annoyance but in terms of the percentage of the exposed who complain or report a certain degree of annoyance. Corresponding figures for workplace noise do not exist and would obviously vary between different types of workplaces.

Finally it should be noted that for some noise sources, especially speech, other qualities than the sound level are likely to be more important. As long as the unwanted speech is intelligible, a lowering of the level has little effect on the annoyance it may cause (see below).

Frequency

There is general agreement on the overall shape of the equal loudness curves, which describe the differential subjective sensitivity of man to sounds of different frequencies. When noise is assessed, consideration is taken to this differential sensitivity by using the A filter described above. The sensitivity of the ear becomes less frequency dependent with increasing level, whereas the A weighting is used at all levels. A consequence of this, which is confirmed by several studies, is that the dB(A) value may grossly underestimate the subjective impression of noise containing strong low-frequency

components (e.g. ventilation noise). The A-weighting therefore may lead to incorrect conclusions when, for example, two machines which emit noise with very different frequency composition are compared.

Another critical aspect of the frequency characteristics of the noise is the presence of pure tones in the noise, which is common in the noise from office machines. It has been repeatedly demonstrated that annoyance is often increased when the tone is clearly audible. This is particularly true for higher frequency tones.

Exposure time

It is commonly believed that in a long-term perspective people will adapt to noise in the sense that they become less annoyed by it. In fact, most evidence from residential areas argues against such an effect [31], at least after the first few weeks in a new environment.

In a shorter term perspective, the question is whether one habituates to a constant noise (e.g. ventilation noise in the office). A common description of the response to that kind of noise is that one rather seldom thinks of it, but that it is very pleasant when it is turned off. This indicates some degree of habituation. However, the absence of direct subjective responses to such a noise does not rule out the possibility that the person is negatively affected by the noise. It is quite possible that an effect of noise on mood or performance is attributed to factors other than the noise.

Temporal variability

Several studies indicate that a variable noise is generally judged as more annoying than a continuous one. This is also true of the repetitive type of noise produced by, for example, computer printers. These types of noise are generally considered more annoying than continuous noise at the same equivalent sound level.

Signal-to-noise ratio

Several studies have shown that noise is especially annoying when it masks speech or other auditory information which is considered important. However, masking may sometimes have a positive effect, by making unwanted sounds less intrusive. Faint intermittent sounds, like dripping water, may become very annoying when heard in an otherwise very quiet environment. In such cases a continuous masking noise would probably decrease the annoyance. The same is true of speech masking. Noise may prevent others from hearing our conversations and thus protect our privacy.

There are several examples of workplaces which have had installed artificial constant background noise ('sound conditioning') to mask annoying noise, primarily speech. It has been found to be very difficult to find an artificial masking noise that is an effective masker and which is not regarded as unacceptable in itself, and there is no consensus on the beneficial effects of such installations [32].

Effects of other noise characteristics on subjective response to noise

As mentioned above, differences in sound level are no good predictor of annoyance. It is evident that others are of greater importance. Unfortunately, research on the influence of such factors on the subjective response is extremely rare from occupational settings [33,34].

Informational content

Irrelevant speech is a major noise problem in many workplaces. Sound level is a very poor predictor of annoyance in such cases. Rather the intelligibility of the irrelevant speech seems to be the main factor determining how disturbing it is.

Predictability and controllability

Results from stress research indicate that an unpredictable and uncontrollable stressor generally yields a stronger stress response than a predictable and controllable event. Accordingly, an expected noise should be less annoying than an unexpected one.

Attitude to noise source and other aspects of the working environment

The response to noise is also influenced by the attitude towards the source of the noise. Thus, the complaints about aircraft overflights were reduced by creating a more positive attitude towards the airforce [35].

It is reasonable to assume that the same mechanisms are at work also in occupational settings. Thus, one would for example expect a secretary who does not like word processors to be especially irritated by the printer's noise. It is also likely that the overall evaluation of the work and the working environment may influence the evaluation of the noise at the workplace. However, systematic studies of such effects have only been reported from residential areas. A conclusion from these studies is that when the basic problem is one of attitudes towards the noise source or to other aspects of the working conditions, a reduction of the sound level is likely to have little effect on the noise problem at the workplace.

Aspiration level and 'necessity' of the noise

A noise level deemed acceptable in a workshop might be regarded as unbearable in an office. The reason probably is that the noise may be regarded as an unavoidable consequence of the activity in a workshop, whereas it would be considered unnecessary in an adjacent office. It was found [36] that, at equal sound levels, persons who judged the possibilities to reduce the noise as good were much more annoyed than those who thought there was no real possibility for an improvement. A conclusion from this and other studies is that a main goal should be to keep the employees protected from noise from sources that have no direct connection with their own job. Another conclusion would be that it is very important to inform workers about measures taken to reduce noise and the problems associated with further reductions.

Effects of ongoing activity on noise annoyance

It is often assumed that the annoyance response depends on the task in which one is engaged. In one respect this is definitely true; one is certainly more disturbed when the noise masks auditory information required for the ongoing activity. The few systematic studies that have reported on the importance of other task characteristics indicate that noise tends to be more annoying when performing more complex tasks, and this is also generally considered in the planning of work-places. Irrelevant speech during a verbal task appears to be the most annoying combination of task and noise. The studies also indicate that a rather small part of the differences between work-places in noise tolerance levels is explained by such task differences.

Individual differences in response to noise

It is obvious that the same noise elicits widely different responses in different persons. Much research has been devoted to these individual differences and has mainly concerned three questions: Are there any stable individual differences regarding the subjective response to noise? If so, is it a case of specific noise sensitivity? And, finally, what characterizes the noise-sensitive persons? Comprehensive reviews of these studies are given in [22] and [37].

The low stability of annoyance ratings indicates that they to a large degree reflect transient states rather than stable traits. Furthermore, there are reasons to doubt that the stable differences in annoyance reflect a specific noise sensitivity. It was found, for example, that a critical tendencies scale (not including any noise questions) predicted noise annoyance as well as the noise sensitivity scale [38].

Research attempting to identify characteristics of the persons most annoyed by noise has not been very successful. The very inconsistent results indicate that noise sensitivity has no clear relation to demographic variables like sex and age. The only group that has been found clearly to deviate from others in their response to noise are those with a hearing impairment, who most often are more annoyed by noise than others.

In conclusion, the research on individual differences shows that one could expect widely different responses to the noise at a workplace and that it is not possible to predict these differences from other known individual characteristics. One important exception, which should be considered at work-places, is that persons with a hearing impairment are likely to be more sensitive to noise.

Performance effects and other behavioural effects

Demonstrations of noise effects on performance are of interest for at least three reasons. They might imply that noise affects productivity, which, of course, would have important implications. They could also indicate an increased risk for errors in noise, which, in certain contexts, could constitute a security risk. Finally, an impaired performance could sometimes be viewed as in indicator of a deteriorated functional state, which should be avoided. It could, for example, be interpreted as an indicator of fatigue.

The research on the effects of noise on performance presents no simple and consistent picture of the effects of noise. One review [39] concluded that no clear effects on performance have been demonstrated of noise below 95 dB. Later research has demonstrated that noise may affect performance at much lower levels. One reason for this has been a shift of interest from sensorimotor tasks (e.g. reaction time and signal monitoring tasks) to verbal tasks.

More comprehensive reviews of noise and performance may be found in [28], [40] and [41].

The effects of noise on performance have been treated within several theoretical contexts. The performance effects may be viewed as a result of masking, distraction, changes of arousal level or changes of the strategy chosen for the performance of the task.

Theoretical explanations of performance effects

Masking

The performance of any task that involves auditory cues may be deteriorated by the masking effects of noise. This, of course, includes all tasks that require speech comprehension, but auditory feedback from the work process is also essential in many tasks that are not primarily of an auditory nature.

Distraction

Any change of the environmental noise may direct attention from the task towards the noise source.

Such distractional effects primarily appear at the onset and offset of noise, but may also be important for the negative effects of other sounds with attention-catching properties (e.g. speech). In many tasks the effect is an inconsequential brief interruption of work; in other tasks the effect is to interrupt a line of thought or a behavioural sequence that is difficult to resume.

Arousal level, allocation of attention

The effects of noise on performance have traditionally been treated within the framework of arousal theory, sometimes supplemented by the hypothesis that attention becomes more selective at high arousal levels. According to this view the effects of noise on performance are seen as consequences of changes along a unidimensional arousal continuum, and noise has generally been assumed to raise the arousal level. The performance effects are often interpreted as a result of the too selective attention accompanying states of overactivation. However, it should be noted that there is reason to believe that repetitive or continuous noise may have the opposite effect; noise, and especially low-frequency noise, sometimes makes people sleepy [42,43]. This unidimensional view of arousal has been criticized on several grounds.

Strategy choice and compensatory processes

One of several problems for explanations of the performance effects in terms of arousal is that small changes in the task or the experimental situation may alter the results dramatically. This indicates that few of the performance effects are unavoidable consequences of the noise exposure in itself.

Such effects have been one of the arguments for a 'strategy choice hypothesis', which states that noise primarily influences the way in which a person chooses to carry out a task. This means, for example, that attentional selectivity is regarded as a way of handling a situation with reduced available information processing resources; attention is directed towards the most important aspects of the task at the expense of the less important ones. In some tasks, such a strategy may be very successful and leave performance unaffected.

The selective intake of information is, therefore, an example of a way of coping with a situation in which the normal way of performing the task requires more resources than those available. However, in most tasks the performance level generally lies well below the person's maximum level. This means that it is usually possible to uphold the performance level in spite of the noise by exerting extra effort. At least this is true for a limited time.

A negative effect of noise on performance is thus attained if the load exceeds the level that can be compensated for, or if for some reason it is not deemed to be worth the extra effort required to keep performance at the level that is normal in a quiet situation.

An unchanged performance level, thus, does not necessarily mean that the environment is without any effect; the performance may have been attained at a higher cost than otherwise would have been the case. This means that performance efficiency, defined as the ratio between performance and its costs, may be affected by noise rather than performance in itself. Another consequence of this view is that work should be more fatiguing in noise than under quiet conditions. The extensive experimental research on after-effects of work in noise indicates that this is also the case (see below).

Field studies of safety and efficiency

The few studies treating the effects of noise on safety and efficiency at workplaces give some support for an association between high noise levels and high accident rates [44] as well as lower productivity or higher error rates [45,46]. All these studies have dealt with factories with very high noise levels. The interpretation of these results is complicated by the fact that the high-noise work settings are likely to be defective also in other respects. The reduced accident rate as a result of wearing ear defenders shown in [47] is less likely to be an effect of such factors.

Noise effects in different tasks

A vast amount of laboratory research on noise and performance has been reported. Most of this research, however, is of little or no relevance for the noise problems in workplaces and the results have not at all been consistent. Another feature that limits their practical interest is that many of the studies have dealt with noise at levels that are far above those that should be avoided for reasons of hearing protection. These studies will only be treated in passing.

Tasks insensitive to continuous meaningless noise

The performance of several types of tasks appears to be unaffected even by very high levels of continuous noise. Examples of such tasks mentioned in [39] are simple reaction time tasks with an easily discriminable and forewarned stimulus, motor performance and sensory tasks such as visual acuity tasks.

Reaction time and vigilance tasks

Complex reaction time tasks are probably the ones used in most noise studies. The typical effect of noise on this type of task is an increased number of errors. Furthermore, this effect of noise, like most other effects on performance, is accentuated with increased time on the task. The increased error rate probably reflects impaired control processes during noise exposure, more specifically a lowered ability to withhold a highly prepared response.

When working in noise with these types of tasks, subjects have also been found to concentrate their attention on the most probable signals at the expense of the less probable ones. Furthermore, if signal probabilities are changed, the adaptation to the new conditions takes a longer time in noise. The results, thus, indicate a more selective and a less flexible information processing strategy in noise.

In many of these studies very high noise levels were used, but when exposure time is prolonged the effect may be obtained at moderate noise levels also.

Rather inconsistent noise effects have been obtained in vigilance tasks, and tasks requiring the monitoring of infrequent and weak signals. Effects of moderate noise levels have only been found in more complex tasks with higher demands on memory.

Memory

The effects of noise on verbal memory have been treated in many studies, which, however, generally have been of greater relevance for information processing theories than for the understanding of noise effects at work. A main finding has been that noise seems to change the learning strategy; in noise, subjects tend, for example, to rely more on rote learning.

Conversations between colleagues or customers are considered a major noise problem in many workplaces. The performance effects of irrelevant speech are therefore of great practical interest. In recent years a large part of the memory research has dealt with such speech effects, which have been found to be unusually consistent. However, the effect seems to be limited to rather special types of memory task, which have very few direct counterparts outside the laboratory. It is possible that the effect in these tasks reflects a disruption of working memory by irrelevant speech, which may be of relevance in several other tasks with a high memory load (see review in [40]).

Proofreading and similar verbal tasks

Proofreading requires abilities that are in one way or another of importance in many real work tasks. Noise has rather consistently been found to impair performance of such tasks [40]. This has been true both when the noise has been recorded noise from office machinery and when it has been irrelevant speech. Similar results have been obtained when the comprehension of the text was tested by asking questions about the content.

Two features of the results from studies of irrelevant speech are particularly important. One is that meaningful speech generally causes the greatest impairment, but meaningless speech and music with lyrics have also been found to impair performance. The other finding is that the sound level of the speech is of no importance for the effect.

Calculation

A diary study [48] indicated that calculation tasks were the ones most sensitive to noise disturbance, according to the employees themselves.

Complex office types of tasks

Schönpflug and Schulz made extensive analyses of office tasks and developed laboratory simulations of more complex office tasks. The aim of these studies has been to analyse how such noise and other loads influence the way such tasks are performed. These studies are reviewed in [49].

In a typical task in these studies, subjects are presented with a problem of a type common for office workers (e.g. the application of a loan) and have to make a choice among alternative decisions. To reach a correct decision the subject needs supplementary information, which he has the possibility to order. Such tasks of varying difficulty have been studied during exposure to different levels of noise. A main conclusion from these studies is that noise constitutes a load while performing these tasks and that subjects cope with this load in two ways. They try either to compensate for the noise load by working harder, or they make more risky decisions. The effect is the same as the fatigue effect found after prolonged work; a shift from a high-effort, low-risk to a low-effort, high-risk strategy.

Under time pressure noise the number of erroneous decisions also increased, i.e. the compensation for the noise effects was sometimes incomplete. Performance efficiency was found to be impaired by the 50–60 dB level, but was more pronounced at 70–80 dB.

After-effects of work in noise

One indication of the increased effort exerted during work in noise is the after-effects of work in noise, which has been demonstrated in a long series of laboratory experiments. A review of these studies is given in [50]. The tasks that seem to be most sensitive to these after-effects of noise do not primarily measure the capacity to perform, but rather the motivation to perform well, for example endurance in insoluble or very dull tasks. In contrast to the acute effects, after-effects have been found to be very reliable. It is also to be noted that an acute effect during exposure is not a prerequisite for these after-effects. The only study demonstrating after-effects of noise at work dealt with groups exposed to very high noise levels [36]. The after-effects are most evident after exposure to uncontrolled or unpredictable noise, whereas they are less dependent on the noise level.

Conclusions

The effects of noise on performance have to our knowledge never been demonstrated in a convincing way on a real work performance, definitely not for noise levels below 90 dB(A). Conclusions concerning the risk for such effects therefore must rest upon laboratory studies. These studies indicate that even moderate levels of noise may impair the performance of many tasks, and that the risk is higher for more complex types of tasks. Many of the effects could be interpreted as the result of an attempt to cope with an increased load and the associated reduction of the available information processing capacity. The strategy chosen is the one that is likely to guarantee an acceptable performance under normal working conditions. The preparedness for deviations from these conditions is likely to be impaired.

The effects of irrelevant speech indicate that speech has a privileged access to our attention, and that it is particularly difficult for us to screen off these sounds. The effects of this intrusiveness of speech are most pronounced in verbal tasks.

The demonstrated effects on performance in the laboratory do not mean that performance in real workplaces is likely to be impaired by the noise, but it is a strong indication that noise constitutes a load when performing some types of tasks. The way in which a person chooses to cope with the increased load caused by the noise, however, is highly dependent on the situation. In some situations one is likely to accept a deteriorated performance, whereas in other situations everything will be done to maintain the performance level.

Critical physical noise characteristics for performance effects of noise

In the studies of performance effects, interest has been concentrated on analyses of how performance is affected by noise and in which tasks such effects are likely to appear. Rather little research has been devoted to studies of the effects of noise characteristics.

Sound level

Sound level is the only physical noise characteristic that has been studied to any extent in connection with performance effects. Broadbent [40] concluded that negative effects on performance were only to be expected at very high levels (> 90–$95\,dB(A)$). This seems to be true for the effects of continuous noise on simple routine tasks. For other types of noise and tasks no such general critical level can be stated. As mentioned above, the effects of speech do not seem to depend on sound level, given that it is high enough for the meaning to be comprehended.

Frequency

Very little is known about how sound frequency affects the performance effects. However, it seems likely that the effects of low- and high-frequency noise on performance are mediated by different mechanisms. Low-frequency noise probably gets its effect by lowering the wakefulness, an effect that takes time to develop. Such an effect should be most evident in repetitive, non-demanding tasks and should primarily lead to slower work. Higher frequency noise is more intrusive and affects performance by competing for attentional resources.

Exposure time

Generally, the effect of noise has been found to increase as a function of time on task. This is not necessarily an effect of exposure time in itself, but is perhaps better described as an effect of working for a long time in noise, i.e. an interaction effect.

Other factors influencing performance effects of noise

Of the factors mentioned in connection with subjective responses, only the individual differences and the information content and predictability of the noise have been the subject of research.

Informational content

As mentioned earlier, the informational content of the speech is probably the main determinant of its intrusiveness and effects on verbal task performance.

Predictability and controllability

Intermittent noise has most often been found to have more a detrimental effect on performance than continuous noise and this effect seems to be accentuated when the time schedule is unpredictable and reduced when the person affected has control of the noise.

Individual differences

The degree of experience with the task at hand is a possible basis for individual differences, which is of interest in the present context. Apparently, noise is more likely to impair the performance of complex than simple tasks. The prevalent explanation of this finding is that the additional load caused by the noise is more critical in a task that demands a great part of the available capacity, than in a task that leaves much spare capacity. This implies that one should be most vulnerable to noise in the early stages of training of a task. This is so, since one important effect of training is that one learns to perform the task with the use of a smaller part of the total capacity. Very little research has, however, been reported on this problem.

Other behavioural effects of noise

Many studies indicate that we behave differently towards each other in noisy environments than otherwise. One obvious reason for this is that noise makes speech communication more difficult, but this does not explain all social effects of noise. Thus, a series of field experiments shows that people tend to be less helpful in noise (a review of these and other studies of social effects is given in [51]). The noise levels used in these studies, however, have in all cases been rather high, and nothing, therefore, is known about possible social effects in offices and other work places with moderate noise levels.

References

1. Malerbi, B. Noise. In *Occupational Health Practice*, 3rd edn. (ed. H.A. Waldron). Butterworth-Heinemann, London (1989)

2. American College of Occupational Medicine Noise and Hearing Conservation Committee. Occupational noise-induced hearing loss. *Journal of Occupational Medicine*, **31**, 996 (1989)

3. National Institutes of Health, Office of Medical Applications of Research, Consensus Conference. Noise and hearing loss. *Journal of the American Medical Association*, **263**, 3185–3190 (1990)

4. Pollak, C.P. The effects of noise on sleep. In *Noise and Health* (ed. T.H. Fay). New York Academy of Medicine, New York (1991)

5. Ashkinaze, B. and Kramer, M.B. The effects of noise on the ear and hearing. In *Noise and Health* (ed. T.H. Fay). The New York Academy of Medicine, New York (1991)

6. Swanson, S.J., Dengerink, H.A., Kondrick, P. *et al*. The influence of subjective factors on temporary threshold shifts after exposure to music and noise of equal energy. *Ear and Hearing*, **8**, 288–291 (1987)

7. Axelsson, A. and Dengerink, A.H. The effects of noise on histological measures of the cochlear vasculature and red blood cells: a review. *Hearing Research*, **31**, 183–191 (1987)

8. International Standardization Organization. *ISO 1999-1990: Acoustics – Determination of Noise Exposure and Estimation of Noise-Induced Hearing Impairment*. ISO, Geneva (1990)

9. Brüel, P.V. and Baden-Kristensen, K. Time constants of various parts of the human auditory system and some of their consequences. In *Time Resolution in Auditory Systems* (ed. A. Michelsen). Springer, Berlin (1985)

10. Axelsson, A. and Barrenäs, M.L. Tinnitus in noise-induced hearing loss. In *Noise-Induced Hearing Loss* (eds A. Dancer, D. Henderson, R.J. Salvi *et al.*). Mosby Year Book, St Louis (1992)

11. Henderson, D., Subramaniam, M. and Boettcher, F.A. Individual susceptibility to noise-induced hearing loss: an old topic revisited. *Ear and Hearing*, **14**, 152–168 (1993)

12. Boettcher, F.A., Gratton, M., Bancroft, B.R. *et al*. Interaction of noise and other agents: recent advances. In *Noise-Induced Hearing Loss* (eds A. Dancer, D. Henderson, R. J. Salvi *et al.*). Mosby Year Book, St Louis (1992)

13. Colletti, V. and Sittoni, W. Noise history, audiometric profile and acoustic reflex responsivity. In *Basic and Applied Aspects of Noise Induced Hearing Loss* (eds R.J. Salvi, D. Henderson, R.P. Hamernik and V. Colletti). Plenum, New York (1986)

14. Casali, J.G. and Berger, E.H. Technology advancement in hearing protection circa 1995: active noise reduction, frequency/amplitude-sensitivity, and uniform attenuation. *American Industrial Hygiene Association Journal*, **57**, 175–185 (1996)

15. Royster, J.D. and Royster, L.H. *Hearing Conservation Programs. Practical Guidelines for Success*. Lewis Publishers, Chelsea, Mich. (1990)

16. Raymond, R.P. Neuroendocrine, immunologic, and gastrointestinal effects of noise. In *Noise and Health* (ed. T.H. Fay). New York Academy of Medicine, New York (1991)

17. deJoy, D.M. The nonauditory effects of noise: review and perspectives for research. *Journal of Auditory Research*, **24**, 123–150 (1984)

18. Rehm, S., Gros, E. and Jansen, G. Effects of noise on health and well-being. *Stress Medicine*, **1**, 183–191 (1985)

19. Abel, S.M. The extra-auditory effects of noise and annoyance: an overview of research. *Journal of Otolaryngology*, Suppl. 1, 1–13 (1990)

20. van Dijk, F.J.H. Epidemiological research on non-auditory effects of occupational noise exposure since 1983. In *Proceedings of the 5th International Congress on Noise as a Public Health Problem*, Vol. 3 (eds B. Berglund and T. Lindvall). Swedish Council for Building Research, Stockholm (1990)

21. Sloan, R.P. Cardiovascular effects of noise. In *Noise and Health* (ed. T.H. Fay). New York Academy of Medicine, New York (1991)

22. Stansfeld, S.A. Noise, noise sensitivity and psychiatric disorder – epidemiological and psychophysiological studies. *Psychological Medicine*, (Suppl. 22), 44pp. (1992)

23. Smith, A.P. A review of the non-auditory effects of noise on health. *Work and Stress*, **5**, 49–62 (1991)

24. International Standardization Organization. *ISO/DIS 9921-1: Ergonomic Assessment of Speech Communication – Part 1: Speech Interference Level and Communication Distance for Persons with Normal Hearing Capacity in Direct Communication (SIL Method)*. ISO, Geneva (1990)

25. International Standardization Organization. *ISO/DIS 9921-2: Ergonomic Assessment of Speech Communication – Part 2: Assessment of Speech Communication by Means of the Modified Articulation Index (MAI Method)*. ISO, Geneva (1990)

26. Pearsons, K.S. Review of relevant research on noise and speech communication since 1983. In *Proceedings of the 5th International Congress on Noise as a Public Health Problem*, Vol. 3 (eds B. Berglund and T. Lindvall). Swedish Council for Building Research, Stockholm (1990)

27. Webster, J.C. Noise and communication. In *Noise and Society* (eds D.M. Jones and A.J. Chapman). John Wiley, New York (1984)

28. Kjellberg, A. and Landström, U. Noise in the office: Part II – The scientific basis (knowledge base) for the guide. *International Journal of Industrial Ergonomics*, **14**, 93–118 (1994)

29. Kryter, K.D. *The Effects of Noise on Man*. Academic Press, New York (1985)

30. Carterette, E.C. and Friedman, M.P. *Handbook of Perception*, Vol. 4, *Hearing*. Academic Press, New York (1968)

31. Weinstein, N.D. Community noise problems: evidence against adaptation. *Journal of Environmental Psychology*, **2**, 87–97 (1982)

32. Keighley, E.C. and Parkin, P.H. Subjective responses to sound conditioning in a landscaped office. *Journal of Sound and Vibrations*, **64**, 313–323 (1979)

33. Graeven, D.B. Necessity, control and predictability of noise as determinants of noise annoyance. *Journal of the Social psychology*, **95**, 86–90 (1975)

34. Kjellberg, A., Landström, U., Tesarz, M. *et al.* The effects of non-physical noise characteristics, ongoing task and noise sensitivity on annoyance and distraction due to noise at work. *Journal of Environmental Psychology*, **10**, 123–136 (1996)

35. Sörensen, S. On the possibilities of changing the annoyance reaction to noise by changing the attitudes to the source of annoyance. *Nordisk Hygienisk Tidskrift*, (Suppl. 1), 76 pp. (1970)

36. Kjellberg, A., Sköldström, B., Andersson, P. *et al.* Fatigue effects of noise among airplane mechanics. *Work and Stress*, **16**, 62–71 (1996)

37. Jones, D.M. and Davies, D.R. Individual and group differences in the response to noise. In *Noise and Society* (eds D.M. Jones and A.J. Chapman). Wiley, Chichester (1984)

38. Weinstein, N.D. Individual differences in critical tendencies and noise annoyance. *Journal of Sound and Vibration*, **68**, 241–248 (1980)

39. Broadbent, D.E. Human performance and noise. In *Handbook of Noise Control* (ed. C.M. Harris). McGraw-Hill, New York (1979)

40. Jones, D. Recent advances in the study of human performance in noise. *Environment International*, **16**, 447–458 (1990)

41. Smith, A. A review of the effects of noise on human performance. *Scandinavian Journal of Psychology*, **30**, 185–206 (1989)

42. Bohlin, G. Monotonous stimulation, sleep onset and habituation of the orienting reaction. *Electroencephalography and Clinical Neurophysiology*, **31**, 593–601 (1971)

43. Landström, U., Lundström, R. and Byström, M. Exposure to infrasound – perception and changes in wakefulness. *Journal of Low Frequency Noise and Vibration*, **2**, 1–11 (1983)

44. Wilkins, P.A. and Acton, W.I. Noise and accidents – a review. *Annals of Occupational Hygiene*, **25**, 249–260 (1982)

45. Broadbent, D.E. and Little, E.A.J. Effects of noise reduction in a work situation. *Occupational Physiology*, **34**, 133–140 (1960)

46. Noweir, M.H. Noise exposure as related to productivity, disciplinary actions, absenteeism, and accidents among textile workers. *Journal of Safety Research*, **15**, 163–174 (1984)

47. Cohen, A. The influence of a company hearing conservation program on extra-auditory problems in workers. *Journal of Safety Research*, **8**, 146–162 (1976)

48. Purcell, A.T. and Thorne, R.H. An alternative method for assessing the psychological effects of noise in the field. *Journal of Sound and Vibration*, **55**, 533–544 (1977)

49. Schönpflug, W. Coping efficiency and situational demands. In *Stress and Fatigue in Human Performance* (ed. R. Hockey). Wiley, New York (1983)

50. Cohen, S. Aftereffects of stress on human performance and social behavior: a review of research and theory. *Psychological Bulletin*, **88**, 82–108 (1980)

51. Cohen, S. and Spacapan, S. The social psychology of noise. In *Noise and Society* (eds D.M. Jones and A.J. Chapman). Wiley, Chichester (1984)

Chapter 19

Psychosocial factors in the work environment – an occupational medicine perspective

T Theorell

Individual and work environment – general models

Psychological and physiological reactions that underlie the association between the psychosocial work environment and health are founded on an interplay between individual and environment. *Figure 19.1* (abbreviated from Levi and Kagan, in [1]) summarizes this interplay. The individual's way of reacting and responding (*individual programme*) to the environment is built both on genetics and on previous experiences during upbringing and adulthood. Furthermore, the way of responding is constantly changing due to his/her experiences. Accordingly, the dynamic interplay between individual and environment is the basis of the individual programme, or *coping strategies*. The most recent twin research has tried to elucidate the relative contributions of genetics, childhood experiences and adult experiences to the individual programme. It has shown that all these categories of factors are important to individual programmes, but also that the relative contributions of the three vary according to which part of the programme we are discussing.

The work environment only represents one part of the total environment of human beings, but a very important part of the societal structure surrounding the individual in western countries has been built around paid work. It could be argued that paid work is performed only during 8 hours a day for 5 days a week, that many days during the working year are holidays and vacations and also that most of us work only between the ages 18 and 65. Quantitatively, therefore, family activities and leisure time should be more important than paid work. However, paid work has such a central

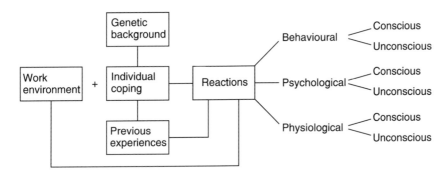

Figure 19.1 Theoretical model of the interaction between the environment, the individual and his or her reactions (from Kagan and Levi [37] and Theorell [38], by permission)

importance to self-esteem and societal roles that the importance of it goes far beyond the proportion of our lives that we spend in it. There are also studies which point at the adverse effects of a bad work situation on parents. According to these observations, a frustrated parent may influence his/her child in a negative way and hence the work situation has an important effect also across generations.

During recent years there have been efforts to describe to what extent and in what ways psychosocial factors at work may influence health. This work has been complicated because there has been no accepted theoretical model according to which the work environment should be described. Recently, however, a few such models have been developed of relevance to the relationship between the work environment and health. Furthermore, evaluations of changes in work conditions, in particular work organization, have been described in the literature. Psychosocial factors are beginning to be incorporated as part of occupational medicine in many countries.

Theoretical models for studying the psychosocial work environment

Several theoretical models for the study of the relationships between psychosocial environment and health have been introduced. Such models could be divided into those which are based upon a general theory and those which are based upon observations in practice. The models in the first group are usually based upon few factors and may be generalized to many different situations. These models may be useful for predictions on a group level and for the assessment of the conditions in a work site, but may be less valuable in individual prediction. One of the first general models was the Person Environment Fit that was presented by the Michigan School of Sociology [2]. Cooper's comprehensive theory for describing the psychosocial aspects of white collar work was based upon factor analyses of a number of questions about working conditions and is accordingly a model belonging to the second group [3]. Another division which could be made is between models which are designed to assess the environment in order to provide information for job design, such as the model proposed by Karasek

described below, and those which are designed to facilitate individual prediction and intervention – including both individual and environmental characteristics – such as the Katz–Kahn and Cooper models and Siegrist's effort-reward model (see below).

This chapter concentrates on one of the general models which is environmentally focused. Its concepts were introduced by Karasek. The factors in it do not cover all aspects of the psychosocial work environment. Karasek introduced his demand–control model which was an architect's synthesis of the demand (= 'stress') and the 'lack of control' (sociological) research traditions (Karasek, 1979, in [4]). In generating the concept 'lack of control', or 'lack of decision latitude' as Karasek labelled it, sociologists had been following their traditions. The question was: Is the worker alienated from the work process? It was assumed that the possibility to utilize and develop skills (*skill utilization*), a concept developed in work psychology, was closely related to *authority over decisions*. In factor analysis of responses to questions about work content these two factors mostly go together, and accordingly they have been added to each other to constitute *decision latitude*. The other dimension, psychological demands, included qualitative as well as quantitative demands.

The demand–control model was never intended to explain all work-related illness. Thus, there was no element of individual variation introduced into its original construction. On the contrary, the model dealt with the way in which work is organized, and the way in which this relates to frequency of illness conditions among workers. This simplicity has made the model useful in organizational work. A model which tries to explain 'all of the variance' has to be more complicated and may be scientifically more but educationally less successful than the simple model that was introduced.

According to the model (*Figures 19.2* and *19.3*), there is interaction between high psychological demands and low decision latitude. If demands are regarded as the *x*-axis and decision latitude as the *y*-axis in a two-dimensional system and the different combinations of high–low demands and high–low decision latitude are regarded, four combinations are recognized. The high demand–low decision latitude combination – *job strain* – is regarded as the most dangerous one in relation to illness development. According to the theory, this kind of situation, if prolonged and repeated for a long time, increases sympathoadrenal arousal and

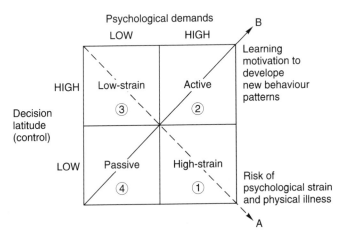

Figure 19.2 Psychological demand/decision latitude model (from Karasek [39], by permission of *Administrative Science Quarterly* © 1979 by Cornell University)

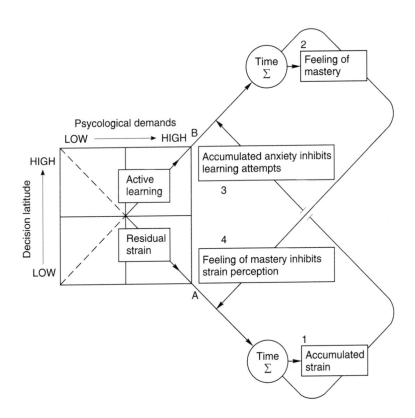

Figure 19.3 Dynamic associations linking environmental strain and learning to evolution of personality (from Karasek and Theorell [4], by permission)

at the same time decreases anabolism, the body's ability to restore and repair tissues.

A combination of high psychological demands and high decision latitude has been labelled an *active* situation. In this situation the worker has more possibility to cope with high psychological demands because he/she can choose to plan working hours according to his/her own biological rhythm and also get good possibilities to develop good coping strategies – facilitating feeling of mastery and control in unforeseen situations. The low demand–high decision latitude situation (relaxed) is theoretically the ideal – *relaxed* – one, whereas the low demand–low decision latitude situation which is labelled *passive* may be associated with risk of loss of skills and to some extent psychological atrophy.

Empirical tests

Karasek's original hypothesis, that excessive psychological demands interact with lack of decision latitude in generating an increased risk of cardiovascular disease, has been tested in a number of epidemiological studies (see [4] and [5]).

A recent epidemiological study in Sweden [6], using one of the aggregated methodologies, is of some interest. In this study a large number of cases of myocardial infarction were identified by means of the nationwide Swedish death register and by means of county registers including hospitalizations. Referents stratified with regard to gender, age and geographical area were selected randomly from the population. Analyses were confined to 'occupationally stable' subjects who stayed in the same occupation during the two most recent censuses (which were 5 years apart) and to those who had a first myocardial infarction (in contrast to subsequent infarctions). *Table 19.1* shows the results for men below age 65 and below age 55 as well as for women below 65. Each of the available questions that are usually included in the demand and decision latitude scores has been displayed separately. The results are typical for this kind of study, with stronger age-adjusted relative risks among the younger men. The expected pattern with the strongest relative risk in the strain quadrant is observed. In men below age 55, relative risks for coronary heart disease development associated with job-strain jobs (inferred indirect measures) between 1.2 and 2.0 have been found. With self-reported data, relative risks in the order

or 1.4–4.0 have been found. Only 4 of 20 studies of men have shown clearly negative results. Three of these studies were made on relatively old men, among whom these associations are inconsistent and weak. One of the reasons for the attenuated relationship in these older men is that many of them have retired during the follow-up period, and accordingly they have not been exposed to the adverse environments during part of the time. The fourth study [7] was based upon a sample of men and women who had gone through coronary angiography. It is difficult to make generalized conclusions from a study of a group that has been recruited in that way.

Women have been less well examined than men with regard to the relationship between job strain and coronary heart disease. A recent study of women employed in health care showed, however, that the combination of self-reported high psychological demands and low decision latitude was associated with high systolic and diastolic blood pressure during working hours (but not during leisure time) – even after adjustment for overweight, moods, age and family history [8]. This finding is in line with other studies of blood pressure during work activities that have been performed with men [9]. For a review, see [5].

A small 5-year clinical follow-up study of men in Stockholm below age 45 who had suffered a myocardial infarction indicated that returning to a job perceived as psychologically demanding and with low decision latitude (particularly low intellectual discretion) may be associated with increased risk of reinfarction death. This was true even after adjustment for biomedical risk factors, degree of coronary atherosclerosis, type A behaviour and education. This finding emphasized the potential importance of this research to cardiovascular rehabilitation.

Research findings with regard to accepted lifestyle risk factors (smoking, diet, etc.) in relation to job strain are ambiguous. Some studies but not all have shown relationships between lifestyle and job strain. One plausible explanation of the relationship between job strain and cardiovascular illness risk may be the effect of a low decision latitude on catecholamine output, and a relationship between deteriorating job strain and decreasing testosterone levels in plasma, possibly reflecting decreasing anabolism, has also been shown. A possible mediating mechanism behind this may be the observed effect of job strain on sleep disturbance – undisturbed deep sleep is of central importance to anabolic processes. In the case of

Table 19.1 Relative risk (RR) with 95% confidence interval (CI) of a first mycardial infarction for participants who did not change type of occupation between 1970 and 1975 in different types of occupations

	Type of occupation[a]							
	Low strain[b]		Active		Passive		High strain	
Hectic work combined with:	RR^c	*95% CI*	RR^c	*95% CI*	RR^c	*95% CI*	RR^c	*95% CI*
Men 30–64 years								
Monotony	1.0	—	1.0	0.9–1.0	1.2	1.1–1.3	1.2	1.1–1.4
Few possibilities to learn new things	1.0	—	1.0	0.9–1.1	1.2	1.1–1.3	1.3	1.2–1.5
Low influence on planning of work	1.0	—	1.0	0.9–1.2	1.2	1.1–1.3	1.3	1.2–1.5
Low influence on work tempo	1.0	—	1.0	0.9–1.1	1.2	1.1–1.3	1.2	1.1–1.3
Low influence on working hours	1.0	—	1.0	0.9–1.1	1.2	1.1–1.3	1.3	1.2–1.5
Men 30–54 years								
Monotony	1.0	—	0.9	0.8–1.1	1.1	1.0–1.4	1.2	1.0–1.5
Few possibilities to learn new things	1.0	—	1.0	0.8–1.2	1.3	1.1–1.6	1.4	1.2–1.7
Low influence on planning of work	1.0	—	1.1	0.9–1.3	1.3	1.0–1.6	1.6	1.2–2.0
Low influence on work tempo	1.0	—	1.0	0.8–1.2	1.1	0.9–1.4	1.2	1.0–1.5
Low influence on working hours	1.0	—	1.1	0.9–1.3	1.1	0.9–1.7	1.5	1.2–1.8
Women 30–64 years								
Monotony	1.0	—	1.4	1.0–2.0	1.3	1.0–1.8	1.4	1.0–1.9
Few possibilities to learn new things	1.0	—	1.2	0.9–1.5	1.4	1.1–1.8	1.3	1.1–1.6
Low influence on planning of work	1.0	—	1.0	0.7–1.4	1.2	1.0–1.6	1.3	1.1–1.6
Low influence on work tempo	1.0	—	1.1	0.8–1.6	0.9	0.5–1.5	1.1	1.0–1.3
Low influence on working hours	1.0	—	1.1	0.8–1.5	1.1	0.8–1.5	1.2	1.0–1.4

Dashes indicate data not available. From 'Job Characteristics and Incidence of Myocardial Infarction,' by N. Hammar, L. Alfredsson & T. Theorell, 1994, *International Journal of Epidemiology*, **28**, p. 281. Copyright 1994 by Oxford University Press. Reprinted with permission.
aThe basis for classficiation of type of occupation was as follows. The job was above or below median in the proportion reporting low strain: below for hectic work and above for decision latitude; active: above for hectic work and for decision latitude; passive: below for hectic work and for decision latitude; high strain: above for hectic work and below for decision latitude.
[b]Reference category.
[c]Relative risk adjusted for age, county, and calendar year.

job strain in bus drivers, it is also possible that frightening traffic with high demands and serious constraint may cause worsening iterated psychophysiological arousal that may contribute to the observed excess risk of myocardial infarction in this occupational group [10].

Introduction of social support to the model

There are two recent developments in this field. First, Johnson and co-workers have included social support in the theoretical models. A study of cardiovascular disease prevalence in a large random sample of Swedish men and women indicated that the joint action of high demands and lack of

control (decision latitude) is of particular importance to blue-collar men, whereas the joint action of lack of control and lack of support was more important for women and white-collar men in this study. The multiplicative interaction between all the three (iso-strain) was tested in a 9-year prospective study of 7000 randomly selected Swedish working men. Interestingly, for the most favoured 20% of men (low demands, good support, good decision latitude) the progression of cardiovascular mortality with increasing age was slow and equally so in the three social classes. In blue-collar workers, however, the age progression was much steeper in the worst iso-strain group than it was in the corresponding iso-strain group in white-collar workers.

Lack of social support has also been shown to have psychophysiological correlates. For instance, those who report low social support at work have a high heart rate throughout the day and night, and furthermore a decreasing social support at work has been shown to be associated with rising systolic blood pressure levels during working hours in a longitudinal study.

Social support and decision latitude at work are two concepts that are closely related. As has been pointed out by Johnson, workers can improve the possibility to control their work situation if they can organize collective action. This is possible if there is good social interaction between workmates – good social support can help collective control. It should be pointed out that social support at work is to a great extent related to work organization. For instance, various ways of remunerating work can facilitate or aggravate social support.

Working life career

Secondly, attempts are now being made to use the occupational classification systems in order to describe the 'psychosocial work career'. Researchers have pointed out that an estimate of work conditions only at one point of time may provide a very imprecise estimation of the total exposure to adverse conditions. Descriptions of all the occupations during the whole work career are obtained for the participants. Occupational scores are subsequently used for a calculation of the 'total lifetime exposure'. The 'total job control exposure' in relation to 9-year age-adjusted cardiovascular mortality in working Swedes was studied. It was observed for men that the cardiovascular mortality differences between the lowest and highest quartiles were close to twofold even after adjustment for age, smoking habits and physical exercise [11]. Furthermore, it has recently been observed that the decision latitude inferred from job titles during each one of the 10 years preceding a first myocardial infarction in 45–54 year old men in Sweden [5] shows a significantly more negative development than in comparable men without myocardial infarction. Decreasing decision latitude could accordingly be associated with increased risk of developing a myocardial infarction in this age when men do not expect to have decreasing decision latitude. Accordingly, the career aspect may be of importance.

Musculo-Skeletal disorders

Another example of a research field that has been exploring the demand–control–support model is that of locomotor disorders. Several studies (unfortunately mostly cross-sectional) have provided data regarding the association between the perceived psychosocial work environment and risk of disorders in neck, shoulders and lower back. The findings are diverging in the sense that in some psychological demands, in others decision latitude and in others social support are important. This may simply reflect the differences in exposure to adverse conditions in different groups. Furthermore, in the case of such disorders we are dealing with less easily defined conditions and it is sometimes difficult to disentangle different levels in a causal chain. In a recent study by our group, psychological demands were shown to be strongly associated with sleep disturbance, high plasma cortisol levels, self-reported muscle tension and with pain in the musculo-skeletal system.

Recent psychophysiological studies of monotonous work have indicated that the ergonomic loads typical of this kind of work elicit increased electrical muscle activity. However, when psychological loads are added, the electrical muscle activity increases considerably [12]. This illustrates that psychological and physical demands may interact in complex ways in generating such disorders.

A recent study by our group has shown that pain threshold may be related to the demand–control–support model in a very complex way. Randomly selected men and women were asked to complete questions about these dimensions in the description of their work. Their pain thresholds were measured on six different points in the neck and shoulders. Our analyses indicated that as expected the pain threshold increased during acute stress, that those who reported a habitually high level of psychological demands at work had higher pain thresholds than others (i.e. were less pain sensitive than others) and finally that those who reported a low level of decision latitude in their habitual working situation had a lower pain threshold during experimental stress than others. The interpretation of these findings is very difficult. It seems plausible that subjects with high psychological demand levels who mobilize energy to be able to meet demands may also repress feelings of pain. This may increase risks of long-term development of pathological changes in locomotor tissues. On the other hand, it is also plausible to assume that long-term exposure to low decision latitude may increase the risk of depression and that this could explain why subjects who describe their jobs in these terms are unable to raise their pain thresholds during periods of acute stress.

Other somatic symptoms have also been investigated in relation to job strain. It has been shown that functional gastrointestinal symptoms increase as job strain increases, and non-ulcer dyspepsia has also been related to job strain in defined populations. A recent study has shown that spontaneous recovery in male patients with non-ulcer dyspepsia is associated with social support at work – those with a good support show spontaneous recovery during a 1-month follow-up to a greater extent than other men [13].

Working hours

Several recent studies have indicated that long-lasting exposure to shift work, in particular constant rotation between day and night work, is associated with an increased risk of developing coronary heart disease. Underlying mechanisms could be direct physiological effects of compensatory arousal of the sympathoadrenal system arising because of chronic lack of sleep, resulting in high catecholamine output, or effects on relevant lifestyle variables (e.g. cigarette smoking). One study has also shown that carbohydrate intake during night shifts has more adverse effects on serum lipoprotein levels than the same intake during day hours. Thus, some of the risk could be due to complex interaction between disturbed circadian rhythm and eating habits.

Long working hours have been suspected of causing increased coronary risk. The risk seems to be different for men and women, respectively. While men in jobs with moderately increased working hours have no increased coronary risk, women have been reported to be at elevated coronary risk when the working week exceeds 50 h/week (see [4]). For men, the risk seems to increase at higher levels of overtime work. The classical work by Hinkle and colleagues [14] showed that men who were working full time in the Bell Telephone Company and at the same time attended night college were running an elevated age-adjusted risk of dying a coronary death. Extremely long working hours have been shown in other studies to be associated with increased risk. Japanese workers (see [15]) frequently have very long working hours and also long commuting distances. Death (in most cases probably coronary deaths) from long working hours, *Karoshi,* has been described. Ongoing research in Japan will show how frequent this mode of death may be.

Social reward

There are several theoretical models that are useful in the study of the psychosocial work environment. In addition to the Person Environment Fit and Cooper's model for exploration of the work environment, Siegrist and co-workers have shown in three different studies that the concept lack of social reward may also be useful in the study of coronary risk in working men. Combinations of excessive individual effort, chronic stressors and lack of social reward are associated with considerably increased coronary risk. According to the theory presented by Siegrist [16], the development of risk should be regarded as a long-term process. In the first phase, in the young worker, *vigilance* is the characteristic feature. The worker wants to show his/her ambition and therefore becomes involved in a large amount of tasks. In the next phase, *immersion,* all the different tasks have started colliding and the worker has difficulties to limit the load which grows exponentially. In the next phase, biomedical risk factors have become evident and in the final phase illness develops.

Work environment and personality

Several researchers have emphasized the importance of individual, more basic psychological characteristics. Ursin and other Norwegian researchers, for instance, have emphasized the importance of psychological defence mechanisms interacting with job stressors in the aetiology of psychophysiological responses. They have tested the relationship between job stressors and self-reported muscle tension and have been able to show that the relationships are different in different occupational groups. Thus, according to these researchers it is not the same job stressors that cause neck and shoulder tension in firemen as in office workers. Other studies from this group show that psychological defence mechanisms influence these relationships. Their interpretations of these findings are made according to cognitive psychology, emphasizing that it is the interpretation of stressors that creates the basis for psychophysiological reactions [17].

Despite the general notion that individual psychological characteristics interact with job stressors in generating psychophysiological reactions, there is no indication that personality in general can 'explain away' the relationships between psychosocial job factors and illness. For instance, it has been shown [18] that the personality traits that are of relevance to the development of coronary heart disease are not more common among subjects who report job strain than in other workers.

Physiological reactions

Apart from the fact that there are effects of the work environment on lifestyle factors and willingness to adopt 'healthy habits' (poor work environment may decrease the willingness among employees to follow health advice), several physiological mechanisms could explain the relationships that have been discussed above between psychosocial work environment and health. A work situation that evokes a feeling of frustration due to 'isostrain' is associated with mobilization of energy – *catabolism* – and at the same time decreased *anabolism*. Anabolic processes stimulate repairing and restoration of bodily tissues and are therefore of central importance to vulnerability to the development of somatic illness. This is a generalized phenomenon since all tissues need anabolism. In the immune system, white blood cells are rapidly worn out and need to be replaced. In the gastrointestinal system, cells in the mucosa are worn out. The muscles are constantly being rebuilt to make it possible for the body to adapt itself to changing patterns in the musculo-skeletal system.

Long-lasting exposure to a given type of job stressors gives rise to a series of regulatory and structural changes. In animal research it has been shown that certain cells in the hippocampus, which is part of the stress regulatory system in the brain, actually show atrophy during long-lasting stress. Certain kinds of gene expression become gradually more obvious when a stressor becomes long lasting. One of the consequences of this is that the synthesis of thyroid hormones may accelerate. Another equally important consequence is that the regulation of cortisol production may change. Normally the corticotrophic releasing factor (CRF) in the hypothalamus stimulates the hypophysis to secrete the adrenocorticotrophic

hormone (ACTH) which influences the adrenal cortex to secrete cortisol. When the blood concentration of cortisol becomes elevated, the secretion of CRF is inhibited. This interplay between positive and negative influences on the hypothalamic pituitary adrenocortical system is of great importance to our survival. Disturbance of it results in serious bodily problems. For instance, the sensitivity to cortisol increases during long-term exposure to severe stressors, as in post-traumatic stress disorders (PTSD). This is due to both an increased number of cortisol receptors on the cell surfaces in the body and to increased sensitivity of each one of the receptors. Perhaps as a consequence of this and the feedback system, the typical finding in PTSD is low blood concentrations of cortisol during 'normal' conditions [19].

In major depression, CRF is secreted in large amounts and the secretion does not seem to be influenced in the normal way by the high plasma cortisol levels that the high CRF activity leads to. In chronic fatigue, one of the problems may be low CRF activity.

In many physiological situations, the stimulation of energy mobilization is paralleled by inhibition of anabolism.

One example illustrating the difference between long-lasting and short exposure is the observation that the concentration of immunoglobulins tends to increase when there is a temporary worsening of the job conditions during a number of weeks – but also decrease when there is chronic exposure to such conditions. A simplified interpretation of these conflicting observations is that some of the physiological systems are activated during periods requiring extraordinary effort. If the adverse conditions become very long lasting (several months), physiological resources may be emptied or some kind of physiological adaptation takes place. This has been observed to be true also for blood pressure reactions – in persons who have been living with long-lasting stressors the magnitude of the blood pressure response to an experimental stressor is attenuated [20].

Physiological measurements

Continuous recording of the electrocardiogram could be made, for instance, during 24 hours. This provides information about heart rate variability and prevalence of cardiac arrhythmias. Both of these parameters reflect the balance between the sympathetic and parasympathetic activity and they have been used extensively in explorations of the work environment (e.g. of the relationship between social support at work and heart rate [21]). By means of diaries it is possible to relate the variations to real events in the working situation.

The electroencephalogram has been used extensively in the study of wakefulness and tiredness during working hours and in studies of the relationship between shift work schedules and quality of sleeping patterns (e.g. [21]).

The electromyogram is used extensively in the study of muscle tensions arising in the working environment. It has been shown that both physical and mental loads in cashiers may contribute to this association. Blood pressure may be recorded during working hours by means of fully automated equipment (which could record blood pressure by means of a portable machine that institutes and stores blood pressure measurements at regular intervals, for instance every 20th minute). It may also be recorded by means of self-triggered apparatus. The fully automated equipment has the advantage that the subjects may not influence the measurements themselves, but on the other hand the disadvantage that subjects may become distressed by the frequent sound and discomfort that is caused by the measurements. This may in itself cause elevation of the blood pressure. It also has the disadvantage that the person should not contract his/her arm muscles during the measurements. Some equipment produces a sound that forewarns of the measurement. This enables the person to avoid muscle contraction during the measurement but may, on the other hand-contribute to the sympathic arousal. The self-triggered measurements may be more subject to measurement bias, since the subject makes the notations himself/herself. We have found, however, that self-triggered measurements may work satisfactorily in many subjects and also that the self-triggered measurements themselves have an educational role.

Endocrinological and metabolic measurements

Blood

The blood is close to many effector receptors and is therefore of great interest as a target for measurements. Blood sampling requires a licensed nurse or similar person. Venous blood is mostly sampled. In order to avoid psychological arousal caused by the blood sampling itself, it is frequently possible to insert a venous catheter. After half an hour of resting the subject is mostly in a sufficiently 'basal' state to make measurements of endocrinological parameters in venous samples taken from the catheter meaningful.

Endocrinological parameters that fluctuate rapidly, such as catecholamines, should be measured on many occasions at short intervals. This is true, for instance, of adrenaline and noradrenaline which fluctuate so rapidly that measurements during work activities in the field are meaningless. Hormones or metabolic factors which fluctuate more slowly are more meaningful to measure. This is true, for instance, of thyroid hormones as well as glycated haemoglobin (Hb A 1 C) which may reflect long-term changes in energy mobilization. Cortisol and adrenocorticotrophic hormone, which reflect reactions aiming at the amelioration of distressing bodily reactions, have intermediately slow reaction patterns. Most endocrine factors show strong circadian variations, which is important to bear in mind when a study is planned in the work site. Cortisol shows peak levels during the early morning hours and reaches relatively low levels in the afternoon. Furthermore, as pointed out above, chronic stress may be associated with lowered cortisol levels.

Immunoglobulins, in particular immunoglobulin G, fluctuate rather slowly. These reflect in a crude way the activity of the immune system (see, for instance, [23]). Measurements of the cellular activity in white blood cells are of more interest biologically, since they mirror in a more direct way the activity in the immune system, but these require more resources and time because fresh total blood has to be taken care of immediately after sampling.

There are also hormones which reflect anabolic activity, for instance testosterone, dehydroandrosterone (DHEA) and oestrogen, that show relatively slow fluctuations and could therefore be studied in a meaningful way in relation to changes in working conditions.

One other hormone which reflects changes in the brain's dopamine and serotonin activity, namely prolactin, has been studied extensively. High levels during adverse psychosocial conditions may reflect feelings of depression and powerlessness (see [24]).

Measurements of the concentration in saliva may sometimes replace the measurement of hormone concentration in blood. In this case, repeated samples have to be taken and only some hormones, mainly steroids (e.g. cortisol and testosterone or immunoglobulins) could be analysed.

Urine has the advantage that the measurements could be integrated over defined time periods. Subjects have to be instructed carefully with regard to the collection of urine. One problem is the large interindividual variation in catecholamine excretion. One way of decreasing the influence of this source of variation in the study of working environments is to make measurements both during work and during leisure. The same hours of the circadian cycle are studied and the measurement during leisure hours is used as a reference. The measurement of the excretion of adrenaline and noradrenaline has been used extensively in the analysis of work environments and has been shown to be useful.

The classical work of Levi, for instance, showed that in particular the excretion of free adrenaline in urine is a very sensitive indicator of sympatho-adrenomedullary arousal. In general, longitudinal changes in relation to changes in the work situation are more easily interpreted than cross-sectional comparisons between two groups on one occasion. Studies by Frankenhaeuser's group [25] have shown that the concomitant study of the urinary excretion of noradrenaline, adrenaline and cortisol is useful. In short-term stress and during laboratory experiments Frankenhaeuser's group has shown that acute stress reactions could be divided according to effort and distress. When subjects react with pronounced effort and distress, a potentially harmful pattern of endocrinological changes occurs with both elevation of catecholamine and cortisol excretion. When a high degree of effort is associated with joy, the reaction is labelled eustress, and this reaction is associated with high catecholamine levels but unchanged or even low cortisol excretion.

Individual and environmental perspectives on the measurements

The psychosocial environment can be recorded in several ways. The conditions may be recorded by external experts who are instructed to observe the conditions either by means of standardized protocols or by means of social anthropological methods. They can also be measured by means of self-reports from the workers themselves. Such self-reports can be recorded either in interviews or in self-administered questionnaires. Both interviews and questionnaires could have fixed-response categories or open-ended questions. Finally, interviews and questionnaires could be standardized on large general populations or adapted to special groups. Interviews may be performed both with individuals and with groups in a work site. Of course, these different forms of measurements provide the researcher with completely different perspectives on the work environment and frequently there is poor correlation between them.

In occupational medicine there is a tradition to work with measures of standard exposures to adverse environmental physical or toxicological factors within different occupations. Such occupational charts have been constructed also for psychosocial factors in Sweden as well as in the USA.

In order to describe how subjects in different occupations with different age and gender and with different duration of exposure to the occupation perceive their work situation, national surveys performed by Statistics Sweden have been utilized [26]. These surveys are based upon interviews with randomly selected working men and women in Sweden. Scores for perceived psychological demands, decision latitude and social support at work have been described for age-, gender- and duration-specific occupational categories. The tables show mean scores for psychological demands, for instance for male carpenters above age 45 who have had 5–19 years of experience in the occupation. Similarly we may find decision latitude means for female licensed nurses below age 45 who have had less than 5 years' experience. This type of background information is of significance in the assessment of stressors that may be common during parts of the career in a specific occupation, but has to be interpreted with due caution when dealing with individuals. In the examples presented it is striking that psychological demands are perceived as high in the beginning of the career for the licensed nurse – this is also the case for other occupations in health care. But it is not true for carpenters, for instance. On the other hand, decision latitude is perceived as good among nurses. Garment stitchers, for instance, perceive their decision latitude as poor.

Observation techniques for the assessment, for instance, of tempo and number of hindrances in a work site have been introduced by German psychologists Hacker [27] and Volpert [28].

These can be used for some kinds of industry work and also in some kinds of offices. In those jobs which include extensive social interaction these techniques are more difficult to use. Number of acts per time unit can reliably be measured, and the tempo in different work sites belonging to the same trade may be compared. The same is true of the number of hindrances, which corresponds to one aspect of lack of authority over decisions. Degree of mental stimulation can also be assessed according to this system. This corresponds to intellectual discretion. In the typical assessment situation, an experienced worker is selected for assessment. He or she is followed in detail during a typical working day, and these observations constitute the basis for the assessment.

In the case of psychological demands, quantitative demands seem to be more objectively measurable than qualitative demands.

When objective measures are compared with questionnaires, the comparison should not be expected to show complete resemblance, since the self-administered questionnaire includes a subjective component. Variables related to decision latitude measured by means of observation and questionnaire, such as the number of hindrances compared to authority over decisions or mental stimulation compared to intellectual discretion, usually show moderate but significant correlations. Several examples of this have been described, such as expert assessments of the work of state employees compared to self-reported decision latitude in England [29], or data based upon national surveys in Sweden indicating inferred decision latitude in the general working population (specific for job title, gender, age and number of years in the occupation). In a recently published study, assessments of decision latitude based upon expert observations and self-reported decision latitude were equally good predictors of sick leave in British civil servants. Thus, the analyses published so far indicate that the objective measurements and the self-reports are related to one another, but that they both reflect relevant pieces of information which are of value in the prediction of health.

For psychological demands, the similarity between objective and subjective assessment seems to be smaller. Significant but small correlations are usually observed. On the whole, several aspects of psychological demands seem to be less robust from the assessment point of view (in comparisons between different work environments).

In case referent studies it may be important to establish whether objective and subjective assessments relate to one another in similar ways among referents and cases. Otherwise recall bias may be a problem.

Some of the dissimilarities between expert observations and self-reports from workers are due to differences in perception between workers. However, another part of the dissimilarities is due to real differences in work contents between individual workers even at the same work site. It is sometimes helpful to separate different work tasks that the individual worker has and to estimate the time spent on each one. Each work task could then be characterized with regard to psychosocial characteristics. The proportion of time spent in these different tasks could differ between workers. A detailed methodology for assessing work contents along these lines has been proposed in [30]. If the components are separated from one another, more reliable observations of work contents could be made than when the total work situation is analysed together. In fact, a high inter-observer reliability has been observed when the work tasks have been separated in this way.

What form of recording/measurement that provides the 'truth' can always be debated. Of course, the individual's own perception of the conditions has the greatest significance to the development of psychosomatic conditions. But on the other hand interviews with individual subjects or self-administered questionnaires may not give the true picture of these perceptions. Denial and other defence mechanisms in the subject as well as social pressure from workmates and superiors and fear of punishment may create systematic errors.

In the preparation for work redesign, the collective function is often the most relevant, and in order to obtain a measure of that function there is need for observations or interviews with groups of subjects. The scientifically most waterproof measurement technique may not always be the one that provides the best starting point in work redesign – in general, interviews with open-ended responses give the employees the most convincing feeling that they are part of the redesign process. This is partly in conflict with a scientifically good recording – to which the employees are not allowed to contribute subjective opinions.

Standardized work environment questionnaires

There are many questionnaires available for the exploration of the psychosocial work environment. Standardized questionnaires have to be supplemented with questions that are specific to the work site and the occupation that is being explored. Furthermore, it has to be determined whether a self-administered questionnaire is really the method of choice in the given situation. Questionnaire information may be meaningless, for instance

- if social pressures are likely ('in this work site we do not complain' or 'those who complain can count on punishment' or 'we have to respond to the questionnaire in such a way that we get rid of this boss')
- if employees are unprepared or unable to analyse their own conditions.

A great advantage of the standardized questionnaires is that it is possible to compare the collected information with that obtained from large reference groups – which may provide answers regarding the relative level of difficulties in the work site studied.

Table 19.2 shows how the indices psychological demands, intellectual discretion, authority over decisions and social support are intercorrelated and how they correlate with a sleep disturbance index and two indices of coping patterns – open and covert coping. For men, a significant albeit rather weak association is observed between demands and decision latitude – when a man has increasing demands he can also expect increasing decision latitude. For women no such relationship is observed. Another gender difference relates to demands and social support. Women who report high psychological demands also tend to report low level of social support at work. This relationship is not seen among men in the study.

It should be pointed out that there are pronounced differences between occupational groups with regard to reported levels of authority over decisions and also for intellectual discretion. Interestingly, both subway train drivers and symphony musicians have very low levels of authority over decisions. Although their work contents are very different and the social context of their working situations is also quite different, they have in common that they are constrained – for the symphony musician music, tempo, inten-

sity and character have been determined by others and for the subway driver there is a time schedule, tracks and very strict rules. The same low level of authority over decisions is reported by men and women. There are also marked (and highly significant) differences between occupational groups with regard to perceived intellectual discretion. Low levels of intellectual discretion are found, for instance, among freight handlers and high levels among physicians. It has been observed that women mostly report lower levels of authority over decisions at work than men – part of this could be due to women's smaller likelihood of becoming promoted to supervising positions [4]. The means for psychological demands also differ significantly between occupational groups, but the differences are much smaller and only a small middle part of the possible range is occupied.

The matrix of psychosocial characteristics of occupations [11] could also be used as an indirect measure of demands, decision latitude and support. Means are available for three-digit occupation codes separately for men and women below and above 45 years of age and for different length of employment (below 5 years, between 5 and 19 years and 20 or more years). An American-constructed matrix similarly is also available [30]. It should be pointed out, with regard to both these matrix systems, that occupations change continuously and that, accordingly, renewal of such tables will become necessary. Furthermore, as the working culture slowly changes, the basic psychosocial concepts may also have to be changed.

A common criticism against the interpretations of the associations between the demand control model and risk of heart disease development has been that the findings actually reflect the well-known differences between social classes with regard to heart disease prevalence. It is true that low decision latitude – the most important component of the model – is a characteristic of low social class jobs. Some of the published analyses have been adjusted for social class and this sometimes reduces the size of the association. It is possible that low decision latitude at work is a key component of low social class. According to this reasoning it is not meaningful to adjust for social class. It should be pointed out that psychological demands follow the opposite social class pattern – high psychological demands are more commonly reported in higher social classes. This may explain some of the inconsistent findings in the field.

Table 19.2   Correlations between self-reported coping patterns and self-reported work environment in randomly selected working men and women in Stockholm ($n = 80$–90 for both groups)

	Open coping	Covert coping	Psychological demands	Intellectual discretion	Authority over decisions	Social support
Men						
Covert coping	−0.16					
Psychological demands	0.07	−0.01				
Intellectual discretion	0.08	0.16	0.28*			
Authority over decisions	0.15	0.07	0.16	0.62*		
Social support	−0.10	−0.13	−0.22*	0.08	0.15	
Age	−0.03	0.13	0.01	0.23*	0.23	0.07
Women						
Covert coping	−0.26*					
Psychological demands	−0.01	0.22*				
Intellectual discretion	0.15	0.17	0.07			
Authority over decisions	0.20*	−0.07	0.01	0.45*		
Social support	−0.04	−0.29*	−0.61*	0.06	0.04	
Age	−0.13	0.16	−0.05	−0.03	0.00	0.05

*Significant at least on the 5% level.
From: 'Flexibility at Work in Relation to Employee Health' by Theorell, T. In *Handbook of Work and Health Psychology*, Schabracq, M.J., Winnubst, J.A.M. and Cooper, C.L. (eds), J. Wiley & Sons Ltd, 147–160 (1996)

Monitoring of medical and physiological consequences of changes in the work situation

Medical and physiological consequences of changes in job conditions can be regarded in several ways. When employees are being followed in a work site and the sequence of changes in the work situation is related to health and physiology, it may be difficult to know what direction observed relationships have. One mostly has to be satisfied with the conclusion that the sequences are parallel. Even so, there are many situations in which the likelihood is great that the changes in the work situation cause the changes in health or physiological state. An effort will be made to illustrate this by means of examples. *Figure 19.4* shows systolic blood pressure levels during working hours and sleep disturbance scores in a group of working men and women who were followed on four occasions during a year. They were asked to fill out questionnaires regarding their working situation. From the responses, the ratio between psychological demands and decision latitude was calculated for every occasion – job strain. Large spontaneous variations were observed. The figures show the average systolic blood pressure (from measures approximately once an hour during working

hours of the studied day) as well as the sleep disturbance score according to the questionnaire for that period. The occasion with the worst ratio (high demands in relation to decision latitude) is to the left and the occasion with the best ratio (low demands in relation to decision latitude) to the right of the diagram. The intermediate occasions are in the middle. A progressive increase in sympathoadrenal activation level as well as in sleep disturbance level is observed with increasing job strain. In this case it is hard to imagine that an elevated systolic blood pressure during activity would cause job strain – the opposite direction seems more likely.

Figure 19.5 shows another example. Plasma prolactin concentrations are shown in male subway drivers who have been exposed to PUT (Person Under Train – a person jumping or falling in front of the train being hurt or killed) experiences 3 weeks, 3 months and 1 year, respectively, following this dramatic accident. This is an event that is unanticipated and impossible to control from the driver's perspective. It causes considerable sleep disturbance during the initial 3 weeks following the event [32] and is associated with temporary elevation of the plasma concentration of prolactin. After 3 months the concentration is lower again. No such changes were seen in a comparison group of drivers who had not been exposed to PUT. Prolactin concentrations in

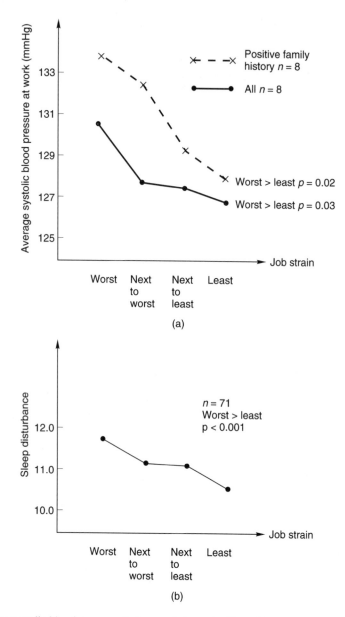

Figure 19.4 (a) Average systolic blood pressure during work hours in 58 working men and women in relation to reported job straining (demand/decision latitude). Observations ranked according to worst–least job strain. Subgroup ($n = 18$) with family history of hypertension (from Theorell [40]). (b) Sleep disturbance index in 71 working men and women in relation to reported job straining (demand/decision latitude). Observations rated according to worst–least job strain (from Theorell [41])

blood co-vary with feelings of powerlessness and passiveness in a crisis [24]. This association is impossible to explain 'backwards' – it is not likely that the person jumped or fell in front of the train because the driver had a high plasma concentration of prolactin. Prolactin in blood is associated with activity in the immune system and with blood pressure regulation. In women, high plasma concentration of prolactin has been found to be associated with high blood pressure during working hours, and an association between job strain and plasma prolactin as well as between job strain and

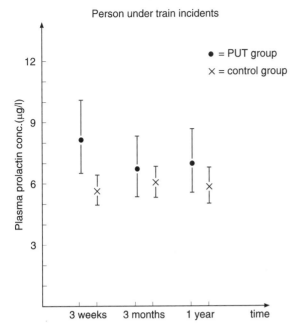

Figure 19.5 Means and 95% confidence intervals of plasma prolactin (µg/l, computations based on logarithms) on each occasion following 'person under train' incidents (PUT) in PUT and control group ($n = 13$ and 15) men who had measurements for all occasions (from Theorell *et al.* [32], by permission)

blood pressure during working hours was also found.

Ways to improve the situation

The ideal sequence of exploration, discussion and improvement of work organization is illustrated in *Figure 19.6* [4]. After consulting key groups (union, management, employees themselves, and occupational health and safety officers), a theory is formulated that is based upon general theory. After exploration of the conditions by means of interviews and/or questionnaires and/or observations, the information is presented to the work site. In the ideal situation there is feedback both to the individuals and to the group. Feedback to the group has to be carefully prepared – if key persons will be criticized they have to be prepared in such a way that they can take the criticism in a constructive way. After this, there will be different opinions regarding what organizational changes should be instituted. If insufficient time and resources have been allotted to this phase, there is considerable risk that no constructive changes will take place and the work site may end up having more conflicts than before the exploration. Accordingly, at the time the exploration is planned the team has to be prepared to devote energy and

time to the process. Follow-up may take a long time – months or years.

Both decision latitude and social support may be improved by means of changes in work organization.

First, improving decision latitude may mean increased job rotation and avoidance of monotonous components in the working process, as well as improved goal formulation resulting in more meaningful work contents (all of these being relevant to intellectual discretion). The possibility of increasing job rotation is well known from practical experiments in the car industry. Instead of traditional assembly line production, which means that every worker is responsible for a very small part of the production, groups are formed that have a collective responsibility for a larger segment of the production of a car. Although such experiments have indicated that productivity may increase and that sick leave rates may decrease (at least in men), there is relatively limited experience so far, and there is no agreement among experts regarding benefits and drawbacks. In the service sector, on the other hand, many practical experiments have been described which indicate the advantages of improved variability and goal formulation.

One example that was evaluated [33] was the experiment at the Enskededalen's home for the elderly, in Sweden. The starting point was the

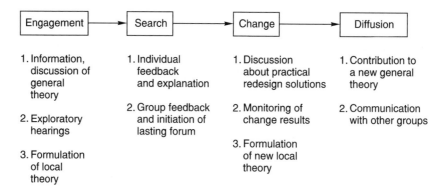

Figure 19.6 Theoretical model of the successful health-orientated job redesign process (from Karasek and Theorell [4], by permission)

work content – how to improve conditions for the elderly tenants? A frequent problem among institutionalized elderly was identified: passivity and social isolation. Part of the reason for this was the way in which the care was organized. The programme consisted of increased emphasis on meaningful social activity. This was achieved by means of the staff's exploration of hobbies and interests in tenants, as well as their exploration of social contacts and discussions between the researchers and the staff regarding the effects of social interaction. The goal was to increase social activity among the tenants. According to the evaluation the tenants increased their social activities more than those in the comparison group. Furthermore, the tenants in the experimental group showed evidence of increasing anabolic physiological activity and decreased energy mobilization (as reflected in carbohydrate metabolism) relative to the subjects in the comparison group. Personnel were followed through this process.

It was shown that sick leave rates and personnel turnover developed more favourably over time in the personnel in the experimental group than in the comparison group (see [4]). Follow-up showed that the personnel in the experimental group had become more focused on social activities and less on instrumental support to the tenants. Therefore, this example could be seen as one piece of evidence that a successful change in goal formulation that was more individualized and perceived as more meaningful by the staff had beneficial effects on turnover and sick leave.

Improving decision latitude may also mean improving democracy by means of decreased hierarchy (relevant to authority over decisions).

Several experiments have been described in which supervisors or foremen changed their function – altering their role from those who made all the decisions to those who had coordinating functions in the interaction between workers and management. One of the most extensively described examples is the Almex study (see [4]). The change in work organization was coupled with a technological computerized change in the work process which made it possible for the workers in the production to be in direct contact with the customers. Thus customers could order, directly from the worker, products that were individually tailored to their needs. This made it possible to change the role of foremen. In this case, the flattened hierarchy resulted in decreased feelings of stress and decreased sick leave despite unchanged workload.

Secondly, one way of improving social support is the institution of organized staff meetings at regular intervals. Such meetings may lead both to improved decision latitude and to improved social support. If the meetings are organized in such a way that the staff are stimulated to find solutions to common problems it may have the effect that mutual understanding increases and thus the social climate improves, but at the same time real improvement in decision latitude may take place. It is necessary, however, for the meetings to be structured – it is not sufficient to devote time to unstructured discussions that may not lead to changes in organizational solutions. An evaluation of the effects of the institution of staff meetings at regular intervals has been published by [34]. Staff meetings were combined with group teaching of problem-solving techniques. Centres at which these changes were started were randomly selected and a group of similar randomly selected wards served as control groups. It was shown that sick leave rates and staff turnover decreased and work motivation increased.

A common experience in organizational work has been that individual focus and collective work should go together. An exploration of the individual's medical and psychological conditions increases the participants' motivation to take part in the collective work. To the contrary, advice regarding individual lifestyle is more likely to be followed by the individuals if the team is also interested in the collective environment.

That mental preparation on all levels in the worksite may be of central importance has been shown in an evaluation of a programme aimed at exploring and subsequently improving collective as well as individual conditions in four different offices. In one of the offices the mental preparation had been good both among supervisors and among personnel. In this group the employees reported good support from superiors both before and during the change process. This worksite was labelled the 'active' worksite. In the other offices the preparation was not as good, and deteriorated support from supervisors was reported during the process. These worksites were labelled 'passive'. Blood concentrations of endocrine factors were followed before, 3 times during and finally 4 months after the end of the change process. *Figure 19.7* shows that the concentration of plasma cortisol rose considerably in the passive group, while decreasing levels were observed as the change process had started in the active group. Since high cortisol levels reflect distress, these findings may illustrate that mental preparation on all levels in the work site may ameliorate distress during the change.

Unemployment

During the present period of high unemployment rates in most countries in the western hemisphere, becoming redundant is one of the major threats of employees. Many research reports were published regarding the effects of unemployment on health during the 1980s. The results of this research have shown that there is pronounced anxiety particularly during the expectancy and the first months of unemployment. The anxiety is reflected in elevated blood concentrations of cortisol and prolactin. There is a slight decrease in anxiety immediately after the start of unemployment, but the level increases again after some weeks. When some additional weeks have passed the prevalence of depression is high, and this is also the phase when suicide rates are elevated. In one study, diminished activity in the immune system has also been shown after a year of unemployment.

Long lasting unemployment has been correlated with elevated blood pressure and lowered blood concentrations of high-density lipoprotein (HDL), the protective cholesterol. There are studies which have shown elevated serum concentrations of total cholesterol after several months of unemployment. In a recent study of shipbuilding workers who became unemployed in Sweden, it was shown that those individuals who reported sleep disturbance and who had a real threat to their financial situation were much more likely than others to have a pronounced elevation of serum total cholesterol [35].

Psychiatric research on the consequences of unemployment has shown that persons who become unemployed often have feelings of shame and guilt even when they have had no role in the redundancy process – for instance when a whole factory has been laid off and all workers became unemployed. It is also evident that the social network is adversely affected by unemployment – this applies even to the social network outside the job. In an unemployment study in southern Sweden in the 1980s, it was found that the contacts with neighbours decreased in subjects who had become unemployed. Obviously persons who do not have an abundance of social contacts in general are more dependent on paid work, since this may be the only social activity of which they may become part. Groups with certain latent problems (e.g. latent alcoholism) suffer more from unemployment than others. Youth unemployment is associated with increased incidence of psychosomatic illness.

During the past 10 years the prevalence of unemployment has been rising in most countries in the western hemisphere. Several studies of the effects of unemployment on health have been published. The development of yearly mortality rates in different countries has shown that rising unemployment is followed by increasing mortality – mainly due to changes in cardiovascular mortality and suicide rates, with or without a delay of one or two years. Opinions are divided regarding the interpretation of such results. It has been emphasized that a rising unemployment rate affects not only those who lose their jobs but also those who

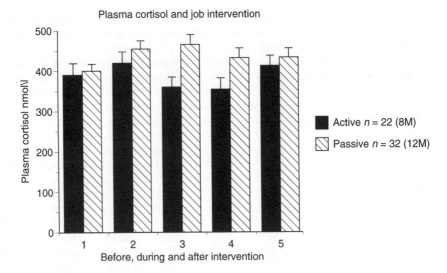

Figure 19.7 Morning levels of plasma cortisol in participants in a psychosocial job intervention on an 'organizationally active' work site (Active) and on three 'organizationally passive' sites (Passive). ANOVA group $p = 0.01$, interaction group time $p = 0.003$ (from Theorell [42], copyright 1993 by John Wiley & Sons, Ltd, England)

remain in the work site. First, those who remain may have to work harder if production is retained with a diminished number of employees, and especially so during a later phase when demands for production increase. This may lead to extreme overload. Secondly, the social climate in the work site may deteriorate, since the decreasing number of jobs enhances the feeling of competition between workmates. This may lead to diminished social support. At the same time, of course, the employees live under the threat of becoming redundant themselves.

Human service occupations

Human service occupations are those in which frequent and/or intense interactions take place between the worker on the one hand and customers, clients or patients on the other. Most workers in these occupations are women (e.g. in the health care sector). Close contacts with other human beings could be regarded both as spice and as poison. According to national surveys of living condition in Sweden, workers in the health care sector, compared to other workers that were comparable with regard to age and gender, perceived their work as psychologically more demanding

and stimulating. The latter finding was mirrored in a low percentage of workers who perceived work as monotonous and non-learning. Long working hours and a high percentage of shift work schedules were reported among health care sector workers. Many human service occupations belong to strict hierarchical organizations, and those in the lower part of this hierarchy (e.g. nursing aides) describe a low possibility of influencing immediate decisions regarding their own work (low authority over decisions).

Close contact with other human beings brings human suffering into focus. In the health care sector, the workers have to take an active, inescapable part in the suffering of others. On the one hand this is stimulating and enables the expansion of coping ability. On the other hand, the close exposure to suffering increases the risk that the worker may develop 'burn-out'.

Burn-out has been described by Maslach as the psychological equivalent of a battery that is not chargeable any more. The worker is not able to become normally engaged in work. Three different components of burn-out have been described:

● *emotional exhaustion*, the inability to experience normal feelings – this results in lack of any kind of emotional reaction to situations that normally arouse depression, anger, anxiety or joy.

- *depersonalization*, the feeling that one is profoundly changed as a person, not the same as one was used to being.
- *lack of personal accomplishment*, the feeling that the person cannot achieve anything.

Emotional exhaustion is more often found in women and the other two components more often in men. An illustration of this was the finding in a study of physicians in Sweden. Three groups were examined by means of standardized self-administered questionnaires, namely female general practitioners, male general practitioners and male surgeons. In general, the demand–control model was applicable to this situation. Physicians with high psychological demands and low decision latitude (job strain) were much more likely to report a high level of emotional exhaustion than others.

Female general practitioners reported both more job strain and more emotional exhaustion than others. The explanation of these findings could be found both in their role as general practitioners and in their role as women. Physicians cannot always leave their work on schedule, simply because a patient may be critically ill. This may create problems with the day care of children. Despite the fact that these women are hard working, they mostly take more of the responsibility for the care of children than their husbands. In a study of blood pressure during activities at home and at work, it was found that female physicians did not have significantly higher blood pressure levels at work than they did at home. This differentiated them from all other occupational groups that we have studied – the rule is higher blood pressure at work than at home. Due to conflicts between the home and work activities, many of the highest blood pressure levels were found when the female physicians came home. In their role as physicians they may have more pronounced expectations from the patients to be emotionally engaged than do their male counterparts, and they may also feel such demands on themselves more frequently than do their male colleagues. This should be a field for research in the future.

According to recent Swedish surveys, the incidence of myocardial infarction is significantly higher in nursing aides than in other working women (40% higher). This difference cannot be explained solely on the basis of differences in smoking habits or other lifestyle differences. A combination of high psychological demands and a small decision latitude may at least partly explain the finding. A high suicide rate has been shown, for instance, in nurses, physicians and dentists.

Prison personnel have been studied extensively in several countries. It has been shown that monotony and lack of authority over decisions is a common problem and that prison guards are often insufficiently educated and informed about the serious problems that they encounter. Personnel in prisons with a very strict hierarchy had higher urinary catecholamine output than personnel in other prisons, in one Swedish study [36]. This was true even when adjustment had been made for alcohol and cigarette consumption as well as overweight and coffee drinking. In a large study of 2000 employees in 63 prisons in Sweden, important findings were that staff in prisons with a high proportion of drug abusers had more health problems than staff in other prisons, and that when the leadership style was considered bad (e.g. that nobody seemed to care about the experiences and opinions about work organization among staff) the prison had a marked elevation of illness rates and sick leave among staff compared to other prisons.

There are many different strategies that could be used for the improvement of conditions for staff in human service occupations. It is possible, for instance, to improve authority over decisions and skill utilization by means of work organization changes. It is also possible to organize so-called 'Balint groups' in order to help staff handle difficult relationships with patients. Balint groups could be organized meetings once every week during several months for the staff. The whole time and energy is devoted to discussions regarding patient–caregiver relationships.

References

1. Levi, L. Introduction: psychosocial stimuli, psychophysiological reactions and disease. In *Stress and Distress in Response to Psychosocial Stimuli*, (ed. L. Levi). *Acta Medica Scandinavica*, Suppl 528, Vol 191 (1972)
2. Katz, D. and Kahn, R. *Social Psychology of Organizations*. Wiley, New York (1966)
3. Cooper, C.L. and Marshall, J. Occupational sources of stress: a review of the literature relating to coronary heart disease and mental ill health *Journal of Occupational Psychology*, **49**, 11–28 (1976)

4. Karasek, R.A. and Theorell, T. *Healthy Work*. Basic Books, New York (1990)

5. Theorell, T. and Karasek, R.A. Current issues relating to psychosocial job strain and cardiovascular disease research. *Journal of Occupational Health Psychology*, 1(1), 9–26 (1996)

6. Hammar, N., Alfredsson, L. and Theorell, T. Job characteristics and the incidence of myocardial infarction. *International Journal of Epidemiology*, 23, 277–284 (1994)

7. Hlatky, M.A., Lam, L.C. and Lee, K.L. Job strain and the prevalence and outcome of coronary artery disease. *Circulation*, 92, 327–333 (1995)

8. Theorell, T., Ahlberg-Hultén, G., Jodko, M. *et al.* Influence of job strain and emotion on blood pressure levels in female hospital personnel during work hours. *Scandinavian Journal of Work and Environmental Health*, 19, 264–269 (1993)

9. Schnall, P.L., Schwartz, J.E., Landsbergis, P.A. *et al.* Relation between job strain, alcohol, and ambulatory blood pressure. *Hypertension*, 19 (5), 488–494 (1992)

10. Belkić, K., Savić, C., Theorell, T. *et al.* Mechanisms of cardiac risk among professional drivers. *Scandinavian Journal of Work and Environmental Health*, 20, 73–86 (1994)

11. Johnson, J., Stewart, W., Hall, E. *et al.* Long-term psychosocial work environment and cardiovascular mortality among Swedish men. *American Journal of Public Health*, 86, 324–331 (1996)

12. Lundberg, U., Kadefors, R., Melin, B. *et al.* Psychophysiological stress and EMG activity of the trapezius muscle. *International Journal of Behavioral Medicine*, 1(4), 354–370 (1994)

13. Westerberg, L. and Theorell, T. Working conditions and family situation in relation to functional gastrointestinal disorders. *Scandinavian Journal of Primary Health Care*, in press.

14. Hinkle, L.E., Jr, Whitney, L.H., Lehman, E.W. *et al.* Occupation, education and coronary heart disease. *Science*, 161, 238–248 (1968)

15. Shimomitsu, T. and Levi, L. Recent working life changes in Japan. *European Journal of Public Health* 2, 76-86 (1982)

16. Siegrist, J. Adverse health effects of high-effort/low-reward conditions. *Journal of Occupational Health Psychology*, 1(1), 27–41 (1996)

17. Ursin, H., Endresen, I.M., Sveback, S. *et al.* Muscle pain and coping with working life in Norway: a review. *Work and Stress*, 7, 247–258 (1993)

18. Landsbergis, P.A., Schnall, P.L., Dietz, D. *et al.* The patterning of psychological attributes and distress by job strain and social support in a sample of working men. *Journal of Behavioral Medicine*, 15, 379–405 (1992)

19. Yehuda, R., Resnick, H., Kahana, B. *et al.* Long lasting hormonal alterations to extreme stress in humans: normative or maladaptive. *Psychosomatic Medicine*, 56, 287–297 (1994)

20. Siegrist, J. and Klein, D. Occupational stress and cardiovascular reactivity in blue-collar workers. *Work and Stress*, 4(4), 295–304 (1990)

21. Undén, A-L., Orth-Gomér, K. and Elofsson, S. Cardiovascular effects of social support in the workplace: 24 hour ECG monitoring of men and women. *Psychosomatic Medicine*, 53, 50–60 (1991)

22. Kecklund, G. and Åkerstedt, T. Sleepiness in long distance truck driving: an ambulatory EEG study of night driving. *Ergonomics*, 36(9), 1007–1017 (1993)

23. Endresen, I.M., Vaernes, R., Ursin, H. *et al.* Psychological stress-factors and concentration of immunoglobulins and complement components in Norwegian nurses. *Work and Stress*, 1, 365–375 (1987)

24. Theorell, T. Prolactin – a hormone that mirrors passiveness in crisis situations. *Integrative Physiological and Behavioral Science*, 27(1), 32–38 (1992)

25. Frankenhaeuser, M. and Johansson, G. Stress at work: psychobiological and psychosocial aspects. *International Review of Applied Psychology*, 35, 287–299 (1986)

26. Swedish Central Bureau of Statistics. *Living Conditions. Appendix 16. The Swedish Survey of Living Conditions*. Central Bureau of Statistics, Stockholm (1996)

27. Hacker, W. *Allgemeine Arbeits- und Ingenieurpsychologie* (General psychology of work and engineering). Huber, Berlin (1978)

28. Volpert, W. Work and personality development from the viewpoint of the action regulation theory. In *Socialization at Work – A New Approach to the Learning Process in the Workplace and Society* (eds H. Leymann and F. Kornbluh). Gower, London (1989)

29. North, F.M., Syme, S. L., Feeney, A. *et al.* Psychosocial work environment and sickness absence among British civil servants: the Whitehall II Study. *American Journal of Public Health*, 86, 332–340 (1996)

30. Waldenström, M., Josephson, M., Persson, C. *et al.* Mental work demands assessed by interview – a useful method? Abstract. 25th International Congress on Occupational Health, Stockholm (1996)

31. Schwartz, J., Pieper, C. and Karasek, R.A. A procedure for linking job characteristics to health surveys. *American Journal of Public Health*, 78, 904–909 (1988)

32. Theorell, T., Leymann, H., Jodko, M. *et al.* 'Person under train' incidents: medical consequences for subway drivers. *Psychosomatic Medicine*, 54, 480–488 (1992)

33. Arnetz, B. and Theorell, T. Longterm effects of a social rehabilitation programme for elderly people: physiological predictors and mortality data. *Clinical Rehabilitation*, 1, 225–229 (1987)

34. Jackson, S. Participation in decision making as a strategy for reducing job related strain. *Journal of Applied Psychology*, 68, 3–19 (1983)

35. Mattiasson, I., Lindgärde, F., Nilsson, J. Å. *et al.* Threat of unemployment and cardiovascular risk factors: longitudinal study of quality of sleep and serum cholesterol concentrations in men threatened with redundancy. *British Medical Journal*, 301, 461–46 (1990)

36. Härenstam, A. and Theorell, T. Work conditions and urinary excretion of catecholamines: a study of prison staff in Sweden. *Scandinavian Journal of Work and Environmental Health*, **14**, 257–264 (1988)

37. Kagan, A. R. and Levi, L. *Society, Stress and Disease. The Psychosocial Environment and Psyosomatic Diseases* (ed. L. Levi). Oxford University Press, Oxford (1971)

38. Theorell, T. In *Health Promotion Research. Towards a New Social Epidemiology* (eds B. Badura and I. Kickbusch). WHO Regional Publications, European Series No. 37. World Health Organisation, Copenhagen (1991)

39. Theorell, T. Personal control at work: a review of epidemiological studies in Sweden. In *Stress, Personal Control and Health,* (eds A. Steptoe and A. Appels). Wiley, New York (1989)

40. Theorell, T. Personal control at work and health: a review of epidemiological studies in Sweden. In *Stress, Personal Control and Health* (eds A. Steptoe and A. Appels). Wiley, Luxembourg (1989)

41. Theorell, T. Medical and physiological aspects of job interventions. In *International Review of Industrial and Organizational Psychology*, Vol. 8 (eds C.L. Cooper and I.T. Robertson). John Wiley, Chichester (1993)

Further reading

Ahlberg, G., Sigala, F. and Theorell, T. Social support at work, job strain and symptoms in the locomotor system in female health care personnel. *Scandinavian Journal of Work and Environmental Health*, **21**(6), 435–439 (1995)

Endresen, I.M. Psychoimmunological stress markers in working life. *Doctoral thesis*, Faculty of Psychology, University of Bergen, Norway (1991)

Hammarström, A. Unemployment and change of tobacco habits. A study of young people from 16 to 21 years of age (manuscript). Department of Community Medicine. Umeå University, Umeå, Sweden (1993)

Janlert, U. Work deprivation and health. Consequences of job loss and unemployment. *Academic thesis*. Karolinska Institute, Stockholm, Sweden (1991)

Johnson, J.V. The impact of the workplace social support, job demands, and work control under cardiovascular disease in Sweden. *PhD diss.*, Johns Hopkins University. Distributed by Department of Psychology, University of Stockholm, Report no 1–86 (1986)

Johnson, J.V. and Hall, E.M. Job strain, workplace social support and cardiovascular disease: a cross-sectional study of a random sample of the Swedish working population. *American Journal of Public Health*, **78**, 1336–1342 (1988)

Johnson, J.V., Hall, E.M. and Theorell, T. Combined effects of job strain and social isolation on cardiovascular disease morbidity and mortality in a random sample of the Swedish male working population. *Scandinavian Journal of Work and Environmental Health*, **15**, 271–279 (1989)

Knutsson, A. Shift work and coronary heart disease. *Scandinavian Journal of Social Medicine*, (Suppl. 44) (1989)

Lennernäs, M. A.-C. Nutrition and shift work. *Academic thesis*. Karolinska Institute, Stockholm, Sweden (1993)

Lichtenstein, P. Genetic and environmental mediation of the association between psychosocial factors and health. *Doctoral thesis*. Karolinska Institute, Stockholm, Sweden (1993)

Markowe, H.L., Marmot, M.G., Shipley, M.J. *et al.* Fibrinogen: a possible link between social class and coronary heart disease. *British Medical Journal*, **9**, 291 (1985)

Marmot, M. and Theorell, T. Social class and cardiovascular disease: the contribution of work. *International Journal of Health Services*, **18**(4), 659–674 (1988)

Theorell, T., Harms-Ringdahl, K., Ahlberg-Hultén, G. *et al.* Psychosocial job factors and symptoms from the locomotor system – a multicausal analysis. *Scandinavian Journal of Rehabilitation Medicine*, **23**, 165-173 (1991)

Theorell, T., Karasek, R.A. and Eneroth, P. Job strain variations in relation to plasma testosterone fluctuations in working men – a longitudinal study. *Journal of International Medicine*, **227**, 31–36 (1991)

Theorell, T., Nordemar, R., Michélsen, H. and Stockholm Music I Study Group. Pain thresholds during standardized psychological stress in relation to perceived psychosocial work situation. *Journal of Psychosomatic Research* **37**(3), 299–305 (1993)

Theorell, T., Perski, A., Åkerstedt, T. *et al.* Changes in job strain in relation to changes in physiological state. *Scandinavian Journal of Work and Environmental Health*, **14**, 189–196 (1988)

Theorell, T. Perski, A., Orth-Gomér, K. *et al.* The effects of the strain of returning to work on the risk of cardiac death after a first myocardial infarction before age 45. *International Journal of Cardiology*, **30**, 61–67 (1991)

Chapter 20

Substance abuse

Ch Mellner

The problem

This chapter deals with the problem of substance abuse in working life. By substance abuse is understood all non-medical use of narcotics or regular use of other drugs leading to psychological, somatic or social complications. Substance abuse should always be suspected when there is frequent absenteeism or changed behaviour and performance in a person at work.

Alcohol is the dominating drug of abuse, but illegal use of narcotics is becoming an increasing problem. Many of the narcotic drugs have been in use for thousands of years, e.g. cannabis, opium, coca and khat. They were used partly for medical purposes, especially morphine, heroin and cocaine. Others were initially synthesized for medical purposes, e.g. phencyclidine (PCP, 'angel dust'), lysergic acid diamide (LSD, 'acid'), amphetamine with derivatives such as methylenedioxymetamphetamine (MDMA, 'ecstasy'). Finally, there are drugs which from the very beginning were designed for illegal use. These drugs are often derived from amphetamine or opiates, e.g. metamphetamine ('ice') and synthetic heroin ('china white').

The use of anxiolytics, sedatives and hypnotics is often common among abusers. Since the beginning of the 1990s anabolic steroids have appeared as a popular drug for abuse. It is important to bear in mind that mixed drug abuse is very common.

Substance abuse is not restricted to certain countries or to certain parts of the population. It appears in all socioeconomic groups, but is more common among young and middle-aged people, i.e. the working section of the population.

Statistics from various countries are incomplete and sometimes based on different definitions. It is therefore difficult to compare the level and pattern of abuse from one country to another. Also, the pattern of abuse changes from time to time.

Increasing demands on quality, cost effectiveness and safety have forced many companies to focus on quality systems such as ISO 9000 and therefore also to take into account various means to handle and refine 'the human resource', i.e. personnel. Thus, employers are becoming increasingly aware of the costs when employees use drugs. The costs derive from frequent absenteeism, increased number of accidents and diminished quality of work, with defective products or services. Employees with a drug problem will cause time-consuming worries to their managers and they will have a high turnover rate which means increased costs for recruiting and educating new personnel.

The absolute level of substance abuse is not of major importance, but the physician has to realize that not only does the problem exist, but it exists in places where it would not be expected. The size of the problem will decide the choice of the strategy.

Responsibility

In many countries, the employers' responsibility for the health of the employees and the standard of their working environment is stipulated in protective laws. Legislation is also becoming more and more internationalized. Moreover, various agreements between the employers' organizations and the trade unions increase the burden upon the employer.

The trade unions, too, have a responsibility to reduce the problem of substance abuse, and the executives of these organizations must be ahead of their members in drug matters, and emphasizing the importance of safe working conditions and a high standard of health if employees are to reach and maintain high productivity.

Moreover, every individual employee is responsible for their sobriety and behaviour at work. It is unacceptable that any workers should cause an increased accidental risk to themselves or to their colleagues as the result of drug abuse. Neither can it be accepted that those who abuse drugs are less productive or have a poor quality of work or make mistakes that will injure the company or its customers. By mistakes is meant not only physical or mental damage, but also direct or indirect economic or social effects.

It is widely accepted that the medical and psychological treatment of the drug addict must be individualized. There is no single treatment to suit all cases. On the other hand, the employer must not take a soft approach regarding the company's policy towards substance abuse at its work sites. It is necessary for every company or organization to have a clear and firm policy, together with a structured programme, with demands and expectations upon the employees.

Company drug programme

The great majority of drug abusers look like ordinary citizens. They have a family, friends and a permanent job. Only late in their drug careers will abusers lose their social networks. It is well known that the chances of a successful rehabilitation are much greater when the abuser still has work as a firm base in an otherwise chaotic life. Therefore, actions early in working life are of particular importance in fighting substance abuse, not only to the company involved but also to society as a whole.

Every company or organization should have a drug programme. It is the duty of top management to have a policy in place which should clearly outline the company's view on substance abuse

and what actions it is prepared to implement in order to reduce the abuse of drugs. The policy should also indicate what measures will be taken when an employee with a drug problem is detected and needs treatment and rehabilitation.

The policy must be written and agreed upon with the local branches of the trade unions. It must be communicated to all employees – everyone must know its details. A policy that is not communicated from top management down to the work sites is a policy in name only.

Role of the Occupational Health Service

The Occupational Health Service (OHS) is organized either as an internal function within a company, which is the form most common in large companies, or as an external consultancy, giving service to many companies, often the smaller ones. The external OHSs may themselves be large service companies with many different specialists, or they may be small organizations with selected specialists working together in a loose network, either small or large scale.

The specialists within the OHS come from many different backgrounds and are commonly physicians, nurses and psychologists who work with the problems of substance abuse. OHSs are organized in various ways in different countries, depending on the surrounding primary health care system and on the historical background of occupational health. However, regardless of their organization, the services provided fall within three main categories:

- *Control of working environment and health status.* The objective here is to support the company to meet the organization relating to the working environment and the health of the employees. Thus, the health screening of certain workers may be obligatory, and requirements for a systematic strategy to make the working environment safer and to support the company's various health programmes may be necessary.
- *Health support.* The care of persons with work-related symptoms and diseases, including accidents, is necessary. This function also includes health education and courses in first aid.
- *Health promotion.* The objective here is to promote health, i.e. to support high-risk groups to increase or maintain their health. Health in this

context means more than the mere absence of disease. From the view of the employer, 'health' is to have highly motivated workers with a good productivity over a long period of time. Health promotion cannot solve all the problems, but it is a very important means by which to get individuals to take responsibility for their own health and to point out what actions the company has to take to get the best 'climate' for its employees.

Prevention

The best strategy is to prevent the problem of drug abuse from arising at work. Therefore, it is important to create and maintain a 'healthy spirit' as part of the culture of the company. Naturally, the illegal use of narcotic drugs is forbidden, but how is the abuse of alcohol, an old and accepted drug, to be tackled? In the author's opinion, alcohol should not be available at conferences or company education programmes – at least an alcohol-free alternative should always be provided.

A prerequisite to a healthy culture within a company is that all managers on all levels have a good knowledge of drugs and abuse. It is the responsibility of the manager to have the skill to deal with an employee who is suspected of having a drug problem.

The OHS should provide whatever support is needed to help create a healthy culture in a company. This is done through health promotion activities. First, however, it is necessary to convince top management of the need for a healthy culture and outline the expected cost savings. When top management is convinced, it is time to formulate the drug policy and it is beneficial if the OHS helps to write it.

Having written the policy, the OHS should help to inform and educate the employees at all levels. Information can be given as a part of various courses, and the appropriate members of local trade unions should also be educated. Brief information may be given at work site meetings and, if possible, the OHS should use corporate newsletters, TV, booklets and so on.

This is not enough, however. Through health promotion activities and through the corporate sports club, if there is one, a positive team spirit should be established – an ethos which does not condone drug or alcohol abuse. The focus here should be on the work group and on risk. This

healthy spirit must be constantly fostered. The preventive work of the OHS must consist not only of enthusiastic campaigns, but be applicable to everyday situations in the workplace. As always, top management must serve as a model to others.

Early detection

The early detection of drug abuse and immediate action thereafter are important. It will send the right signal to everyone, preventing further spread of the abuse. It is easier to rehabilitate an individual when the abuse is detected early.

The available diagnostic 'tools' do not give an easy and distinct answer to the question of whether substance abuse is occurring or not. There are anamnestic errors (lies, denials) and technical laboratory errors, together with the fact that many drugs are metabolized very quickly and therefore cannot be traced in the blood or in the urine. The possibility of interference with samples also exists.

The various anamnestic methods are the most important tools to detect early substance abuse. The OHS must select the most appropriate methods, rather than have them all in use. It is better to have a good understanding of a few tools and how to use them, than to use all at random.

Medical history-taking is the primary tool. It includes a general medical history, with focus on somatic and psychological symptoms, but social factors must also be investigated. After the initial interview, a directed interview regarding the use of alcohol or other drugs follows. This part of the medical history-taking must be performed in a structured manner to be reliable and to avoid the possibility that the individual will manipulate the interviewer.

There are several structured questionnaires and exit scales, but only those in common use are mentioned here. The Michigan Alcoholism Screening Test (MAST), developed by Seltzer in 1971, consists of 24 scored items and is very suitable for screening purposes. Another screening questionnaire which is frequently used is the CAGE, with four simple questions, which give a general idea of the status of the patient. Under the guidance of the World Health Organisation the AUDIT questionnaire, containing nine items, has been developed.

In order to get a substantial diagnosis (chemically dependent or high consumer) it is necessary to proceed to further tests. One such is the Substance Use Disorder Diagnostic Schedule (SUDDS), which consists of a series of structured questions based on DSM-III.

The Minnesota Assessment of Chemical Health (MACH) is a clinical interview incorporating three tests – the MAST, the Mortimer–Filkins and the MACH Drug Involvement Scale. The MACH protocol emulates clinical decision-making and produces a tentative diagnosis according to DSM-IV. The MACH method is computerized and the patient is guided through the program, which has a branching technique, by a specially trained interviewer, often the occupational health nurse.

Physical examination by the physician should always be included in the investigation, although it is rare for this procedure to issue any findings in the early stages of substance abuse. For instance, an enlarged liver, tremor or spider naevi are relatively late signs of alcohol abuse. On the other hand, a slight elevation of the blood pressure should alert the physician. With narcotics, it is even more difficult to reach a conclusion. The size of the pupils and other 'textbook signs' will not be of any help in detecting regular abuse as they are found only in acute cases of intoxication.

Laboratory tests are important, but there is no single test giving the ultimate answer to the question of abuse or not. However, it is the pattern of several tests that will give the clue.

It is well known that persistent high consumption of alcohol might affect the traditional liver tests, i.e. alanine aminotransferase (ALAT), aspartate aminotransferase (ASAT) and gamma-glutamyltransferase (gamma-GT). However, these tests are also affected by factors other than alcohol. Moreover, studies show that only about a third of heavy drinkers have an increased level of gamma-GT and only about half of chronic alcoholics will have an increased level of ASAT. In other words, these tests can only be used as relatively faint indicators, especially in the early stages of alcoholism, but they can be used to follow an individual during rehabilitation to monitor progress.

In recent years, the measurement for carbohydrate-deficient transferrin (CDT) has become a promising test. CDT reflects the consumption of alcohol during the 10–14 days before the sample was drawn. The test reacts at a consumption of 50–60 g alcohol per day or more. However, 10% of high consumers will have normal levels of CDT.

A new indication of alcohol intake is 5-hydroxytryptophol (5-HTOL) in urine. This is an extremely sensitive marker and will react to a small amount of alcohol intake and is therefore suitable for follow-up during a transient programme.

For drug abuse other than alcohol, urine tests should be chosen, although precautions may be taken to protect the sample from interference and the analysis must be made by a qualified laboratory to ensure that the test results are admissible in court. In some countries, Sweden for example, when the employer wishes to dismiss an abuser it is necessary to have an accurate test result. For this reason, analyses performed by simple drug kits at the OHS centres are not valid without confirmation.

The occupational physician has to make his decision based on the findings in the interview with the patient, laboratory data and on the findings on physical examination. The author's experience is that the MACH interview is of major help in most cases and will give a good indication of the likelihood of abuse.

In addition, the investigation should also include management's opinion of the patient's performance at work and behaviour towards colleagues and customers. The pattern of absenteeism from work should also be available.

The OHS may be involved in drug screening or in the investigation of suspect cases, e.g. in health screening as a part of the employment procedure, in multiphasic screening among the employees, following accidents or when clinical suspicion is aroused. In some companies, tests for drug abuse are performed on a random basis in the same manner as in the sports world.

Treatment

First, it should be pointed out that treatment of individuals who are dependent on drugs or alcohol is not the task of the OHS. Such treatment requires special skills and experience beyond the responsibilities of the OHS team. Instead, the task of the OHS is to give professional support to employers and help them refer patients for appropriate treatment. Therefore, the OHS must have knowledge of methods or treatment currently in use and which institutions to recommend.

For substance abuse without chemical dependency, the OHS could counsel the employee to help him or her reduce the consumption of the substance. In the case of abuse with a drug other than alcohol, it is necessary for the patient to quit completely. Well-defined regimens of patient visits and methods of control are required to support the abuser. An example of a method of control is the Feedback, Responsibility, Advice, Menu and Empathy (FRAME) system, which emphasizes the central elements in a support programme.

A treatment contract should be drawn up between employee and employer, the content of which will depend on the moral and ethical issues of collective rights of that society. The contract should state what demands are put on the individual and what commitments the employer is willing to accept. When the individual does not accept treatment or refuses to sign the contract, appropriate actions should be stipulated in the policy.

The treatment of an individual who is drug dependent should be given in an institution which provides inpatient care. There are several treatment strategies, one being the Minnesota model which has become widely used not only in the USA but also in Northern Europe. In this model, the treatment period is usually 4–6 weeks, and consists of group seminars, literature studies and personal interviews with a chosen therapist. The treatment is based on the 12 Steps in the programme of Alcoholics Anonymous (AA). After the first 4–6 weeks, almost a year of weekly outpatient visits follows. During this period, and for the rest of his or her life, the patient is encouraged to attend the meetings of AA regularly.

In early cases, and especially if the diagnosis of dependency is in doubt, outpatient treatment may be tried. Experience shows, however, that such treatment will often result in the requirement for a period of care as a inpatient.

Follow-up

An important role for the OHS is to have close contact with the patient after the initial treatment period. In the company programme at the Pripps Brewery Corporation, in Sweden, the OHS team will meet the patient once a month, or more if necessary. The pattern of absenteeism will be followed. Now and then, on an irregular basis, blood or urine samples are taken for analyses of the drugs previously abused. When everything is working well, the follow-up will be ended after a year. If there are any problems, the follow-up is extended for a further year.

Follow-up should be performed in a structured manner and in accordance with a follow-up contract, designed in a similar manner to the previous treatment contract. The follow-up contract should state very clearly what will happen if the employee relapses into abuse or does not follow the recommendations of the OHS team.

Results

The most important elements in the successful rehabilitation of individuals with substance abuse are rules within the company, early detection, professional treatment at a specialized institution and long-term follow-up. At the follow-up stage it is important to have close cooperation between the employer, the OHS and the treatment centre. The importance of the OHS in these procedures cannot be overestimated.

When the substance abuse is handled as described above, 75% of patients are expected to be treated successfully.

In a study from the Pripps Brewery (1995, unpublished), it was shown that the costs of institutional treatment of alcoholics were recouped in less than a year by the decreased costs of sickness absence. Similar results have been found by other major Swedish companies.

The outcome of a good drug programme will be enhanced work performance, diminished problems for the managers and a better quality of life for the individuals who are treated. The OHS team has an enormously important role to play in supporting companies or organizations which have a problem with substance abuse, whether they know it or not.

Chapter 21

Preventing occupational injury

N Carter and E Menckel

Acute occupational injuries continue to be a major public health problem throughout the world. Occupationally related fatalities prior to age 50 are most often due to acute injury. Although the majority of acute occupational injuries are unintentional, these injuries are not accidental in the sense that they are random or inevitable. Occupational injuries are a consequence of interactions between the physical and social environment and the individual, and many injuries are potentially foreseeable and preventable. To the extent that we can learn about injury risks, develop measures to prevent their occurrence or recurrence and motivate the consistent use of such measures, we will have contributed to safer occupational environments. Each of these three areas will be dealt with further in what follows.

This chapter discusses how occupational health service (OHS) personnel can contribute to the primary prevention of occupational injuries. The techniques described can, however, be readily applied by others with an interest in injury prevention. Described here are the way to make use of records and other forms of documentation, how to organize and promote participation in general prevention activities and how to supplement employee training with techniques designed to maintain safe work practices.

The current view of acute injuries is that they occur as part of an extended process made up of multiple stages or parts [1]. *Figure 21.1* shows the relationship of various factors to an acute injury, in schematic form. An injury was formerly viewed as a single, isolated, unforeseeable and uncontrollable event, but *Figure 21.1* indicates that injuries result from series of events and conditions, some immediate and temporary, others more distal and enduring or permanent. Situational factors are those temporally and physically close to the injury that influence the sequence of events; for example, an employee's knowledge of relevant safety instructions or the presence of guards on a machine. Structural factors refer to more enduring and encompassing conditions, such as company commitment to safety, safety policy and the organization of prevention activities throughout the company. Personnel from occupational health services have a role to play in each of these areas.

The unique competence of occupational health services

Occupational health services are available throughout the world, although their prevalence and form vary considerably. Some occupational health services are provided directly by larger corporations, the so-called in-house OHS, but smaller enterprises are frequently compelled to share services, here called OHS centres. Health services organized for specific branches or occupations constitute another form. Occupational health services have come to devote more attention to the prevention of injury and disease prior to occurrence rather than predominantly diagnosing, treating and rehabilitating individuals already injured.

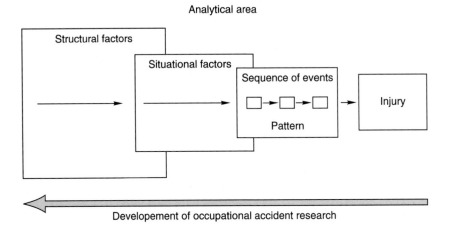

Figure 21.1 An overview of the development of accident and injury prevention research: from dealing with injuries as single, isolated events to treating them as one outcome of an extended process. Attention has come to focus upon situational and structural factors in addition to the sequence of events immediately preceding an injury

Regardless of form, OHS personnel are for several reasons especially suited to work with primary injury prevention. They normally have an excellent knowledge of local conditions at participating companies and often have an integrated position in company safety organizations. Furthermore, OHS staff are often multidisciplinary and may, for example, include doctors, nurses, safety engineers, behavioural scientists, physiotherapists, ergonomists and industrial hygienists. OHS personnel, by contrast with union or management representatives, are in a unique position since they play an independent and advisory role.

In order successfully to contribute to the prevention of occupation injuries, OHS personnel must assist others in learning about injury risks, contribute to developing preventive measures and help to motivate participation in injury prevention activities. *Figure 21.2* describes the interrelated nature of these three areas. Examples of how different OHS professionals have collaborated with others are given below.

Learning about injuries – investigation and analyses

Injury prevention is, of necessity, based upon knowledge about injuries that have already occurred. Consequently, investigation, analysis and documentation of what has occurred are cru-

cial to developing preventive measures. Adequate documentation of injuries that have occurred also makes it possible to transfer knowledge across time and space, to people not directly affected by the injury.

All investigations and analyses are based upon a conceptual framework of how acute injuries occur. The questions asked about the causes of a specific injury are related to a general model or conceptualization of what factors are involved in the causal chain. Andersson and Menckel [2] performed a comparative analysis of 11 conceptual frameworks and found major compatibility among the frameworks. Their synthesis of the common dimensions encompassed in the individual frameworks serves as a background for the presentation.

Investigating injuries

Once an injury has occurred, it is important to learn as much as possible about the causal events and conditions in order to influence these and prevent further injuries. Investigations of injuries normally begin with the individual case and are based on interviews. Investigations include the following general questions; Why? Who? By whom? When? Where and How? Each of these questions is dealt with from the perspective of OHS. More detailed questioning related to these general issues is required in the investigation of a specific injury.

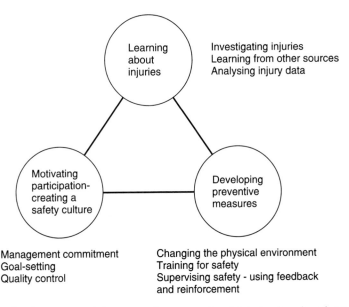

Figure 21.2 Three interrelated areas essential to preventing occupational injuries: learning about injuries, developing preventive measures and motivating participation

Why?

Injury investigations are often conducted for more than one reason. Issues of blame and negligence will rarely be the primary concern for representatives of occupational health services. Rather, the purpose of an investigation is to identify potential points for correction and prevention. Towards these ends, those conducting an investigation should avoid placing blame and should encourage the forthright participation of those being interviewed. Those investigating should, however, be aware that legal and insurance issues may be relevant and can influence how events and conditions are reported.

Who?

Besides the person or persons injured and direct witnesses, it is important, and usually beneficial, to interview the responsible supervisor and union safety representative. In order to obtain more information about the influence of structural factors, interviews with those responsible for production, training and company safety policy, e.g. upper level management, are recommended.

By whom?

OHS personnel, if they have an independent organizational position, are well suited to conduct interviews. Interviews can, however, be conducted by supervisors, safety representatives or others who are able to convey the goal of the interview, which is to obtain information important for prevention.

When?

Investigations should be conducted as soon as possible following the injury. As time passes, those who are interviewed and others involved in the investigation may tend to provide consistent but inaccurate reports of what occurred.

Where?

The site where the injury occurred is in most instances the best place to perform the investigation. In many cases the victim and witnesses are most readily accessible at the injury site. A reconstruction of events and conditions is more realistic when created at the injury site.

How?

Occupational health service personnel both can and should collaborate with on-site personnel. They can, for example, suggest that the company create a special group to assist with investigations. Such a group should include representatives from production, the local safety organization and occupational health services. Investigation groups that met promptly at the injury site were found to produce better documentation and contributed to reductions in injury rates [3,4]. These groups were made up of a union safety official and a nurse and a safety engineer (from an in-house OHS) who met with supervisors and the injured.

Recording a reconstruction with video or photographs can provide more detailed material for analysis. Pictures, photographs, videos and written descriptions can all be used to document investigations so that knowledge can be transferred to other people and across time and location.

Learning from other sources

In addition to interviews and the accompanying documentation of the current injury, there are several other potential sources of relevant information. Other documentation associated with the injury site may provide information about factors contributing to the injury. Examples of such documentation include written instructions, records of repairs, work orders, operation records, and records from safety inspections or safety committee meetings. Other injury investigations from the same workplace or company can also be helpful.

Critical incident or near-accident reporting can be an effective means of identifying hazardous conditions at a work site prior to the occurrence of an injury [5]. It is crucial that near-accident reporting be viewed as part of injury prevention and that the knowledge obtained be used to develop preventive measures.

Reports about incidents can be obtained through interviews or written descriptions. Interviewing employees at their work sites during a limited period (e.g. daily during a 2-week period) can increase knowledge about injury risks. It is important that interviews are conducted by non-biased, trusted individuals familiar with conditions at the workplace, i.e. OHS personnel.

National and branch statistics can provide information about injury risks that may be found at individual sites. Information about some injury types, hand injuries, for example, may also be useful. Information about injury patterns, such as fall injuries or falls on stairs, regardless of branch, can be transferred to prevention at the company level. Various computerized databases and sites on the Internet can also be useful sources of information.

Analysing injury data

The purpose of an analysis is to identify what combination of events and conditions were necessary and sufficient to produce the injury, and what situational and structural factors interacted to contribute to the injury? Commonly, an analysis starts at the endpoint (an injury) and proceeds backwards in time with the sequence of immediately preceding events. The analysis continues with the factors determining the immediate situation in which the injury occurred (see *Figure 21.1*).

While analyses can be performed by specifically trained safety experts alone, OHS personnel may normally desire to achieve more than the analysis of a single case. For OHS personnel, an investigation and analysis of an injury provide an opportunity to train on-site personnel, and their participation is thus encouraged. An analysis can also provide information applicable to other sites served by OHS personnel.

OHS personnel who analysed and reviewed injury investigations together with members of company safety committees contributed to a reduction in the frequency and severity of injury. The members of these groups represented production, management and union interests in addition to OHS. The groups met monthly to analyse injuries that had occurred since the previous meeting and to discuss the likelihood that similar risks existed elsewhere within the company. This form of analysis has been tested at several companies with similar positive results [3,4,6].

Developing preventive measures

The purpose of analysing the mixture of conditions and events contributing to an injury is to identify potential points for change. For any given injury type, changes can most probably be made at several points. There are good reasons for attempting to identify more than one potential point for change. The possibility that an effective solution to a safety problem may require change at more than one point must be considered. Further, constructive discussion can be promoted by developing two solutions, both of which are believed to be reasonable and effective and which are acceptable to those concerned. Presenting alternatives and asking those concerned which they prefer makes compromise easier.

Changing the physical environment

The general strategy for injury prevention involves a hierarchy of measures: elimination, reduction and use of personal safety equipment. Eliminating the risk entirely is the most preferable and effective measure, assuming that eliminating one risk does not entail creating another. Banning and removing certain machines or chemicals from occupational settings, for example, eliminates the opportunity to become injured. In practice, the complete elimination of injury risk is not always feasible. If elimination is not possible, then prevention activities should focus upon changing physical and social conditions in order to reduce the risk of injury. To prevent unintentional acute injuries, it is often sufficient to remove or alter one of the multiple factors which contribute to the injury in an acceptable way. Acceptability thus becomes a key concept in creating safety.

If safety and acceptability can successfully be designed directly into the product or environment, those otherwise exposed to risk will not be required to change their individual behaviour. To the extent that safety and acceptability are inherent features of the environment or product, the need for personal safety equipment, special instructions, training or supervision is reduced or eliminated. Built-in safety appears preferable if it does not depend upon continuous monitoring and supervision. Axelsson and Carter [7] describe how collaboration with OHS personnel, manufacturers, inventors and others has led to several safer products in the construction industry. Problems identified at individual construction sites served as the impetus for changes in products used industry-wide.

If no single measure eliminates an injury risk, then a combination of changes in physical and social/organizational conditions seems justified.

The direct 'cause' of the injury may not always be the most appropriate point at which to intervene. For example, a burn injury might be prevented by reducing the risk of fire rather than by reducing the heat of the fire.

The use of personal safety equipment is an option to be considered when other attempts to eliminate or reduce injury risk have not been completely successful. However, we propose that personal protective equipment should be viewed as a complement to other prevention activities and measures rather than as a sole and sufficient countermeasure. For example, the use of hard hats in the construction industry can never be accepted as the sole means of protecting workers from the danger of being struck by falling objects.

Personal safety equipment generally presupposes both training and supervision. Those expected to use the equipment must understand why the equipment is necessary and be trained as to how, when and where the equipment is appropriate. Employers must also arrange a system of supervision to ensure that use is consistent with training. Since personal safety equipment can, despite attempts to individualize, be uncomfortable and cumbersome, employees may avoid using it without close supervision. The topics of training and supervision of safety are dealt with in separate sections below.

Training for safety

Most employers expect to devote some time and effort to training employees about the tasks they will be expected to perform. Occupational health service personnel should attempt to ensure that on-the-job training and other job-related training done by employers incorporates and integrates safety issues. Prior to suggesting new training programmes, an evaluation should be made of those in current use. Are safety issues integrated into training? Is what is said realistic and valid? Do workers actually do what is suggested? If yes, fine. If no, why? (interferes with job, uncomfortable, supervisors and foremen don't comply, older and/or more experienced workers don't comply). Sulzer-Azaroff and colleagues [8] provide a thorough analysis of how to achieve and maintain improved safety performance. The major points of that analysis are presented here.

Choosing important behaviours

Important and valid safety-related behaviours can be selected from epidemiological data for the industry and job, on-site injury records and safety audits, from interviews with personnel and from direct observation. Those expected to perform safely must be aware of the exact times, places and conditions for which certain behaviours are safe or unsafe. Specifying what is desired and what is to be avoided is a prerequisite of training.

Using instructions

Instructions can take several different forms: lectures, readings, films, demonstrations, signs or displays. Demonstrations and opportunities to practise under supervised conditions are suggested. Role-playing and simulation provide opportunities to model and correct performance. Reliance upon written instructions alone is not to be recommended. Although widely used, written instructions are rarely preferred by users and are seldom adapted to individual user skills.

Prompting and fading

On occasion, simple instructions and demonstrations are not sufficient to achieve an acceptably safe level of performance. Temporary, artificial methods (prompts) may be required to improve performance. Physical guidance and reminders are two means of prompting desired performance in naturally occurring occupational conditions. For example, a hearing protection programme may initially require the use of reminders to get employees to use noise abatement equipment and personal hearing protection. Fading (gradually withdrawing) the use of artificial prompts is a method to eliminate reliance on reminders.

Teaching complex skills

In many cases, safety involves performing several separate and sometimes complicated behaviours. For example, protecting oneself from noxious gases may demand following detailed operating procedures and the correct use of personal protective equipment. Teaching complex skills may require a preliminary task analysis in order to separate the complicated whole into simpler parts. The separate components can then be taught individually and in sequence until the complex behaviour can be performed correctly. In training new and complex behaviours, it is essential to provide praise for gradual improvements towards the final, desired performance.

Assisting fluency and generalization

Smooth and expert-like performance characterizes fluency. Fluent performance occurs despite distractions and changes in the environment. Conducting rapid and thorough preoperational checks and following emergency procedures are examples of situations requiring immediate, precise, apparently automatic performance. Fluency is best achieved by providing feedback and reinforcement for performance that is both unhesitating and correct.

Training in one situation does not guarantee that performance will occur in others [9]. Classroom training does not necessarily transfer (generalize) to the natural occupational situation in which it is expected to occur. Rather, effective training requires inclusion of the various situations and conditions in which safe performance is expected to occur. Training for a variety of situations using real-life conditions increases the likelihood that generalization will take place. Performance that is fluent and that has generalized to a variety of settings may still deteriorate over time. Consequently, a system for supervising safe performance is suggested.

Supervising safety – using feedback and reinforcement

Safe performance may or may not be its own reward. In occupational settings a system of supervising safe performance will most likely improve a company's safety record. This section emphasizes the use of positive methods to increase and maintain safe performance. Reviews of the occupational injury prevention literature have repeatedly found feedback and reinforcement to improve safety [10–13].

Feedback

In this context, feedback refers to information provided to individuals about the quantity or quality of their past performance [14]. Feedback has been found to be most effective when used in combination with goal-setting and/or rewards [15]. Feedback can have numerous characteristics; the source (e.g. supervisor), content, method of presentation (e.g. chart, memo), frequency and who receives feedback. Research has yet to provide clear guidelines concerning which combination of characteristics produces optimal results or if there are specific characteristics to be avoided.

Providing information feedback to personnel has been shown to stimulate employee participation in prevention activities [16]. Physiotherapists fed back information about acute exertion injuries to personnel groups at more than 100 wards in order to stimulate discussion and prevention in Swedish health care settings. Feedback has also been shown to improve different behaviour-based measures of safety and to reduce injury statistics (see reviews in [8,10–12,17].

Reinforcement

Reinforcement is a technical term; it is a process in which performance is strengthened as a function of an event that occurs as a consequence of the performance. The regular and consistent use of reinforcers indicates that injury prevention is desirable to management. The events used to reinforce performance can take many forms [18]. One of the most important characteristics of a reinforcer is that it is meaningful to the individual. Reinforcement immediately following performance is more effective than providing consequences following delays. Providing reinforcers for safety was an integral part of a comprehensive programme developed for two open-pit mining sites [19]. Major reductions in accident frequency were obtained rapidly and maintained throughout a 15-year follow-up.

Decreasing blatantly unsafe performance can on occasion become an issue. While reprimands and formal actions should not be excluded, it may be important to identify the reasons why 'unsafe' behaviour is more attractive to the individual than 'safe' performance. Temporary or permanent changes to make safe performance attractive may be more effective than reprimands and sanctions.

Motivating participation – creating a safety culture

The ultimate goal of injury prevention activities is to minimize the frequency and severity of injuries. However, for many individual businesses injuries are rare and may not present obvious patterns even when they do occur. Although management and employees readily agree as to the ultimate goal of injury prevention activities, they may not be motivated to participate in specific safety-related activities. We propose that OHS personnel should assist companies in creating a safety culture. A safety culture promotes and recognizes safe performance as a means of achieving reductions in injury statistics. Geller [20] proposes the concept of actively caring as characteristic of a culture devoted to safety. In creating a safety culture it is important to obtain management and employee commitment and to develop a system of goal-setting and quality control.

In their efforts to create a safety culture, OHS personnel may be more effective in the role of adviser rather than expert. In taking the role of adviser, OHS personnel emphasize that safety depends upon active management and employee participation. An advisory role promotes management and employee involvement and responsibility. On occasion, opposition to change can be encountered which can require trouble-shooting skills on the part of those involved in the process of change.

Management commitment

It is essential that management commitment be seen at the highest level and that it is consistent and enduring. Management commitment should manifest itself both in what is said and in what is done. Management should produce clear and specific policy statements on the topic of safety and safety goals, i.e. what is expected of employees and what is forbidden, and what the consequences of compliance and non-compliance are.

Upper level management must demonstrate through behaviour that safety is an essential part of the organization. Management should participate in meetings, set aside resources (time and money), attend courses and educational programmes, include material in staff newsletters and so on. Management must also be scrupulous in following policy. If policy requires hard hats for personnel and visitors, then management, at all levels, must wear hard hats when on the shop floor.

Goal-setting

Determining a clear and specific description or standard of performance is called goal-setting. A goal should specify who will be doing what by a given date. The process of determining safety goals should be participative, i.e. management, employees, worker organizations and other concerned parties should be involved. Participative goal-setting is recommended for both ethical and practical reasons. Goals determined in cooperation with those affected is non-coercive and more likely to receive their active support. Goals that are not acceptable to those affected tend to produce negative reactions, such as non-compliance or outright sabotage. Goals phrased in positive terms describing what is to be done or achieved are preferable to goals using negative terms. For example, 'Always wear a hard hat on construction site' is better than 'No one without hearing protection permitted on shop floor'.

Goals should be achievable but challenging. If employees are currently using personal hearing protection 40% of the time, then an increase to 60% might be a reasonable initial goal. If the 60% level is reached and maintained, then a newer and higher goal can be agreed upon.

It is essential that goals be measurable on some agreed dimension. Unless the goal can be measured, it will be impossible to determine if it has been reached. Including a time limit or date when setting a goal can be crucial. For example, 'As of March 1, 1997 all employees will wear safety glasses when on the shop floor'.

Selecting valid, meaningful goals can be problematic. For example, the goal of 2 million injury-free working hours during the coming year is probably not desirable if it is the sole goal. The goal might be achieved at the expense of individuals failing to report injuries that should have been reported.

Quality control

As with production, safety requires review, refinement and renewal. Injury prevention policies and activities are often readily integrated with quality control systems, e.g. ISO 9000. Methods used to improve product and service quality are usually applicable to safety issues. Since most safety issues also concern production, there are obvious advantages to integrating the systems, techniques and methods used in their management. The role of OHS personnel can be to assist company staff in incorporating safety issues into quality control activities.

Measuring safety – structure and outcome

While injury statistics – an outcome measure – are essential to determining if the ultimate goal of preventing injuries has been achieved, they cannot be made the sole measures of the effectiveness of a safety programme. Safety programmes should be evaluated with respect to both structure and outcome.

Structure refers here to the presence or absence of organizational systems that deal with safety-related issues. Are there systematic arrangements for safety and health at the company? Is there a safety committee at the site? Does the company plan to conduct regular safety inspections? Are the services provided by OHS adequate to meet the needs of the company? Structural aspects provide a framework and serve as prerequisite for safety activities without guaranteeing that the activities take place or that they achieve the intended goals.

Outcome measures refer to both behaviour and results. Measures of behaviour focus upon what is actually done. Are safety inspections carried out as planned? Are corrective measures carried out or implemented? How many employees wear hearing protection when required? Is lifting done in a safe manner?

The results of structure and behaviour are another form of outcome measure. For example, pathways clear of hindrances can be measured without having to observe and measure the behaviour that produced the final result. Various forms of injury statistics are the most recognizable form of result-oriented outcome measure. The number of hand injuries per year, lost work days, injuries per million work hours or per 1000 employees and injuries meeting reporting characteristics, e.g. OSHA reportable injuries, are all examples of result-oriented outcome measures.

Measuring both permits and promotes comparison. At individual sites, comparisons with measures compiled from previous years are often the most appropriate. Although conditions at individual companies usually make each site unique, comparisons with other companies of similar size in the same branch are sometimes feasible. To the extent that data are available, comparisons with comparable companies, enterprises and branch or national statistics are also recommended.

Reviewing

Measuring should not be done solely for its own sake. Data that have been collected must be inspected, summarized and analysed. The responsibility for these activities should always lie with those with a formal, legal responsibility for safety and health. Management may turn to OHS personnel for advice as to how these activities can be organized and may even commission these services from OHS. Reviewing injury records and documentation regarding safety on a regular basis – monthly or quarterly – is recommended. Regardless of who inspects, analyses and summarizes data, the goals are to determine if the procedures and countermeasures are operating as planned and if they are applicable at other times or places or for other groups. Those involved in the review should have a mandate to take corrective actions when procedures and countermeasures do not match expectations.

Planning for maintenance

Maintaining safe work practices is also an issue for management. Change is the constant of life. Success in preventing the occurrence of occupational injury comes from constant, consistent, systematic effort and adaptation, not simply from creating retrospective solutions to current problems.

In order to maximize the likelihood that safety-related structures and activities will survive change at the company, it is important to ensure that these are not dependent upon the interest or qualifications of a single individual or position. The examples of investigation and review group routines [3,4,6] were designed to be robust in

nature. Each survived changes in management and original participants. In order to minimize their vulnerability, each routine was adapted to complement existing routines and structures at the sites.

Trouble-shooting

Despite a willingness to accept the general proposition that injury prevention is desirable, both management and employees may on occasion oppose specific preventive measures. Rather than be surprised that people do not always act in what might be considered their own best interests, OHS personnel should prepare themselves for factors which can supersede safety as an issue of importance. The list below is not exhaustive, but does include likely and commonly occurring reasons for opposition. At worst, several of these reasons may be operating simultaneously. For each reason for opposition, a suggestion for surmounting – if not eliminating – the cause is provided.

Uniqueness

Opponents to change commonly cite the uniqueness of their organization or conditions as a reason for resisting a proposal. This argument usually masks other reasons for resistance. Attempting to determine what these other reasons are will probably be more fruitful than spending time analysing and describing similarities between the current organization and others. By acknowledging uniqueness, it may also be possible to suggest that changes be evaluated during a trial period.

Novelty

Newness as such creates opposition among some people; promoting active participation of those involved and repeatedly informing them may reduce this problem. Change may also be threatening to some individuals since it will entail new duties or alterations in their authority or status. It is important to consider these possibilities.

Familiarity

Most prevention measures are multifaceted. Resistance may occur when people recognize some part of a proposed change as having previously been unsuccessfully implemented. The criticism may be valid and, if so, the proposed solution should be revised. The alternative is to demonstrate that current conditions are different and that these justify the proposed solution.

Cost (time, effort, complexity or money)

Those affected have legitimate reasons for considering the costs of proposed improvements in safety. Changes that entail increases in the time taken or effort required to perform a task, economic cost or complexity of a task will almost assuredly meet with opposition. Employees may be unwilling to reduce the hazard level of a task for which they have traditionally received extra compensation based upon their willingness to take risks. Involving those affected in discussions about how to evaluate changes can ensure that important dimensions are included. A willingness to participate despite potential costs can be encouraged by suggesting a trial period with an ensuing evaluation period.

Other, more pressing problems

Safety may not be ignored, but will not be foremost in people's minds during a reorganization or when there is a threat of job loss. For OHS personnel, drastic changes actually increase the need for attention to safety issues since established routines may be disrupted.

A continuation of other conflicts

Disputes between management and employees, departments or employees about other issues can on occasion influence safety activities. It may be necessary to wait until these other issues are resolved before proceeding with efforts to improve safety. During such conflicts OHS can best maintain their credibility by remaining neutral with respect to other issues.

Mandatory safety

People resent and oppose change that is forced upon them. Again, active participation of those affected reduces the problem. Mandatory change

can be expected to produce negative side-effects for a period, but these can be minimized by making the new procedure or condition as attractive as possible. If other methods can be used to increase the acceptance level to 40–50% of a population, the remaining individuals are more likely to accept mandatory safety.

Solutions to the wrong problem

The world is full of solutions that need to be accurately matched to appropriate problems. Taking a bag of solutions and looking for suitable problems is probably less successful than developing a solution on the basis of the problem at hand. For example, near-accident reporting is appropriate when knowledge about risks is lacking. Employee enthusiasm for near-accident reporting was found to be minimal at sites where management failure to implement agreed safety measures was identified [5].

Final comments and recommendations

Society, management and labour representatives and others can readily subscribe to the goal of safety in occupational settings. Although this ultimate goal may never be permanently achieved, the systematic application of techniques and principles described in this chapter can lead to reductions in the number and severity of injuries. Improvements at individual companies and work sites will contribute to the achievement of the ultimate goal. Small-scale attempts at improvements are thus to be encouraged.

Occupational health service personnel can play a crucial role in initiating and implementing prevention activities. During the initial stages of change, the involvement of one or a few enthusiastic individuals may be essential to success. The continued survival of effective procedures should, however, not be made dependent on the presence of one or a few enthusiasts. Programmes should be designed to be able to function beyond a change in persons filling key functions. This can best be achieved by involving groups of individuals representing several functions within a company or site.

Introducing changes that are adaptations of current practices rather than entirely new programmes increases the likelihood of acceptance and survival. Regardless of the extent of the proposed changes, the use of trial periods that include agreed upon evaluation measures is recommended. A trial period permits those concerned to test changes and become involved without forcing a permanent commitment. Trial periods also imply that changes can either be modified or removed entirely.

Continued involvement in safety activities can be encouraged in several ways. The use of outcome measures that focus on increases in safe behaviours are preferable to measures of decreases in unsafe behaviour. The use of positive feedback and reinforcement is recommended to achieve increases in safe behaviour. Outcome measures that can detect short-term improvements in performance are desirable since they permit small successes to be acknowledged, which encourages continued involvement. Efforts and activities that produce more immediate, tangible and visible results are also to be encouraged. These and other techniques that promote cooperation between management, employees, OHS personnel and others contribute to safety and the prevention of occupational injuries.

References

1. Menckel, E. and Kullinger, B. (eds). *Fifteen Years of Occupational Accident Research in Sweden.* Swedish Council for Working Life Research, Stockholm (1996)
2. Andersson, R. and Menckel, E. On the prevention of accidents and injuries. A comparative analysis. *Accident Analysis and Prevention*, **27**, 757–768 (1995)
3. Carter, N. and Menckel, E. Group routines for improving accident prevention activities and accident statistics. *International Journal of Industrial Ergonomics*, **5**, 125–132 (1990)
4. Menckel, E. and Carter, N. The development and evaluation of accident prevention routines: a case study. *Journal of Safety Research*, **16**, 73–82 (1985)
5. Carter, N. and Menckel, E. Near-accident reporting: a review of Swedish research. *Journal of Occupational Accidents*, **7**, 41–64 (1985)
6. Menckel, E., Carter, N. and Hellbom, M. The long-term effects of two group routines on accident prevention activities and accident statistics. *International Journal of Industrial Ergonomics*, **12**, 301–309 (1993)
7. Axelsson, P.-O. and Carter, N. Achieving safer products: general lessons from case examples. In *Work Environmental Safety Series*, vol. 2 *Occupational Safety in Various Industries* (eds D. Brune, G. Gerhardsson, G. Crockford *et al.*). Scandinavian Science Publisher, Oslo and International Labour Office, Geneva (1997)
8. Sulzer-Azaroff, B., Harris, T.C. and Blake McCann, K. Beyond training: organizational performance management techniques. In *Occupational Safety and Health Training, Occupational Medicine: State of the Art Reviews* (ed. M.J. Colligan). Hanley and Belfus, Philadelphia, PA (1994)
9. Stokes, T.F. and Baer, D.M. An implicit technology of generalization. *Journal of Applied Behavior Analysis*, **10**, 349–367 (1977)
10. Carter, N. Behavior analysis and the primary prevention of occupational injuries. *Scandinavian Journal of Behaviour Therapy*, **21**, 89–103 (1992)
11. Saari, J. Feedback som medel för säkra arbetsmetoder – en litteraturöversikt (Feedback as a method of achieving safer work practices – a literature review. In Swedish). *Arbete, Människa, Miljö*, no. 3, 159–168 (1986)
12. Sulzer-Azaroff, B. Behavior approaches to occupational health and safety. In *Handbook of Organizational Behavior Management* (ed. L.W. Frederiksen). Wiley, New York (1982)
13. Sulzer-Azaroff, B. The modification of occupational safety behavior. *Journal of Occupational Accidents*, **9**, 177–197 (1987)
14. Prue, D.M. and Fairbanks, J.A. Performance feedback in organizational behavior management. A review. *Journal of Organizational Behavior Management*, **3**, 1–16 (1981)
15. Balcazar, F., Hopkins, B.L. and Suarez, Y. A critical, objective review of performance feedback. *Journal of Organizational Behavior Management*, **7**, 65–89 (1986)
16. Menckel, E., Hagberg, M., Engkvist, I.-L. *et al.* The prevention of back injuries in Swedish health care – a comparison between two models for action-oriented feedback. *Applied Ergonomics*, **28**(1), 1–7 (1997)
17. *Successful Accident Prevention: Recommendations and Ideas Field Tested in the Nordic Countries.* Final report of the Nordic Cooperative Program of Effective Accident Prevention Methods. Project of the Nordic Council of Ministers. Institute of Occupational Health, Helsinki (1987)
18. Nelson, B. *1001 Ways to Reward Employees.* Workman Publishing, New York (1994)
19. Fox, D.K., Hopkins, B.L. and Anger, W.K. The long-term effects of a token economy on safety performance in open-pit mining. *Journal of Applied Behavior Analysis*, **20**, 215–224 (1987)
20. Geller, E.S. *The Psychology of Safety. How to Improve Behaviors and Attitudes on the Job.* Chilton Book Company, Radnor, PA (1996)

Chapter 22

Rehabilitation and prevention of work-related musculoskeletal disorders

K Ekberg

Introduction

Musculoskeletal disorders, in particular those affecting the back, neck and shoulders, are a major source of disability in many countries. Back symptoms are the most common cause of disability in those under 45 years of age and cause the largest consumption of health care resources in the western world, leading to early retirement and compensation claims. Low back pain accounts for roughly 25% of all sick leave in western countries. Most of those suffering from acute low back pain will recover within 6 weeks without help from the health care system. A small number, between 2% and 10% in western countries, consume about 80% of the resources due to health care needs and in particular due to compensation for long-term sick absenteeism. Pain in the neck and shoulders contributes similarly to a huge consumption of resources.

Work-related musculoskeletal disorders appear to be on the increase. Evidence continues to accumulate supporting the view that disability due to occupational musculoskeletal illness or injury is the consequence of a complex interaction of medical condition, physical capabilities, ergonomic demands, conditions due to work organization, and individual behavioural and psychological resources such as coping ability, ability to manage pain and psychosocial conditions. The interaction of these factors appears to contribute to the development and maintenance of disability.

The difficulties involved in diagnosing musculoskeletal disorders contribute to the problems of understanding and exploring the causes of the symptoms and how they should be treated. As a consequence, the clinician is faced with a bewildering array of treatment methods, e.g. exercise, relaxation, physical therapies, medication and cognitive–behavioural therapies. The methods used most likely reflect the opinion of the researcher or clinician on the causes of the disorder, and possibly also on the goals established for rehabilitation. A strictly medical perspective on the aetiology of the disorder may narrow the treatment methods to physical and medical therapies that are primarily aimed at restoring mobility and strength, and at reducing pain. A multi-causal perspective may initiate a wider range of treatment methods, and the goals for rehabilitation may be more far-reaching and involve measures of work ability, psychological wellbeing and social activities. This, of course, has implications for studies of the outcome of rehabilitation, since different perspectives produce different aims and treatment methods. A successful rehabilitation, given one perspective, may be considered less successful from another.

Snook [1] suggested that an efficient rehabilitation programme should ideally combine efforts to prevent the first occurrence of the disorder, to reduce the length of a disability, and to hinder or reduce the risk of relapse. For work-related musculoskeletal disorders, primary prevention must obviously focus on the workplace, as well as on the interplay between the employee and the conditions at the workplace. To shorten the duration of the disorder, rehabilitation may involve not only treatment of the symptoms, but also efforts to improve the ability of the individual to cope with the symptoms and, in addition, to change those aspects of the working conditions that contribute to or maintain the disorder. Finally, in order to reduce the risk of relapse, those aspects of the work that once contributed to the development of the symptoms should be changed, i.e. interventive changes may reduce the risk of relapse and prevent others in the workplace from developing musculoskeletal problems. In essence, there must be a multifactorial approach to rehabilitation.

The literature is dominated by studies on the rehabilitation of low back pain, but there are few controlled studies of rehabilitation of pain and symptoms in the neck and shoulders. Ideally one should differentiate between these symptom areas, as the aetiology may be different. As there are also similarities between certain diffuse painful conditions in the low back and in the neck, respectively, a combined discussion may be justified in this context.

Rehabilitation of individual health variables

Physical rehabilitation

Rehabilitation that focuses on individual health aspects is often designed to improve overall physical fitness, strength, cardiovascular fitness, mobility and endurance. The long-term effects of these methods have been evaluated in a few controlled studies. In a review of rehabilitation involving manual therapy and physiotherapy of neck pain patients, of four studies the two with the highest methodological scores were negative, and the other two were positive with regard to rehabilitation outcome in terms of pain [2]. In a randomized clinical trial of therapy for back and neck complaints, physiotherapy, manual therapy, treatment by a general practitioner and placebo treatment were compared. After a period of 1 year, manual therapy appeared to be slightly more successful than physiotherapy with regard to the main complaints and the physical functions of individuals with chronic conditions (> 1 year) and those under 40 years of age [3]. No difference was noted between the groups when considering how the patients themselves rated the 'global effects' of the two types of treatment.

In the Clinical Practice Guideline by the US Department of Health and Human Services [4] it is stated that 'for patients with acute low back symptoms without radiculopathy, the scientific evidence suggests spinal manipulation is effective in reducing pain and perhaps speeding recovery within the first month of symptoms. For patients whose low back problems persist beyond 1 month, the scientific evidence on effectiveness of manipulation was found to be inconclusive'. The same committee states that physical modalities, such as ice, heat, massage, ultrasound, cutaneous laser treatment and electrical stimulation, in the treatment of acute low back problems are of insufficiently proven benefit to justify their cost. Transcutaneous electrical nerve stimulation (TENS), spinal traction, acupuncture and biofeedback are not recommended by the committee for treatment of patients with acute low back problems.

Exercise at the workplace is frequently employed as a means to rehabilitate or prevent musculoskeletal disorders. Lahad and colleagues [5] reviewed 16 studies of treatment and prevention of low back pain with exercise. They found support for a short-term benefit from exercise intervention in terms of days of work lost because of back pain, or fewer days with back pain, compared with controls. Leisure activities have been associated with a lower degree of back pain in other studies, but several prospective studies indicate that strength in the back muscles is not predictive of later disorders in the low back. In general, it appears that exercise by itself does not prevent musculoskeletal problems, but wellbeing effects of physical fitness may be beneficial.

Education is often used as a tool to increase the individual's knowledge about proper lifting techniques, to increase the interest in physical training and/or to increase the individual's ability to cope with pain. Individual variations in work technique are large. A few studies have shown a positive association between type A behaviour and neck and shoulder symptoms. The pattern of behaviour may influence working technique, proneness to take rests, the number of movements made to accomplish a task, and the ways movements are made. The more dynamic the working technique, the fewer the symptoms, indicating a positive effect of a work organization that stimulates more movements and changes in posture at the workplace. Attempts to prevent disorders by vocational training indicate that it may be possible to teach appropriate techniques to newly employed workers, but experienced workers are less able to relearn work techniques. Education and training is often used as a combined primary and secondary preventive action, but there are few if any controlled studies that show long-term effects in terms of lower incidence of low back pain after training in lifting techniques.

Sometimes efforts are made to select physically fit employees to some physically demanding work tasks in order to prevent symptoms developing. Selection may be based on strength tests, radiography or previous history of musculoskeletal disorders. The predictive value of such selection of the workforce is low with respect to later disability. In a population of 1500 individuals with low back pain who were followed for 20 years, only 7–8% of young employees who later developed pain could be identified from medical history and examinations [6]. The best predictor for the development of musculoskeletal disorders is a previous musculoskeletal problem. Since low back pain and pain in the neck and shoulders is very common in any population, it does not appear reasonable or realistic to select out all those who once had musculoskeletal pain.

To summarize, it is not possible to determine clearly if one physical treatment is significantly superior to others in terms of return to work, sick leave, pain or symptoms. Manual therapy may improve physical health condition during the acute phase. Physical training in order to improve muscular strength or to improve health functions does not reduce the incidence and duration of low back pain. Selection of physically fit individuals to certain work tasks is not likely to reduce the incidence of musculoskeletal problems.

Multidisciplinary rehabilitation

There is a growing interest in multidisciplinary rather than single-modal action for the prevention and treatment of musculoskeletal pain. Despite the widespread growth of programmes and services that provide multidisciplinary rehabilitation of work-related disability in the upper extremities, few controlled outcome studies have been published. The majority of studies focus on the chronic low back pain patient. Many multidisciplinary programmes consider some or all the somatic, affective, behavioural and cognitive aspects. Some of the most popular strategies

are those involving cognitive behavioural programmes.

It is now commonly recognized that psychological factors play an important role in chronic pain. Gamsa [7] gave an excellent overview of the different psychological theories on this problem. From about 1940 to the mid-1960s the psychological approach was dominated by psychoanalytic theory. Studies aimed to show that patients with chronic pain suffer from unresolved conflicts and that their pain expresses this unconscious conflict. In the 1970s, behaviour theory and cognitive theories were advanced to explain the role of psychological factors in pain and to provide a conceptual framework for treatment. Fordyce and colleagues [8] were the first to apply the behavioural model to pain. Behaviour theory is the basis of operant pain management programmes which aim to extinguish pain behaviour and thereby also the pain itself. Pain contingent reinforcers are eliminated and the reinforcement of healthy or active behaviours is introduced. Successful treatment outcome is defined by, for example, a decrease in pain behaviour. Behaviour management programmes are criticized because they disregard a number of variables in the patient's real life, which may contribute to or preserve pain.

Since the 1970s cognitive approaches of pain have studied how the meaning of pain influences the patients, and coping styles have gained increased attention. Cognitive strategies attempt to change the way patients think about pain and to increase the patient's feeling of control over pain. Interventions that combine cognitive and behavioural approaches aim to help patients restructure the way they think about their pain and to change their behavioural limits due to the pain by increasing their day-to-day activity. Pain is not eliminated, but the impact of pain on the individual's life is diminished. In essence, psychological models for treatment and intervention have developed from linear to more comprehensive and multi-causal models of pain.

An example of this approach was provided by Lindström [9]. In her studies, the rehabilitation programme is tailor-made for each patient in terms of the kind and number of professionals informed, the number of treatments and the rehabilitation time. The rehabilitation programme starts with a careful medical examination and most of the patients see a physiotherapist. About one-third of the patients meet a psychologist individually or in a group working with stress and coping. About a quarter of the patients see a social worker and about 10% see the vocational counsellor. In addition, a workplace visit is made by the physiotherapist, the patient and his or her supervisor. All patients remain in the rehabilitation programme until they are working full time, and they keep in touch with the rehabilitation team for at least 4 weeks after they have left the programme.

The rehabilitation programme has five components:

- measurements of individual capacity in physical performance to show the patients that they are able to perform physical tests and to provide feedback about later improvements
- measurements of complaints of low back pain to be used for later positive reinforcement of improved function
- determination of individual physical work demands at the workplace
- a modified version of the Swedish Back School principles, with information based on ability rather than on disability due to low back pain
- an individually graded exercise programme with a behavioural therapy approach, based on individual capacity and individual physical demands at work. Fordyce's model of exercise to quota, not to pain, is used: each patient has their individually graded exercise programme 3 days a week until they return to their ordinary work.

This programme was reported to be superior to traditional rehabilitation in terms of the proportion of patients who returned to work, the proportion on sick leave up to 1 year later, and in terms of the total number of sick days during the first follow-up year.

Linton [10] proposed a similar model that integrates operant activities training and relaxation as coping. The operant approach considers problems of physical activity in terms of learning theory. This involves two learning models: avoidance and reinforcement of passive behaviours. The programme essentially selectively reinforces active behaviours rather than the passive lifestyle patterns that are part of the sick role. It is important that the patients are willing to participate in increasing their activity levels. Overall treatment goals are discussed and a key aspect of the programme is that the method is based on teamwork between the patient and the health care provider. To increase the patient's motivation, target activities are selected that are relevant to the patient and that may occur frequently. The first goal is selected close to a baseline level, so that the patient

cannot fail. Gradually the demands are increased and reinforcement is made, for example, by providing feedback on the activity increases, or by special benefits. In addition to the activities programme, Linton suggests applied relaxation training as a coping strategy. Applied relaxation aims to increase the patient's ability to cope with pain by disrupting the connections between anxiety, despair and pain. The training programme preferably involves conditioned relaxation, differential relaxation and rapid relaxation, so that the patient has tools to handle different situations involving pain.

In essences, the methods described not only focus on improving the physical capacities of the patient, but also attempt to improve the internal, mediating resources of the individual in terms of coping ability and lifestyle. Apparently the internal, mediating resources are of major importance for a successful rehabilitation programme.

Some rehabilitation programmes deal only with internal resources by providing group cognitive therapy or relaxation training [e.g. 11]. The basic assumption is that differences in ability to handle stress and to develop efficient coping strategies for pain management largely contribute to the differences in adjustment between patients with musculoskeletal pain. Patients who believe they can control their pain, who avoid agonizing about their condition, who have stronger internal beliefs and who believe they are not severely disabled appear to function better than those who do not.

Education and training

Group education is an intervention strategy that has been used to improve the recovery of people with low back pain. The content, administration and clientele of back schools vary, but most aim to motivate the individual to improve his or her lifestyle and to increase the understanding of how to care for the body. Back and neck schools may involve information on healthy behaviour, back and neck care, physical fitness, nutrition, stress and so on. In a review of group education interventions for people with low back pain [12], only one of four quality studies with chronic back pain patients found a positive short-term effect on one of the outcome measures considered, namely pain intensity. In one of two studies with acute cases, the programme reduced pain duration and short-term sick leave duration. After 1 year there was no evidence in any of the six studies of clinically important benefits. In general, it appears that traditional education and information has little impact on the incidence and duration of musculoskeletal problems.

Rehabilitation and intervention at the workplace

Case management programmes at the workplace

Battié [13] describes several intervention programmes at the workplace that are based on case management or employer interventions. An example of this type of programme was given by Fitzler and Berger [14]. In a shoe factory the company started a programme that aimed to change the attitudes and response of management to back pain reporting and to encourage prompt, appropriate medical care. The needs of employees were recognized and responded to emphatically. Attempts were also made to modify work tasks to allow the employee to continue working during recovery. Back pain reporting, work loss and associated medical and compensation costs were compared for the 3 years before adopting the programme and the following 3 years. There was a substantial decrease in lost time and costs after the initiation of the programme, although the rate of reported back pain was unchanged. This was considered to support the intentions of the programme, i.e. not to decrease the rate, but rather to reduce the consequences of the incidents.

Several other studies have shown considerable positive health and cost reduction effects of case management programmes involving changes of management attitudes, improved communication networks at the workplace, and a change in the communication to a more empathetic and positive approach. There are also several promising reports on educational programmes for managers to improve their insight and understanding of the problems facing employees when returning to work after rehabilitation. Employees who suffer from musculoskeletal disorders, and who may have difficulties in fulfilling their duties due to the pain, may be regarded as less desirable at the workplace both by managers and colleagues, as they may be less productive. Returning to work

after rehabilitation may, in some cases, reactivate negative attitudes and expectations from colleagues and managers and may, in the worst case, force people back into sickness absence.

Workplace interventions

An increasing number of studies emphasize the importance of work organization and psychosocial factors at work as important contributors for the development and maintenance of musculoskeletal disorders and long-term sickness absence. Follow-up studies after rehabilitation indicate that among the factors that contribute most to long-term sickness absence are work organizational factors such as decision latitude, opportunities for stimulation and development in the job, in addition to ergonomic conditions and a previous history of musculoskeletal pain. Some studies indicate that low intellectual discretion in the job may lower the pain threshold, which may result in an increased tendency to report pain symptoms.

There are few studies on work environment interventions that comprise both physical and organizational or psychosocial aspects. Most intervention studies hitherto tended to focus on reduction in static muscle strain. Westgaard and Aarås [15] evaluated an ergonomic adaptation programme designed to reduce static muscle load. After the introduction of height-adjustable work-stands, chairs with armrests and other measures to improve working postures, the static load on the trapezius muscle was reduced. Work organizational changes such as flexibility in working hours was introduced with a fixed pay system. Sick-leave statistics decreased by 33% and labour turnover also diminished. Ratings by the workers indicated that the ability to alter the position of the work table and to change the work posture, along with change of the fixed pay system contributed most to the improvement in health.

In an effort to evaluate the health effects of changed work organization, Parenmark and colleagues [16] compared an old plant with traditional assembly work and a new plant with the same equipment and hardware in which the workers were taught how to use the equipment properly. In the new plant all work tasks were based on group organization which involved quality control, external contacts and production planning. Extra work places were introduced to allow for rehabilitation needs, on-the-job training to reduce muscular load, and training of newcomers. The work pace was set to about 75% of the production at the old plant. The wage system was adjusted to compensate for age-related reduction of physical capacity, and working hours were flexible to adjust for individual preferences. The sick-leave rate decreased by 5% and labour turnover decreased from 35% to about 10%. The production quality increased, providing a diminished total production cost of about 10% compared to the old plant during the first year.

The results may be an overestimate due to the attention that employees at a new plant will get, and by a possible bias in the selection of the workforce between the old and the new plant. In spite of these possible drawbacks, the study points to several important organizational features at the workplace that appear to influence the incidence, duration and prognosis of work-related musculoskeletal disorders. As important though is the fact that the studies on workplace interventions show that worker health and productivity are influenced by the same aspects of work organization.

Less extensive intervention programmes are more common. Organizational changes which involve an increased number of short breaks and shortened continuous working hours in repetitive work are associated with a decreased prevalence of occupational cervicobrachial disorders. When comparing three intervention strategies in paced monotonous work with regard to muscular activity in the trapezius muscle, shortened work hours were superior to lower work pace and increased number of breaks for the outcome measure of muscle fatigue [17].

Today, much evidence points to the fact that, in order to be effective, rehabilitation and prevention of work-related musculoskeletal pain must involve work organizational and psychosocial improvements in addition to ergonomic improvement. In a consensus paper for the prevention of work-related musculoskeletal disorders, Hagberg and co-workers [18] suggest flexible equipment and lifting aids, job rotation, job enlargement, flexibility in production planning and increased responsibility of the employees. The authors also suggest that employees should have opportunities to increase their skill and knowledge and that wages should be organized so that they encourage job enlargement and development of competence and responsibility. In the previously cited empirical studies, intervention at the workplace was multifactorial and comprised in some cases several of the aspects suggested by Hagberg and colleagues. As such

intervention is complex in character, it is not always possible to specify more precisely what has determined the outcome. Lack of appropriate control conditions in some studies may cause overestimation of effects, since the mere attention provided to a subject may have positive health effects, as long as attention is maintained.

Work-related factors affecting length of a disability and risk of relapse

An individual's cognitions or perceptions are of importance for the outcome of re-entry after rehabilitation. Job dissatisfaction has been shown to increase the risk for back pain and dissatisfied people tend to attribute the cause of their pain to the work environment. Time-management factors and psychosocial aspects of the work environment are important factors which hinder a return to work [19]. It also appears that those who have obtained a new job or new work tasks after rehabilitation have a higher job satisfaction than those who return to their former work tasks. Several studies have shown that rehabilitation of those already suffering from musculoskeletal pain is more successful if the rehabilitation also involves changes at the workplace or even reallocation to new jobs. It is not advisable to return to any new work task however, as low quality of work content, in terms of low influence on the job and low opportunities for development in the job, in addition to physical demands, are predictors of a requirement for more days off sick during the first year after rehabilitation [20].

Interplay between individual resources and work conditions

At all levels, prevention and rehabilitation appear to be more successful if not only external factors, but also internal, mediating factors such as perception of work conditions, perception of health and appropriate coping resources, are appreciated as important parts of the process. The importance of acknowledging the patient's disorder, rather than neglecting it, must be stressed. Scepticism from doctors, supervisors and colleagues may force patients into a pattern of credibility seeking, which possibly maintains and prolongs their illness. Sickness absence has been suggested to be a coping behaviour which is directed against stren-uous working conditions and perceived ill health. In accordance with this reasoning, work and psychosocial conditions that allow for efficient coping strategies at the workplace when the demands are perceived to be too high, would be crucial for a positive health outcome. Social support and recognition by supervisors have been observed in several studies as being impor-tant for primary prevention and for facilitating re-entry after rehabilitation.

Compliance

The negative outcome of many rehabilitation pro-grammes may be due partly to the lack of control of compliance with the activities of the pro-gramme, as lack of adherence or compliance, which is a common problem in particular in reha-bilitation programmes of longer duration, is often considered as a lack of motivation from the patient. It may, however, be more fruitful to iden-tify typical circumstances that are barriers to com-pliance to the rehabilitation programme. Some common barriers have been discussed by McIntosh and colleagues [21], pointing out the importance not only of focusing the rehabilitation on the pain itself, but also considering if the goals for the programme are realistic. A return to unchanged work may be a less desirable goal for a patient who strongly dislikes the job, who has no job, or who is involved in conflicts at work. Similarly, scheduled activities in the rehabilitation programme may seem inadequate, irrelevant or not possible to follow for some patients.

A general problem in most rehabilitation and intervention programmes appears to be the absence of a participative approach for establish-ing the individual's specific goals for the rehabili-tation, as well as for the strategies to reach these goals. In organizational psychology, participative models have been demonstrated to improve worker motivation and productivity. It has been argued that participative goal-setting, as opposed to assigned goals, yields increased performance. Participation, and proper involvement from the management, are powerful tools for utilizing employee expertise to achieve high-quality solu-tions, for gaining employee acceptance of deci-sions and for motivating employee compliance with the solutions. A similar perspective may be applied to rehabilitation, i.e. patient participation in goal-setting and a high degree of involvement

from the management may promote successful rehabilitation. If the goals of rehabilitation are predetermined by experts, mechanisms enforcing passivity and alienation may be activated and the process may produce a patient who feels worse and more helpless than when started.

Problem-based rehabilitation

A heuristic model of the essential components of a rehabilitation process has been outlined elsewhere [22]. The model suggests three levels of action that appears necessary to approach in the rehabilita-tion of work-related disorders: the work situation, the mediating resources of the individual, and the health outcome including physical, social and psychological functions. In this perspective, the aspects of the work situation and of individual mediating resources are considered as equally important for a successful rehabilitation process as are reduction of pain, increased muscular strength and other physical outcome measures.

The theoretical basis is found in the demand–control–social support model described by Karasek and Theorell [23]. Their model essentially outlines important aspects of work organization that promote health and prevent stress-related dis-orders. The model has gained extensive support in epidemiological studies on work-related stress dis-orders. Of particular importance for a positive health outcome is a high decision latitude at work in combination with demands that do not exceed the individual's resources, and good social support. The combination of high demands and a low decision latitude at work promotes strain. It is suggested that a work situation inducing high strain may inhibit learning through accumulated anxiety. The other side of the coin, high decision latitude in combination with demands that are possible to cope with, will rather stimulate the ability and willingness to accept challenges and new learning. New learning leads to a reduction of perceived stress and to improved coping, and eventually a feeling of mastery may develop as a global behavioural orientation. Such health-promoting aspects of work are hypothesized to have similar positive effects if implemented in the rehabilitation realm.

One important aim of rehabilitation is to sup-port the development of efficient internal mediat-ing resources such as high self-esteem, efficient strategies for coping with strenuous situations, and to develop the patient's social ability to interact and communicate at work and outside work. It is also important that the patient learns not to avoid challenges but rather to try to master them. By using a problem-based methodology, the advantages of a high degree of control and influence, individually adjusted demands and an extensive social support can be fulfilled.

A basic assumption of problem-based rehabilitation is that the patient is the best expert on how the rehabilitation process should proceed and which goals for the rehabilitation should be given priority in the short and long run. It is considered essential that the patients themselves formulate the goals for their rehabilitation and develop individual strategies to reach these goals. It is also assumed that individuals who return to the workplace after rehabilitation with high intrinsic motivation to handle strenuous work conditions and who dare to apply constructive coping strategies for excessive demands will become 'change agents' at the workplace and provide good examples for others.

The methodology of problem-based rehabilitation is founded in problem-based learning [24], but adapted to the present context. Patients with musculoskeletal problems work in groups for about 2 hours every week during 4 months. At each meeting the group-work follows the problem-based method. First the group decides on a theme to discuss during the meeting; themes may focus on the work situation, the situation outside work or on internal problems. Examples of such themes are stress at work, hindrance factors for work, self-esteem, health, exercise, etc. The group then has a brainstorming session on the selected theme, and the outcome of the brainstorming process is structured into content areas. This process gives rise to many new ideas and associations for the group members. Each group member then decides on an individual goal that is related to the selected content area. If, for example, the originally selected theme was 'hindrances to work', and the resulting content area of the brainstorm-structure session became 'supervisory behaviour', each patient decides on an individual goal to accomplish until the next group session. Such an individual goal may be 'to initiate discussions with supervisor about instructions given to perform a work task'. At the next group meeting the group discusses how their subgoals were accomplished, internal and external barriers, and other experiences while attempting to manage the goal. Experiences and hints are shared in the group, and usually the social support within the group is extensive.

A cornerstone in the problem-based approach is that the patient must be responsible not only for determining the subgoals during the rehabilitation process, but also for finding strategies to reach the goals. Patients may have different hindrance factors and different goals for their rehabilitation, and some patients may need more time than others to obtain their goals. Such differences do not create problems for the group. The source of motivation is intrinsic and built upon the participative approach.

In addition to the problem-based group meetings, the patients may select to participate in other activities, such as physiotherapy, relaxation training, physical activities, stress handling, etc. These activities are not mandatory, but are offered as a supplement. It is assumed that in time patients will selectively enrol in those activities they find appropriate for their improvement.

To facilitate the goals of improving work conditions and the attitudes at the workplace, supervisers or managers of the patients enrolled in the problem-based group are actively enrolled in another group which meets monthly to discuss rehabilitation matters, aspects of the work, and to get support for a more active approach with regard to workplace changes. The experience of the problem-based strategy is that if supervisers or managers are involved from the start of the rehabilitation period, their interest and involvement will be maintained throughout. The meetings also help the supervisers and managers to identify problems at their workplace, rather than solely to focus on the individual employee and his or her problems, hence rehabilitation and prevention are integrated in the same process.

Conclusion

There are several views on the aetiology of work-related musculoskeletal disorders. The perspective of causality naturally affects which strategies are chosen for rehabilitation and prevention. Improved physical strength and mobility, or reduced pain, do not necessarily imply that a treatment has led to better health in terms of improved ability to work or function in normal life. Improved physical health may be a necessary, but not a sufficient condition for improved work ability and quality of life. There is now much evidence to suggest that a multidisciplinary approach to rehabilitation is most effective. Today, many such programmes involve cognitive behavioural programmes. It also appears necessary to merge the present knowledge on aetiological aspects and knowledge on prognosis into the same frame of reference, as there is a lack of studies encompassing the workplace as a significant component of rehabilitation programmes. In general, integration of rehabilitation and prevention is not well developed. A change of focus from the clinical, pathological view of the individual to an integrated multidisciplinary view, comprising both internal and external aspects of the individual and the work conditions, is required for successful rehabilitation and prevention.

References

1. Snook, S.H. Approaches to the control of back pain in industry: job design, job placement and education/ training. In *Back Pain in Workers* (ed. R.A. Deyo) *Occupational Medicine: State of the Art Reviews*. Hanley & Belfus Inc., Philadelphia, PA (1988)
2. Koes, B.W., Assendelft, W.J.J., van der Heijden, G.J.M.G., *et al.* Spinal manipulation and mobilisation for back and neck complaints: a blinded review. *British Medical Journal*, **303**, 1298–1303 (1991)
3. Koes, B.W., Bouter, L.M., van Mameren H. *et al.* Randomised clinical trial of manipulative therapy and physiotherapy for persistent back and neck complaints: results of one year follow up. *British Medical Journal*, **304**, 601–605 (1992)
4. Bigos, S., Bowyer, O., Braen, G. *et al. Acute Low Back Problems in Adults*. Clinical Practice Guideline No. 14. AHCPR Publication No. 95-0642. Agency for Health Care Policy and Research, Public Health Service, US Department of Health and Human Services, Rockville, MD (1994)
5. Lahad, A., Malter, A.D., Berg, A.O. *et al.* The effectiveness of four interventions for the prevention of low back pain. *Journal of the American Medical Association*, **272**, 1286–1291 (1994)
6. Rowe, M.L. *Backache at Work*. Perinton Press, Fairport, NY (1983)
7. Gamsa, A. The role of psychological factors in chronic pain. I. A half century of study. *Pain*, **57**, 5–15 (1994)
8. Fordyce, W.E., Fowler, R.S., Lehmann, J.F. *et al.* Some implications of learning in problems of chronic pain. *Journal of Chronic Diseases*, **21**, 179-190 (1968)
9. Lindström, I. A successful intervention program for patients with subacute low back pain. *Doctoral dissert.*, Göteborg University (1994)
10. Linton, S.J. Chronic back pain: activities training and physical therapy. *Behavioral Medicine*, **20**, 105–111 (1994)
11. Turner, J.A. and Jensen, M.P. Efficacy of cognitive therapy for chronic low back pain. *Pain*, **52**, 169-177 (1993)
12. Cohen, J.E., Goel, V., Frank, J.W. *et al.* Group education interventions for people with low back pain. An overview of the literature. *Spine*, **19**, 1214–1222 (1994)
13. Battié, M.C. Minimizing the impact of back pain: workplace strategies. *Seminars in Spinal Surgery*, **4**, 20–28 (1992)
14. Fitzler, S.L. and Berger, R.A. Chelsea back program: one year later. *Occupational Health and Safety*, **52**, 52–54 (1983)
15. Westgaard, R.H. and Aarås, A. The effect of improved workplace design on the development of work-related musculo-skeletal illnesses. *Applied Ergonomics*, **16**, 91–97 (1985)
16. Parenmark, G., Malmkvist, A-K. and Örtengren, R. Ergonomic moves in an engineering industry: effects on sick leave frequency, labor turnover and productivity. *International Journal of Industrial Ergonomics*, **11**, 1-10.
17. Mathiassen, S.E. and Winkel, J. Physiological comparison of three interventions in light assembly work: reduced work pace, increased break allowance and shortened working days. *International Archives of Environmental Health*, **68**, 94–108 (1996)
18. Hagberg, M., Kilbom, Å., Buckle, P. *et al.* Strategies for prevention of work-related musculoskeletal disorders: consensus paper. *International Journal of Industrial Ergonomics*, **11**, 77–81 (1993)
19. Linton, S.J. and Bradley, L.A. An 18-month follow-up of a secondary prevention program for back pain: help and hindrance factors related to outcome maintenance. *The Clinical Journal of Pain*, **8**, 227–236 (1992)
20. Ekberg, K. and Wildhagen, I. Long-term sickness absence due to musculoskeletal disorders. The necessary invention of work conditions. *Scandinavian Journal of Rehabilitation Medicine*, **28**, 39–47 (1996)
21. McIntosh, G., Melles, T. and Hall, H. Guidelines for the identification of barriers to rehabilitation of back injuries. *Journal of Occupational Rehabilitation*, **5**, 195–201 (1995)
22. Ekberg, K. Workplace changes in successful rehabilitation. *Journal of Occupational Rehabilitation*, **5**, 253–269 (1995)
23. Karasek, R. and Theorell, T. *Healthy Work. Stress, Productivity, and the Reconstruction of Working Life*. Basic Books, New York (1990)
24. Barrows, H.S. *How to Design a Problem-Based Curriculum for the Preclinical Years*. Springer, New York (1985)

Appendix

Occupational medicine resources on the Internet

The number of sites on the Internet dealing with occupational and environmental medicine is small at present but is increasing rapidly, as is the size and scope of the Internet itself. The list of resources given here is not complete and should be looked upon as an example of what can be found on the Internet, and could serve as the starting point for further exploration of the Internet and the World Wide Web. As the Internet is constantly changing, some of the links mentioned in this list may no longer be operational by the time this book is published. All the links have been tested and were functioning as of July 1997 however. Consider them as starting points for further investigation of the Internet.

Agency for Toxic Substances and Disease Registry

http://atsdr1.atsdr.cdc.gov:8080/

Among other things you find some useful databases and FAQs on this site, such as HazDat, ATSDRs Hazardous Substance Release/Health Effects Database, a scientific and administrative database developed to provide access to information on the release of hazardous substances from Superfund sites or from emergency events and on the effects of hazardous substances on the health of human populations, and ToxFAQ, short, easy-to-read summaries about hazardous substances that have been excerpted from the ATSDR Toxicological Profiles.

Duke Occupational and Environmental Medicine

http://152.3.65.120/oem/

The World Wide Web home for the Occ-Env-Med-L Mail-list.

ECDIN – Environmental Chemicals Data and Information Network

http://ulisse.etoit.eudra.org/Ecdin.html

ECDIN is a factual databank, created under the Environmental Research Programme of the Joint Research Centre (JRC) of the Commission of European Communities at the Ispra Establishment. The databank is designed as an instrument which will enable people engaged in environmental management and research to obtain reliable information on chemical products.

ERGOWEB

http://www.ergoweb.com.

This is a goldmine for people interested in ergonomics, and contains much information on analytical tools and checklists, case studies, standards and guidelines, ergonomic trends and concepts, and OSHA-related material. Contains links to many sites. A detailed index and keyword search is available.

Health and Safety Executive, HSE

http://www.open.gov.uk/hse/hsehome.htm

HSE is the UK agency responsible for health and safety at work. The web site contains a list of HSE's activities, their publications, current interests and research.

National Institute of Occupational Safety and Health, NIOSH

http://www.cdc.gov/niosh/homepage.html

NIOSH is part of the Centers for Disease Control and Prevention. The home pages give links to NIOSH's activities, their database, publication and research. It is also possible to get information on health hazards and on the NIOSH evaluation program. There is a comprehensive link to other web sites of interest.

National Institute for Working Life, NIWL

http:/www.niwl.se

The National Institute for Working Life is Sweden's R&D centre for occupational health and safety, working life and the labour market. Other important tasks are the dissemination and application of knowledge through education and training, publications and international collaboration. You can search the National Library for Working Life, and also order articles on-line.

Occupational Safety and Health Administration, OSHA

http://www.osha.gov/

This US government site gives information on regulations and standards, technical information and publications. There are many links to other web sites.

Occupational Safety and Health WWW Board

http://turva.me.tut.fi/~tuusital/ bulletinboard/

From the Institute of Occupational Safety Engineering at the Tampere University of Technology in Finland, a bulletin board system for discussions in the occupational medicine field.

OSHWEB

http://turva.me.tut.fi/~oshweb/

Another resource from the Institute of Occupational Safety Engineering at the Tampere University of Technology in Finland. This is one of the best lists of Internet resources in the field of occupational medicine.

Safety Related Internet Resources

http://www.mrg.ab.ca/christie/safelist.htm

From Christie Communications, a company that develops health and safety training materials. Contains links to virtually everything on the Internet that deals with occupational health: web sites, mailing lists, electronic publications, etc. A must on any 'hotlist' for occupational medicine resources on the Internet.

Index